BHG
MAIN LIBRARY
STO

ALLEN COUNTY PUBLIC LIBRARY

ACPL ITEM
DISCARDED

D1550332

617.632 AL5P   2317479
ALLEN, DON L.
PERIODONTICS FOR THE DENTAL
HYGIENIST

ALLEN COUNTY PUBLIC LIBRARY

FORT WAYNE, INDIANA 46802

You may return this book to any agency, branch,
or bookmobile of the Allen County Public Library.

PERIODONTICS
FOR THE
DENTAL HYGIENIST

PERIODONTICS
FOR THE
<u>DENTAL HYGIENIST</u>

Don L. Allen, D.D.S, M.S.
Dean and William N. Finnegan III Professor of Dental Science
Department of Periodontics
University of Texas
Health Science Center
Dental Branch
Houston, Texas

Walter T. McFall, Jr., B.S., D.D.S., M.S.
Professor and Acting Chairman, Department of Periodontics
The University of North Carolina at Chapel Hill
School of Dentistry
Chapel Hill, North Carolina

Joyce W. Jenzano, R.D.H., B.S., M.S. (Oral Biology)
Assistant Professor, Department of Dental Ecology (Dental Hygiene Program)
The University of North Carolina at Chapel Hill
School of Dentistry
Chapel Hill, North Carolina

FOURTH EDITION

Lea & Febiger

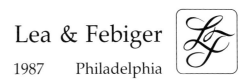

1987   Philadelphia

Lea & Febiger
600 Washington Square
Philadelphia, PA 19106-4198
U.S.A.
(215) 922-1330

Allen County Public Library
Ft. Wayne, Indiana

First Edition, 1968
  Reprinted 1970, 1972
Second Edition, 1974
  Reprinted 1975
Third Edition, 1980
Fourth Edition, 1987

Library of Congress Cataloging in Publication Data

Allen, Don L.
  Periodontics for the dental hygienist.

  Includes bibliographies and index.
  1. Periodontics. 2. Dental hygiene. I. McFall,
Walter T. II. Jenzano, Joyce. III. Title. [DNLM:
1. Dental Hygienists. 2. Periodontal Diseases.
WU 240 A425p]
RK361.A37   1986   617.6'32   86-7305
ISBN 0-8121-1047-1

Copyright © 1987 by Lea & Febiger. Copyright under the International Copyright Union.
All Rights Reserved. This book is protected by copyright. *No part of it may be reproduced
in any manner or by any means without written permission from the publisher.*

PRINTED IN THE UNITED STATES OF AMERICA

Print number: 5 4 3 2 1

2317479

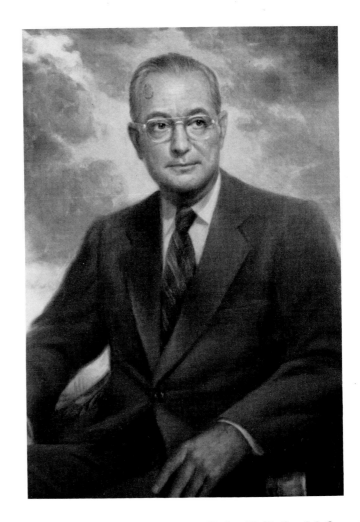

To Grover C. Hunter, Jr., B.S., D.D.S., M.S.,
Educator, Author, Mentor and Friend.

PREFACE

In 1968 when the first edition of *Periodontics for the Dental Hygienist* appeared, the authors were convinced that the dental hygienist would occupy a strategic position in the prevention and treatment of periodontal disease. During the intervening years ample evidence has proven the validity of that concept. Today the hygienist is recognized as being vital to the successful control of periodontal disease. We remain convinced that expanding duties of dental hygienists should be in the area of periodontics. The authors strongly support the concept of the dental team because we believe the public is best served by that approach. The dental hygienist is an important part of that team. We would like to believe that knowledge gained from previous editions of this book has helped contribute to the essential role that hygienists occupy in peridontal therapy.

Exciting discoveries have occurred in periodontics since 1968, and previous editions of this book have chronicled these improved methodologies and new developments. This fourth edition extends and expands on efforts of the previous editions.

Addition of a hygiene editor to the list of authors brings to this edition a fresh perspective and a rich source of new information. An expanded chapter arrangement has permitted a more in-depth examination of basic cellular phenomena, microbiology, immunology, clinical techniques, epidemiology, and long-term maintenance. All chapters contain new subject matter as well as revision and enhancement of previous material. Many new illustrations supplement the text. As with previous editions, we continue to present the hygienist reader with challenges to stimulate and enrich the mind.

We are grateful for suggestions from dental hygiene educators from many schools. We particularly appreciate the valuable secretarial support of Ms. Kathy Dodson, Ms. DeeAnn Shull, and Ms. Gloria Y. Martel; the additional photography by Mr. Tom Edwards; and new illustrations by Mr. Peter G. Bedick.

Houston, TX Don L. Allen
Chapel Hill, NC Walter T. McFall
Joyce W. Jenzano

CONTENTS

Techniques of Periodontal Surgery
Reconstructive Surgery
Role of the Hygienist in Periodontal Surgery

THE DENTAL HYGIENIST AND PERIODONTICS

Periodontal disease, a term used to designate pathologic changes in the supporting structures of the teeth, apparently has affected humankind since the dawn of history. Studies of the skulls of ancient humans indicate rather severe periodontal bony destruction even though the life span of early man is considered to be much shorter than it is today.

Although there have been many epidemiologic studies of periodontal disease conducted, our knowledge of the incidence, prevalence and severity of the disease is still somewhat limited. It is generally accepted that periodontal disease is universal and that over 70% of the adults in all countries are affected (Striffler, Young, and Burt, 1983).

An estimated 22 million people in the United States are completely edentulous. The major cause of tooth loss in the age group over 35 is periodontal disease. In the 45 to 54 year age group approximately 17% are toothless, whereas, among those 65 or older as many as 1 in every 2 has lost all of his or her teeth. This latter age group, of course, is the fastest growing group of people in the world.

The incidence of periodontal disease in young people appears to be much greater than was previously thought. As classified by the Periodontal Index, an estimated 9.2 million children in the United States (approximately 39%) age 6 to 11, have inflammatory diseases of the gingivae or a more advanced form of periodontal disease. Among youths age 12 to 17 years, an estimated 15.4 million or 68% of this age group in the United States have gingival or periodontal disease. A study of 2,409 15-year-old Norwegians showed that 11.3% have bone loss with boys being affected more than girls. Twenty-eight percent of 264 Nigerian boys age 18 to 20 years demonstrated bone loss. In Sweden 20% of the subjects in a study showed periodontal disease by age 15.

In the 55 to 64 years age group an approximately 85% of individuals in the United States have some manifestation of periodontal disease. As would be expected the incidence and severity of the disease increases with age. In Great Britain it was reported that 99% of people with natural teeth had periodontal disease with 4 out of every 10 so severely affected that they were about to lose their teeth (Sheilham, 1979). In the same study, it was reported that 99.7% of Swedes between 45 and 49 years of age had periodontal disease. In another Swedish study (Hugoson and Gordan, 1982), no subjects in the 40, 50, or 70 year age groups were free of gingival or periodontal disease, but only 8% had severe destructive periodontal disease. In a study conducted in South Australia, 85% of the subjects had periodontal disease with it being severe in 25% of the 680 subjects examined.

Millions more people will become edentulous if periodontal disease is not prevented or treated. It is the responsibility of the dental hygienist and other members of the dental health profession to provide the prevention and treatment needed.

As with most good things, the dental hygiene profession has grown out of a need. Some of the early leaders of dentistry in this country realized that the ultimate goal of dentistry should be to prevent dental diseases from occurring. They astutely observed that dental caries and periodontal disease occur in an environment of oral uncleanliness. They also observed that the majority of their colleagues were more intent on treating oral diseases than in attempting to prevent them.

Dr. Alfred C. Fones stands out as a major pioneer in preventive dentistry and in the development of the dental hygiene profession. Mainly through his efforts, the first school of dental hygiene was established in 1916. He strongly felt that it should be a profession for women. In 1912 he wrote, "A woman is apt to be conscientious and painstaking in her work. She is honest and reliable and in this one form of practice, I think, she is better fitted for the position of a prophylactic assistant than is a man." He further stated that the major duties of the hygienist should be those of performing oral prophylaxis and giving oral physiotherapy instructions to patients.

While the duties and responsibilities of the dental hygienist are expanding and will continue to do so, it would be most unfortunate if the basic ideas of Dr. Fones were forgotten. The primary clinical activities of the hygienist are to remove deposits from the teeth and to teach patients how to best take care of their dental and oral tissues. While these procedures are beneficial in the prevention of dental caries, their greatest impact is in the prevention of periodontal disease.

Because of the significant roles of the hygienist in the prevention and, in the future, possibly the treatment of periodontal disease, it is extremely important that she possess a working knowledge of the nature of the disease, the causes, and the methods available to treat it. It is not possible to appreciate the service which the hygienist renders for patients unless she understands the mechanisms and destructive potential of the disease processes. It is not possible to know how to prevent periodontal disease in general, or especially in individual situations, unless she understands what causes the disease. It is not possible to work most effectively with the general practitioner or dental specialist unless she understands the rationale of, and techniques available for, the treatment of periodontal disease. In order to educate patients as to the part they must contribute to prevent periodontal disease, it is necessary that the hygienist have a thorough understanding of the major aspects of the problem. All patients cannot be approached or managed in the same way. A wealth of information is needed to be most effective when dealing with various clinical problems. The objective of this book is to present the information needed to best practice clinical dental hygiene.

PEOPLE AND TEETH

The value people place on their teeth varies. The value is individual and depends on the educational level of the patient, his past dental experience, and his relationship with people in the dental profession.

The hygienist has many opportunities to inform and influence people in regard to the meaningfulness of their teeth.

In general, however, it would seem that more people are placing a higher value on retaining their natural dentition. This apparently is related to an overcoming of the negativism that existed in regard to the permanency of the teeth. Most informed people no longer believe that the loss of the permanent teeth is inevitable as part of the aging process.

People are placing more importance on their teeth in relation to their general body health and psychologic health. The role of the teeth in the ingestion of food, the preparation of food for digestion, in speech, and in facial appearance is better appreciated by the general public. People have more confidence in the ability of the dental health team to maintain and retain the natural dentition. The dental profession understands the mechanisms of oral diseases better than before. The teeth and their supporting structures (periodontium) are appreciated as living tissues which are an integral part of a living organism. The disadvantages and discomfort of dental prostheses undoubtedly are positive motivating factors for patients wanting to preserve the natural dentition.

The demands for periodontal services will increase in the future. As a result of the increase in the dental educational level of the public at large through school activities and mass media, as well as directly from the dental and medical professions, more people will seek periodontal care. Schools are graduating dentists with a better knowledge of preventive periodontics. As a result, more patients will receive periodontal care before destructive periodontitis occurs. The progressive expansion in the size of the population and the increase in the expected life span of individuals will increase the need for periodontal care. The availability of prepaid and other forms of third party dental health insurance will make it feasible for more people to receive periodontal care. These increases in the demands for preventive periodontics will not be met unless the hygienists play a significant part with the rest of the dental profession in meeting it.

PREVENTIVE DENTISTRY

In the broadest and most appropriate sense, preventive dentistry is not a specific entity in itself but relates to all areas of dentistry. The term is used to designate the measures used to stop the initiation of oral diseases and also those measures employed to stop or retard the progression of oral diseases which have already started.

The effects of the various diseases of the hard and soft tissues of the mouth may predispose the patient to developing other diseases of the mouth. Proximal dental caries destroys the contact relationship of the involved teeth. In addition to the damage to the teeth themselves, food impaction and bacterial plaque formation occur in the interproximal area. These cause gingival inflammation and lead to loss of periodontal support of the teeth. The loss of a tooth due to caries or periodontal disease without its proper replacement usually results in drifting and supraeruption to the other teeth in that area. The resultant malalignment of teeth may cause malocclusion, food impaction, plaque formation, caries, and periodontal disease.

Periodontal disease is a general term used to designate any entity which is characterized by injury to the gingival or periodontal tissues. The most frequent periodontal diseases are those of an inflammatory nature. In most cases, the inflammation is caused by bacterial plaque and dental calculus which form on the tooth surfaces. The primary clinical responsibility of the dental hygienist is to remove these deposits from the teeth and to teach patients how they can best prevent the deposit from re-forming. In some situations this is a simple technical task. In most situations, it requires the highest caliber of clinical proficiency and a sincere enthusiasm for motivating people.

DENTAL HYGIENE AND PERIODONTICS

Since the fundamental clinical activities of the hygienist are primarily those of removing from the teeth irritating deposits that are known to cause periodontal disease, it is obvious that her relationship in dentistry is closest to periodontics. Periodontics is the area of dentistry that is concerned with the prevention and treatment of diseases affecting the tissues that surround and support the tooth (gingiva, cementum, periodontal ligament, and alveolar bone).

The degree to which a hygienist is effective in the prevention of oral diseases is dependent on her knowledge of the diseases and on her clinical abilities. Of course, there are legal and ethical limitations on what she can do.

Within the past few years dramatic changes have been made in the dental practice acts of many states, authorizing the dental hygienist to perform clinical tasks and treatments under the supervision of a dentist which, heretofore, she had been unable to do. This simply reflects the dynamic period that currently exists relative to the practice of clinical dental hygiene.

In 1972 the Inter-Agency Committee published an interim report in reference to attitudes and policies on the utilization of dental auxiliary personnel. In the area of expanded functions for dental auxiliaries the following statements were made: "On the basis of research and practice, each of the following functions has been accepted by one or more states as appropriate and logical for assignment to auxiliaries. However, not all functions are performed by auxiliaries in all states. Therefore, the guidelines have been constructed to enable states to use the information that relates to

Table 1–1. Number of States with Provisions for Delegating Specific Functions to Hygienists July, 1985

Take impressions for study casts	45/48
Place periodontal dressings	40/48
Remove periodontal and surgical dressings	45/48
Remove sutures	44/48
Administer local anesthetic agents	15/48
Place rubber dam	46/48
Remove rubber dam	46/48
Place matrix	38/48
Remove matrix	34/48
Place temporary restorations	35/48
Remove temporary restorations	27/48
Place amalgam restorations	11/48*
Carve amalgam restorations	10/48
Polish amalgam restorations	44/48
Place and Finish composite, resin, or silicate cement restorations	9/48
Apply pit and fissure sealants	42/48
Apply cavity liners and bases	17/48
Root planing	41/48
Closed soft-tissue curettage	30/48

The number on the right of the (/) is the total number of jurisdictions that provide information on the specific functions. The number on the left of the (/) is the total number of jurisdictions that permit delegation of the function. Information from Indiana, Maine and Rhode Island was not available.
*Three of the eleven states required condensation by the dentist. (American Dental Association, Division of Educational Measurements).

provisions for dental practice in the particular state." (See Table 1–1.)

Many of these duties have been part of the practice of dental hygiene for some time. Others are new. Some may not be the most appropriate duties for hygiene practice. We recommend that dental hygiene practice be expanded exclusively in the fields of preventive and therapeutic periodontics and that other auxiliaries expand their functions in restorative dentistry. However, the significant factor is that they represent a trend—a trend that may broaden the scope of dental hygiene practice even more in the future. As more dentists are treating periodontal patients, the hygienist's duties as a surgical assistant will increase. Certainly a great deal of what the hygienist will be doing in the future is dependent on the ambitions of the profession itself.

Preventive dentistry is dynamic with new concepts, techniques, and procedures continuously available. We cannot determine with any degree of certainty the benefits that will be derived from present and future research in bacterial plaque inhibitors, calculus inhibitors, and caries prevention. The role of the hygienist in preventive periodontics in the future can only increase. However, it is certain that it must be based on a clear understanding of the characteristics of the periodontal tissues and the mechanisms of periodontal diseases.

Unlike the days of Dr. Fones, all modern dental practitioners incorporate preventive dentistry as an important aspect of the care they provide. The dentist is concerned with the total health of the patient. The taking of a medical history and vital signs, nutritional analysis, laboratory tests, and evaluation of general health are routine procedures in many offices. Comprehensive dental treatment and preventive dentistry recalls on a routine and periodic basis are characteristic of dental practice today. The dental hygienist plays an important role in all of these activities.

BIBLIOGRAPHY

Allen, D.L.: The implications of changing patterns in oral health for dental education, Int. Dent. J., *35*:83, 1985.

Douglas, D., et al.: The potential for increase in the periodontal disease of the aged population, J. Periodontol., *54*:721, 1983.

Fones, A.C.: The necessity for the training of a prophylactic assistant, Dent. Cosmos., *54*:284, 1912.

Fones, A.C.: The origin and history of the dental hygienist movement, J. Am. Dent. Assoc., *13*:1809, 1926.

Hansen, B.F., Gjermo, P., and Berowitz-Larsen, K.R.: Periodontal bone loss in 15-year-old Norwegians, J. Clin. Periodontol., *11*:125, 1984.

Hugoson, A. and Jordan, T.: Frequency distribution of individuals aged 20–70 years according to severity of periodontal disease, Community Dent. Oral Epidemiol., *10*:187, 1982.

MacGregor, I.D.M.: Radiographic survey of periodontal disease in 264 adolescent school boys in Lagos, Nigeria, Community Dent. Oral Epidemiol., *8*:56, 1980.

National Center for Health Statistics, Edentulous persons. U.S. DHEW, PHS Publications. Series 10, No. 89, June 1974.

National Center for Health Statistics, Periodontal disease among youths 12–17 years. U.S. DHEW, PHS Publication. Series 11, No. 141, June 1974.

Sheilham, Aubrey: The epidemiology of dental caries and periodontal disease, J. Clin. Periodontol., *6*:7, 1979.

Srikano, T.W. and Clarke, N.G.: Periodontal status in South Australian industrial population, Community Dent. Oral Epidemiol., *10*:272, 1982.

Striffler, D.F., Young, W.O., and Burt, B.A.: *Dentistry, Dental Practice and the Community*, Philadelphia, W.B. Saunders Co., 1983, pp. 512.

Chapter 2

ANATOMY AND PHYSIOLOGY
OF THE PERIODONTIUM

Natural teeth are primarily responsible for the mastication of food and thus aid in digestion, but they also contribute to speech, facial esthetics, emotional well-being, the grasping of objects, and as an aid in swallowing. The tissues which support the natural teeth and enhance their beauty and functions are collectively termed the periodontium.

The periodontium consists of the gingivae, periodontal ligament, cementum and alveolar bone (Fig. 2–1). The gingival tissues cover alveolar bone and have a firm fibrous attachment to underlying bony surfaces. The attachment of the gingiva to the tooth is mediated by epithelial cells and connective tissue fibers and is referred to as the dentogingival junction. Periodontal ligament fibers are apical to the gingival fibers and are connected to cementum and to the bone of the tooth socket. This suspensory mechanism is referred to as the attachment apparatus and provides the major support to the tooth. These tissues are interrelated both as to their function and their health, and are tissues of primary concern to the dental hygienist.

Mucous membrane is the tissue that lines all body cavities that open externally. The oral mucous membrane lines the mouth, and it is modified in various parts of the mouth dependent upon the physiologic demands placed upon it. Basically, oral mucosa may be divided into three types based upon functional and histologic characteristics.

1. *Masticatory mucosa.* This consists of the gingival tissues and the covering mucosa of the hard palate. These oral tissues are subjected to heavy stress and friction.

2. *Lining mucosa.* Other portions of the mouth are overlaid with a protective surface termed lining mucosa. Further subdivision of lining mucosa occurs dependent on location. Totally it consists of the mucosa of lips and cheeks, floor of the mouth, inferior surface of the tongue, soft palate, uvula, and the alveolar mucosa. Alveolar mucosa is apical to the gingiva and forms the vestibule between lips or cheeks and alveolar ridge. The mucosa at the base of the vestibule is sometimes referred to as vestibular mucosa.

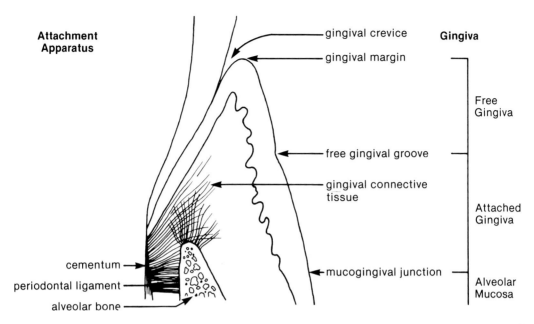

Figure 2–1. Anatomic Relationships of the Periodontium. The major anatomic components of the periodontium are illustrated.

3. *Specialized mucosa.* The dorsum of the tongue is covered with tissue that is especially modified for the sensation of taste.

THE GINGIVA

The gingiva consists of those portions of oral masticatory mucosa that attach to the teeth and alveolar bone and which surround the cervical areas of the teeth (Fig. 2–2). The bulk of gingival tissues is firmly anchored to underlying structures and is termed attached gingiva.

The unattached coronal portion of the gingiva (free gingiva) is comprised of marginal gingiva on facial and lingual surfaces and interdental papillae that fill the gingival embrasures between the teeth. Free gingiva contains numerous fibers that in health adapt it firmly against the tooth. The area between the inner aspect of the free gingiva and the adjacent tooth surface is the gingival crevice (sulcus). In health, the gingival crevice represents only a potential, not an actual, space since the tissue is

firmly adapted to the tooth. Measurable depth of this potential space should ideally be less than 1 millimeter. It usually is greater than that on proximal surfaces. The relevance of this measurement to the clinical assessment of gingival health will be discussed in Chapter 6. On the outer gingival surface a shallow groove, the free gingival groove, that approximates the base of the crevice may be observed in some mouths (Fig. 2–3). The presence of gingival grooves is apparently related to masticatory forces and neither their presence nor absence is an indicator of health.

On the facial aspect attached gingiva meets the alveolar mucosa at a wavy line termed the mucogingival junction. A similar junction occurs on the inner surface of the mandible where the tissues of the floor of the mouth meets the gingiva. No such line occurs in the hard palate, where a smooth transition between gingival tissue and palatal mucosa ensues.

Clinical Features of the Gingiva

COLOR. Classically, healthy gingival tissues are described as light pink or coral

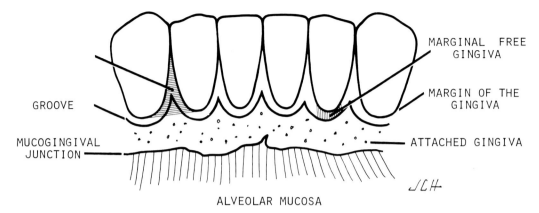

Figure 2–2. Clinical Characteristics of Normal Gingiva. This drawing illustrates the normal clinical characteristics of gingiva. The free gingival groove is a variable finding (after Orban).

pink. The color of the gingiva is dependent on the thickness of the epithelium and upon the richness of the blood vessels in the deeper connective tissue layers. Within the range of normality there are, however, rather wide variations in gingival color. Primarily these color changes are related to differences in complexion and racial differences. The gingival tissues of dark-skinned individuals tend to be of a deeper hue than those of individuals with fair complexions. Members of the black race and certain Mediterranean and far eastern races may exhibit mottled color changes (pigmentation) ranging from grayish pink to purplish. All of these color distinctions are considered normal.

Gingival color is lighter in children than in adults. The color does not vary with the sex of the individual. In adults, gingival

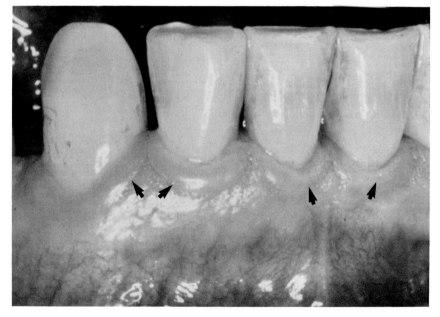

Figure 2–3. Free Gingival Groove. Gingival grooves (arrows), when present, approximate the base of the gingival crevice (Courtesy of Dr. Ike Aukhil).

color does not change with aging as long as the tissues remain healthy.

Gingival color changes often are indicative of early periodontal disease. In more acute disease stages dramatic color shifts occur in gingival tissues.

TEXTURE AND TONE. In a state of health the adult gingivae are pitted with a myriad of tiny depressions (Fig. 2–4). This results in the gingivae appearing stippled, similar to the texture of an orange peel. These stippled areas may be minute rounded depressions or oval-shaped craters or even linear dips. Stippling occurs in the greatest amount in the attached gingiva, but also may be noted in the central portion of the interdental papillae. Marginal gingiva is not stippled by any significant degree.

Apparently age plays some role in the stippling phenomenon. Young children exhibit little or no stippling (Fig. 2–5). Stippling is most prominent in adults but tends to decrease with old age. Another aspect of gingival texture as well as color relates to the degree of keratinization of surface epithelium. Typically, outer surfaces of gingival tissue are almost fully keratinized reflecting their stress-bearing function. The keratin layer imparts a dull or matte appearance to the gingiva as well as making the color light pink in contrast to the redder nonkeratinized alveolar mucosa.

The tone of the gingivae refers to their firm and resilient nature. Except at the free gingival margin this tissue is securely anchored by a dense connective layer to tooth and bone. Such an arrangement lends to this tissue an immobility and toughness. This is in marked contrast to the smooth, mobile, and highly elastic alveolar mucosa. Free gingiva is well adapted against the tooth and if the tone is firm, it cannot be easiy displaced from this position.

TOPOGRAPHY AND CONTOUR. Considerable variation occurs between individuals in the bulk, width, and contour of the gingiva. The approximate apicocoronal width of the gingiva varies between 2.5 and 5 millimeters. Widths greater or lesser than this can exist and still be considered within normality. Many factors influence gingival width, including underlying osseous morphology, contour of tooth crown, and prominence of the tooth roots. Character-

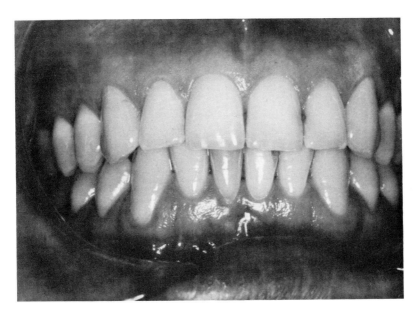

Figure 2–4. Normal Gingiva in the Anterior Region of the Mouth. The gingiva is characterized by pointed interdental papillae, knife-edged margins, and stippling.

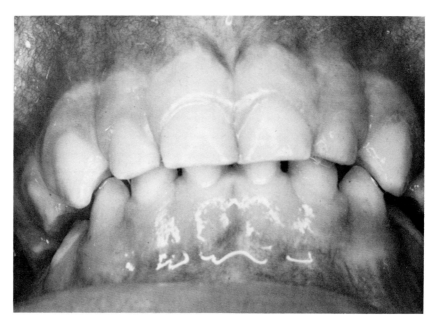

Figure 2–5. Normal Gingiva in Child. Appearance of normal gingiva in a four-year-old child. There is a relatively wide zone of attached gingiva and little stippling. Vertical grooves between the teeth are a prominent feature.

istically, a more narrow band of gingiva can be found in the mandibular arch when compared with the maxillary arch. This is particularly true for the mandibular premolars and canines.

Gingival width is particularly important in that a sufficient zone of attached gingiva is necessary to resist masticatory stress and act as a buttress against the pull of the elastic alveolar mucosa and muscle attachments.

Contour of gingival tissues can be influenced by size, shape, and position of the teeth; the relationships of the tooth contact areas to one another; spacing of teeth; and the gingival embrasure pattern found between the teeth.

The topography of the gingivae of children, as long as they retain their primary dentition, is different from that of the adult. The size and shape of the teeth and the spacing between the teeth cause the gingiva to appear more bulbous. Fully developed papillae may be lacking and vertical grooves in the gingivae between the teeth may be especially prominent in the anterior region of the mouth. The spacing of the teeth and their small size often makes the child appear to have a great deal of gingival tissue relative to the adult (Fig. 2–5).

Healthy marginal gingiva is firmly adapted to the teeth terminating in a thin, slightly rounded edge. When viewed clinically, the marginal tissues present a smooth, undulating outline from tooth to tooth. The level of this tissue is just apical to the height of tooth contours. Tooth position in the arch plays a significant role in the form of these tissues. Teeth which are prominently placed facially usually have a gingival margin located more apically than on adjacent teeth. Conversely, lingually positioned teeth may have a gingival margin that is considerably more coronal than on neighboring teeth. Often this marginal gingiva becomes a flattened tissue shelf.

Prominence of roots also determines to some degree the topography of attached gingiva. Where roots are prominent, vertical folds in the attached gingiva occur interdentally. This is also dependent upon the bulk of the tissue, and these grooves are defined less clearly when the gingiva is thick.

The interdental papillae fill the gingival embrasures. Consequently, their form is determined by the size and location of contacts as well as the shape or contour of the teeth. The shape of the interproximal bone also may have an influence.

Anteriorly in the mouth the papillae assume a pointed, triangular, or cone-shaped configuration (Fig. 2–4). Generally the roots of the incisor and canine teeth are close together and the contact areas small faciolingually, and this plays a role in the arrangement of the papillae.

Posteriorly, in the premolar and molar areas, the papillae are more flattened. Here the interseptal bone is also flatter than anteriorly. The teeth are wider faciolingually and the contact areas broader. All of these features are reflected in the shape of the interdental papillae (Fig. 2–6). The papilla is actually separated into facial and lingual

peaks joined by a depression in the region of the contact area. The depression is termed the col (Fig. 2–7). Although this arrangement may occur anteriorly, it is more prominent posteriorly because of the wider faciolingual dimension of the teeth. The epithelium of the interdental col is thin and not covered by a protective layer of keratinized cells. This anatomic characteristic of the col may predispose the interproximal area to increased susceptibility to the effects of plaque accumulation.

Where diastemas occur between the teeth, the interdental gingiva is firmly attached to the interproximal bone and no papillae exist. This does not compromise gingival health in this area and may in fact result in better health because of better access of self-cleaning mechanisms.

Microscopic Features of the Gingiva

All mucous membranes basically consist of an epithelial component resting on a basement membrane which separates the epithelium from the connective tissue portion of the mucosa. Considerable morpho-

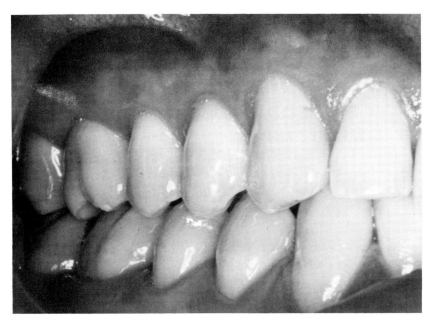

Figure 2–6. Normal Gingiva in Posterior Region of Mouth. Note that the interdental papillae become progressively flatter in the molar area.

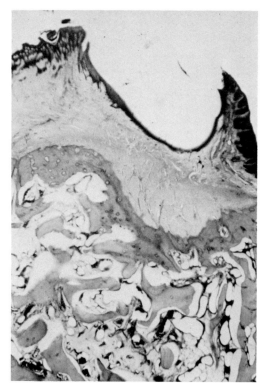

Figure 2–7. Interdental Col. This histologic section shows the interdental col with facial and lingual gingival peaks. In this specimen a similar anatomic arrangement occurs in the bone. (Courtesy of Dr. D. Walter Cohen.)

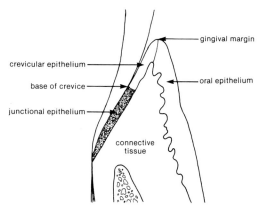

Figure 2–8. Gingival Epithelium. Oral epithelium covers outer gingival surface. Crevicular (sulcular) epithelium lines the gingival crevice. Junctional epithelium forms the epithelial attachment to the tooth and the base of the crevice.

(1) oral epithelium which covers the outer surfaces of free and attached gingiva, (2) crevicular or sulcular epithelium which lines the gingival crevice and (3) junctional epithelium which attaches to the tooth and forms the epithelial attachment (Fig. 2–8).

Oral epithelium is stratified squamous epithelium in which cells are arranged in a series of layers, representing a pattern of

logic variation occurs in the mucous membranes dependent on the location. Many of these features are established prior to birth. Since the gingival portion of the oral mucosa is subjected to particularly heavy masticatory stresses, these tissues are structurally adapted to resist these pressures and serve their unique oral function of protecting subjacent structures.

The histologic features of the gingivae were established originally with the use of the light microscope. The use of the electron microscope and other cytologic methods have facilitated a more detailed examination of the fine structure of the various components of the oral mucous membranes.

Gingival epithelium can be divided functionally and structurally into three areas:

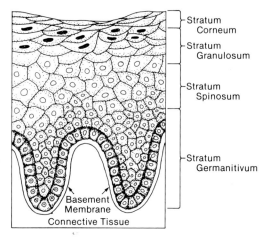

Figure 2–9. Cell Layers of Oral Epithelium. Cellular morphology in the various layers of keratinized oral epithelium is illustrated at the light-microscopic level. Compare with Figure 2–13.

cell birth, development, maturation and death (Fig. 2–9). That is, cells originate in the inner layer adjacent to connective tissue and undergo functional and structural changes as they move to the surface and are eventually desquamated. The cell turnover rate for oral epithelium has been estimated to be 10 to 12 days.

Nearest to the basement membrane is located a layer of cells termed the stratum germinativum. The cuboidal shaped cells of this basal layer possess a high degree of mitotic activity. A constant germinative process is required to replace mature cells being desquamated from the surface of the gingiva. The vast majority of these cuboidal cells, termed keratinocytes, are thus engaged in cell reproduction. These cells contain a well-defined cytostructure or cellular skeleton. They are connected to the underlying basement membrane by an arrangement known as a hemidesmosome. Also located between the keratinocytes in the basal layer of the epithelium are special pigment-producing cells, melanoblasts. Melanin pigment elaborated from these melanoblasts is stored in the cytoplasm of the cuboidal keratinocytes and accounts for gingival pigmentation observed in dark-skinned individuals.

The stratum spinosum is situated above the basal cell layer. Well-developed, polyhedral-shaped cells known as prickle cells comprise this thickened layer. When viewed through the light microscope, these cells appear to be connected by so-called intercellular bridges giving the cells a spiny appearance. Actually these intercellular bridges consist primarily of layers of keratin protein between the cell boundaries. Studies with the electron microscope have revealed that the cells are held together at junctional boundaries termed desmosomes.

As epithelial cells mature they become more flattened. Nuclei may become shrunken and chromatin in the nuclei clumps together. Such a nuclear arrangement is termed pyknosis. Within the cytoplasm,

granules of keratohyalin appear. Keratohyalin plays a role in the cornification of gingival epithelium, but the exact mode of action has not been fully determined. This flattened, granular layer is the stratum granulosum.

The stratum corneum of gingiva oral epithelium is most commonly parakeratotic or keratotic in contrast to lining mucosa, which lacks a cornified exterior. When the squamous cells lack nuclei, the surface is keratotic. If remnants of nuclei remain, a parakeratotic surface is found. The presence of keratotic epithelium is reflective of greater functional demands, e.g., from a coarser diet, than is a parakeratotic surface.

BASEMENT MEMBRANE. A wavy, well-developed basement membrane is interposed between the basal epithelial cells of the stratum germinativum and the underlying dense connective tissue of the gingiva (lamina propria). This interface between epithelium and lamina propria provides a tight continuity of tissue layers. The epithelium is folded into a series of projections into the connective tissue. These epithelial folds are called rete pegs or rete ridges and the connective tissues interdigitating between them are connective tissue papillae. Such an arrangement provides for tissue stability and enhances fluid exchange across the basement membrane by increasing the surface area of this interface. This is particularly essential since epithelium lacks blood vessels.

The stippling phenomenon noted clinically may be explained by the arrangement at the junction of epithelium and connective tissue. The stippled depressions occur over the rete pegs and may be related to the papillae pushing up the tissue, leaving the area over the rete pegs depressed. It is also possible that desquamation of cells may be more pronounced over the rete pegs due to greater distance of these surface cells from the blood supply in the connective tissues. Such desquamation may be reflected as stippling.

Electron-microscopic studies have revealed that the basement membrane is more complex in its arrangement than previously reported with the light-microscopic observations. The basement membrane in the electron-microscopic photographs is divided into a light layer, termed the lamina lucida, near the basal cells of the epithelium and a darker layer, the lamina densa, near the connective tissue. Apparently both the epithelium and the connective tissue cells contribute to the formation of the total basal structure. The basal cells of the epithelium are attached to this basal lamina through their hemidesmosomes and fine fibrillar loops from connective tissues. This intimate relationship of epithelium to connective tissue enhances the exchange of nutrients from connective tissue to epithelium. It also creates a junctional boundary that may become involved in certain disease states affecting these tissues.

Crevicular epithelium is similar in stratification to oral epithelium except that it is not keratinized. There is a tendency towards parakeratinization especially near the gingival margin. The junction between crevicular epithelium and underlying connective tissue tends to flatten as it extends apically with rete ridges being evident though not pronounced towards the gingival margin. These differences reflect a transition to an area subjected to less functional stress. Cells are desquamated into the gingival crevice.

Junctional epithelium is distinctly different from oral and crevicular epithelium (Fig. 2–10). Cells originate in a basal layer and migrate toward the tooth surface but do not exhibit any tendency toward maturation into granular or keratinized layers. Cells in the suprabasal layer do become flattened longitudinally as they approach the tooth surface. The thickness of this epithelial layer varies from 1 to 2 cells at its most apical point to 15–18 cells at the base of the gingival crevice (Fig. 2–11). Cells migrate obliquely towards the gingival crevice and are eventually sloughed there exhibiting a turnover rate of 3–6 days.

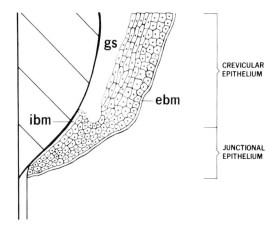

Figure 2–10. Junctional Epithelium. The most apical portion of the gingival crevice is occupied by junctional epithelial cells. (ebm) external basement membrane, (ibm) internal basement membrane (lamina), (gs) gingival sulcus (crevice).

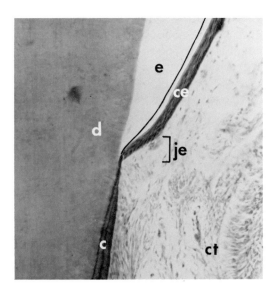

Figure 2–11. Gingival Crevice. Nonkeratinized epithelium lines the gingival crevice. The epithelial attachment is located at the cementoenamel junction. (e) enamel, (ce) crevicular epithelium, (d) dentin, (je) junctional epithelium, (c) cementum, (ct) connective tissue.

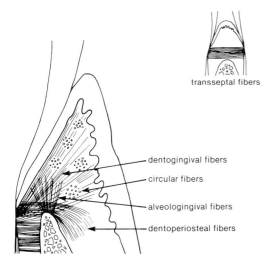

transsseptal fibers

dentogingival fibers

circular fibers

alveologingival fibers

dentoperiosteal fibers

Figure 2–12. Gingival Fiber Groups. The major connective tissue fiber groups are illustrated schematically.

CONNECTIVE TISSUE. The gingival connective tissue is referred to as the lamina propria and is composed of a dense assemblage of collagen fibers and interfibrillar ground substance and cells. There is no submucosa and elastic fibers are absent. Consequently the collagen fibers firmly bind the attached gingiva to underlying cementum or bone and hold the free gingiva firmly against the tooth.

A rather definite pattern of collagen bundles arranged into fiber groups occurs in the gingiva. This arrangement reflects the multidirectional functional stress that the gingival tissues are subjected to and accounts for their relative immobility when healthy. The orientation of these fiber groups are illustrated in Fig. 2–12. The *dentogingival* fibers originate in cementum and extend laterally or coronally terminating just beneath the epithelium. The *dentoperiosteal* fibers extend facially and lingually from cementum over alveolar crestal bone and bend apically to merge with fibers arising from the outer aspect of bone.

Supplementing these fiber groups in maintaining the gingiva firmly against the tooth is a group of fibers passing circularly around the tooth. This fiber group, the *circular* fibers, is so designed that it has a purse-string effect that results in keeping the free gingiva close to the tooth.

Passing from one tooth to the next across the bony interdental septum is an important gingival fiber group, the *transseptal* fibers. These transseptal fibers insert in the cementum of adjacent teeth and provide a barrier to apical migration of the epithelium of the gingival crevice.

Also distinguishable as a fiber group are those fibers taking their origin in crestal alveolar bone and passing coronally into the lamina propria. These are the *alveologingival* fibers. Other gingival fibers may partially encircle a tooth, insert into the free gingiva of adjacent teeth, or extend across facial or lingual free gingiva from tooth to tooth.

The ground substance is composed predominantly of proteoglycans, especially chondroitin sulfate, hyaluronic acid and serum-derived glycoproteins. It is highly hydrated and provides a gelatinous matrix in which fibers and cells are embedded.

Between the fibers of the connective tissue and located within the ground substance is a multiplex of cellular elements. This consists primarily of fibroblastic cells that manufacture both the collagen fibers and the components of the ground substance. Also located here are lymphocytes, plasma cells, mast cells, macrophages, and polymorphonuclear leukocytes derived from the vascular circulation. Apparently these cells are either normal inhabitants of gingival tissue or they indicate that there is always some degree of gingival irritation present, for these cells are part of the body's defense system.

A rich vascular system is found in the lamina propria of the gingiva. Numerous small vessels pass throughout the connective tissue and anastomoses are common. A submucosa, found in mucosal tissues, is lacking in the gingiva, and thus the blood supply passes directly into the lamina propria. Primarily the vessels arise on the outer aspect of alveolar bone. Additional blood is supplied from intra-alveolar vessels and vessels penetrating the osseous septum. Anastomoses with vessels supplying the periodontal ligament also occur. The complex arrangement of the small arterioles, venules, and capillaries thus provides a rapid and abundant mechanism for supply of nutrients and for defensive purposes.

Gingival tissues are well innervated. Free nerve endings transmit pain sensation. Special nerve receptors are modified for pressure and temperature. Most nerve endings terminate in the connective tissue papillae in close association with the basement membrane (Fig. 2–13). An unusual type of free ultraterminal nerve ending in gingival epithelium has been demonstrated. In these instances, the nerve fiber crosses the basement membrane and ends in the epithelium.

Dentogingival Junction

The dentogingival junction represents a unique relationship between a calcified tissue, the cementum of the tooth, and a soft tissue, the gingiva. This has been cited as a weak point in the defensive arrangement of the oral tissues. While this is true, it also must be noted that nature's defensive mechanism in this area is surprisingly effective. Both epithelium and connective tissues participate in forming the defensive barrier in their attachment to the hard structure of the tooth. Connective tissue forms the firmer attachment, and it supports the epithelium. The connective tissue fiber groups of the gingiva provide for great resistance against stress and, when intact, prohibit the apical migration of junctional epithelium.

EPITHELIAL ATTACHMENT. A zone of attachment of junctional epithelial cells to the tooth surface comprises the epithelial component of the dentogingival junction. In the initial formation stage the epithelial attachment is mediated by reduced enamel epithelium. At eruption of the teeth and thereafter junctional epithelial cells originate from the basal layer of gingival epithelium. These cells differentiate into attachment cells instead of keratinocytes and subsequently migrate towards the tooth

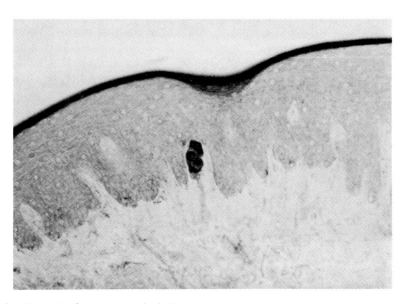

Figure 2–13. Nerve Ending in Attached Gingiva. Special stains demonstrate nerve endings in connective tissue papillae. Note the relation of epithelium with lamina propria. (Courtesy of Dr. Thomas McNeely.)

surface. Undifferentiated basal cells have the continuing capacity to specialize into attachment cells and consequently the potential for regeneration of destroyed junctional epithelium is always present.

For many years there has been debate as to the exact mode of this epithelial interface with tooth surface. Some investigators believed that there was a true organic or cellular union between tooth structure and epithelial cells—an epithelial attachment. Others contended that there was only a firm adhesion of epithelial cells against the tooth—an epithelial cuff.

With the use of modern techniques the controversy over the manner of attachment is now somewhat clarified. The junction between epithelium and tooth surface is similar to that which exists between epithelium and connective tissue. Junctional epithelial cells synthesize substances, primarily mucopolysaccharides, which form a cementing layer called the basal lamina on the tooth surface. Attaching epithelial cells possess hemidesmosomes and fibrillar extensions which insert into the basal lamina and provide a firm physical attachment mechanism. The ultrastructure of this juncture is quite complex and represents a high degree of cellular specialization in the formation and maintenance of this biologically unique association between hard and soft tissues.

A relatively stable distance exists between the base of the crevice and the height of the alveolar bone. In health this distance of 1 to 2 millimeters is occupied by the gingival fiber groups of the connective tissue and by the junctional epithelium.

PASSIVE ERUPTION. As a tooth erupts through the gingiva, the crevice is established. The occlusalward movement of the tooth to meet its antagonist is active tooth eruption. Even when the erupting tooth reaches the occlusal plane the coronal portion of the tooth is still partially covered by soft tissue. Further exposure of the crown from the subsequent apicalward move-

ment of the epithelium is termed passive eruption.

Several stages occur in the passive eruptive process (Fig. 2–14). Initially, the apical border of the junctional epithelium is located at the cementoenamel junction, and the bottom of the gingival crevice is coronal to this. Some investigators contend that the depth of the crevice is at the cementoenamel junction as soon as the tooth erupts through the gingival epithelium. In the second stage of passive eruption, the junctional epithelium migrates partially onto cementum, but the base of the crevice remains located on enamel. A third stage occurs when all cells of the junctional epithelium are on cementum and the depth of the crevice is at the cementoenamel junction. A fourth stage of passive eruption is reached when both the junctional epithelial cells and the base of the gingival crevice are located on cementum, often with the associated exposure of the root. Although this fourth stage of passive eruption is frequently seen in older individuals, this does not imply that this stage is physiologic. While the first and second stages are normal phases of passive eruption, it is believed that the fourth and probably the third stages are reflective of pathologic processes.

In the process of eruption, the epithelium that is adjacent to the tooth must adjust to a variety of hard surfaces—enamel, the cementoenamel junction, cementum, and, in some instances, exposed dentin.

MUCOSA OF THE HARD PALATE

Because of the rigors of food passage and tongue movements, the hard palate is modified to resist stress. Many of the general features relating to the attached gingiva may also be noted in the palatal mucosa. This mucosa is tightly attached to the palatal surface of the maxilla and thus is nonmobile.

Anteriorly, the palate is thrown into ridges termed rugae. Along the midline a

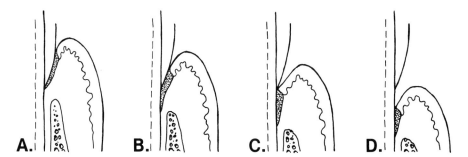

Figure 2–14, A–D. Passive Eruption. A, At eruption, junctional epithelium and the base of the crevice are on enamel. B, In the second stage, junctional epithelium is on cementum (c) and enamel; the base of the crevice is still on enamel. C, In the third stage, junctional epithelium is on cementum and the base of the crevice is at the cementoenamel junction. D, In the fourth stage, junctional epithelium and the base of the crevice are on cementum reflecting alveolar bone loss.

narrow band, the median raphe, can be noted. Just lingual to the central incisors a small elevation, the incisive papilla, covers the foramen of the nasopalatine nerve and vessels.

Palatal epithelium contains the same cell layers as previously noted in attached gingiva. The stratum corneum is uniform and thickened. Large, long rete pegs penetrate a dense lamina propria. The connective tissue shows some distinction dependent on location. These differences are most prominently displayed in the submucosa, a tissue layer not found in the gingiva. The submucosa is also lacking in the gingival portion of the palate and along the midline raphe. Anteriorly and laterally, the palatal submucosa contains variable amounts of fat. Posteriorly, numerous small accessory salivary mucous glands are located.

LINING MUCOSA

Mucosa lining the remaining portions of the mouth is characteristically smooth, shiny, and mobile. Lining mucosa is usually reddish-blue in color. This color distinction is in dramatic contrast to the pink keratinized gingiva.

The clinical characteristics are reflected in the arrangement of the anatomic structures. All parts of the lining mucosa have a fairly thin epithelium without a keratinized surface. Rete pegs are broad and shallow. Fewer collagen bundle groups are found here than in gingival tissue and are more scattered. A rich blood vascular supply interlaces the connective tissue. The thin, nonkeratinized epithelium and the wealth of blood vessels account for the color of these tissues. The shallowness of the rete pegs and lack of cornification explain the smoothness of these mucous membranes.

Gingiva is attached firmly to bone and tooth, but the mode of connection of lining mucosa is different. A submucosa of loose areolar tissue penetrated by large nerves and blood vessels is a prominent feature. Collagen fibers provide connection to deeper fascia and musculature. Elastic fibers occur in abundance. Some portions of the lining mucosa, notably lips and soft palate, contain large numbers of accessory salivary glands.

The alveolar mucosa and mucosa of the floor of mouth, at the point where they blend with the attached gingiva, are the areas of lining mucosa of primary importance in relation to periodontics. Because of their lack of keratinization and easy retractability, these tissues are unsuitable as a protective covering around the cervical area of the teeth.

SPECIALIZED MUCOSA

The dorsal surface of the tongue has been designated as specialized mucosa due to its physiologic adaptation for taste reception. Though not a part of the periodontium, physiologically the tongue plays a significant role in the health of the periodontal tissues. A high degree of self-cleansing of the lingual surfaces of teeth is achieved by the tongue. Also muscular forces exerted by this organ can produce movement, particularly on periodontally diseased teeth.

Simply, the tongue consists of a mass of muscle bundles covered by a keratinized epithelium modified as lingual papillae. The most numerous of the papillae are the thread-like filiform variety. These give the tongue its furry or velvety appearance. Less numerous and scattered among the filiform papillae occur the red, mushroom-shaped fungiform papillae. Separating the anterior two-thirds of the tongue from the posterior base is a V-shaped line of about ten large, circumvallate papillae. Although all papillae may contain taste buds, the circumvallate are especially adapted to transmit taste perception. This is due to a fluid derived from glands placed deep in trenches surrounding the circumvallate papillae. Foliate papillae are located in the posterolateral aspects of the tongue.

THE ATTACHMENT APPARATUS

A tooth maintains its functional position primarily through the mode of its attachment. This consists of a relationship established between the cementum of the tooth, the periodontal ligament, and the alveolar bone forming the socket. Such an arrangement allows for eruption as the coronal tooth surface is lost through attrition and for a repositioning of the tooth in a mesial direction from wear at the contact areas. In addition, the attachment apparatus permits the tooth to absorb repeated occlusal contacts with little damage to itself. It is this design of soft and hard tissue connection which permits orthodontic movement of teeth.

Periodontal Ligament

Filling the space between the surface of the root and the wall of the alveolus is the periodontal ligament. Although the width of this soft connective tissue varies from tooth to tooth and from area to area even on the same tooth, it is approximately 0.1 to 0.3 millimeter. The periodontal ligament has also been termed the periodontal membrane, but because of the anatomic arrangement of the fibers, periodontal ligament is the name best applied.

The periodontal ligament blends with the gingiva that it supports. Further it serves the functions of maintaining the tooth in its socket; building and maintaining cementum, alveolar bone, and itself; and transmitting vessels for nutrition and nerves for sensation (Fig. 2–15).

Morphologically, the periodontal ligament is composed of various fiber bundles and of an interstitial connective tissue that winds its way between the fiber groups. These fiber bundles are composed primarily of collagen fibers and follow a wavy path from cementum to bone. At their insertion into the cementum and bone these bundles are termed Sharpey's fibers. Other types of fibers, much fewer in number, are also found in the ligament. Reticular and elastic fibers are found in association with the vascular channels. Oxytalan fibers can be detected scattered among the collagen fibers, but their exact function is unclear.

PRINCIPAL FIBER GROUPS. Collagen fiber bundles are assembled into groups arranged to resist mechanical force on the tooth. These functional groups, termed principal fibers, are in turn made up of smaller fibers. It should be understood that although different fiber groups are given specific names, they actually merge into one another (Fig. 2–16). The gingival fiber groups are listed under the section on gingival connective tissue.

The principal fiber groups of the periodontal ligament are as follows:

1. *Alveolar Crest Group.* The fibers take

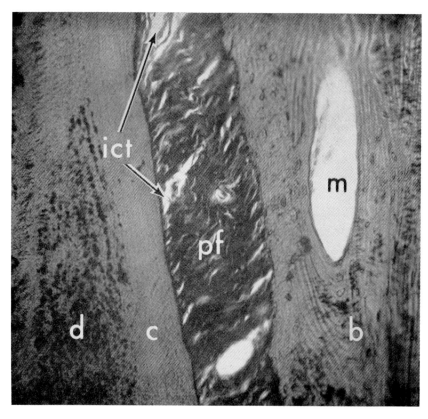

Figure 2–15. Attachment Apparatus. A histologic view of the tooth attachment to bone. (d) dentin, (c) cementum, (pf) principal fibers, (ict) interstitial connective tissue, (m) marrow, (b) bone.

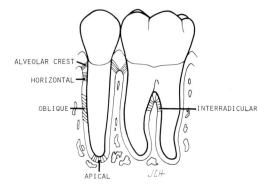

Figure 2–16. Periodontal Ligament. The principal connective tissue fiber groups of the periodontal ligament are represented.

their origin at the crestal portion of alveolar bone and pass slightly coronally, and insert into cementum apical to the junctional epithelium.

2. *Horizontal Group.* Fibers extend horizontally from cementum to alveolar bone. They aid in resistance to lateral stress.

3. *Oblique Group.* This is the major fiber group. The attachment occurs more coronally on the alveolar bone surface than on the cementum. This group of fibers is responsible primarily for resistance to vertical forces applied along the long axis of the tooth.

4. *Apical Group.* Radiating outward from cementum to the base of the tooth sockets are overlapping groups of apical fibers.

5. *Interradicular Group.* In multirooted

teeth the fibers pass from cementum to the interradicular bone septum.

Wavy collagen fibers of the principal fiber groups may extend the entire distance from cementum to bone. There is evidence that some fibers may even pass from the cementum of one tooth through the interalveolar bone to the cementum of an adjacent tooth. These have been termed transalveolar fibers.

Interposed with the principal fibers are shorter segments of collagen fibers. These may serve in a splicing capacity. The concept of an intermediate group of fibers has been advanced. This envisions some fibers inserting in bone and others in cementum with a splicing occurring somewhere in between. This intermediate plexus has been demonstrated in rodent teeth and in developing human teeth. It has not been definitely established in functioning human teeth. The presence of an intermediate plexus would aid in the explanation of fiber rearrangement during eruption and orthodontic movement. It is probable, however, that the rapid replacement rate of collagen fibers partially explains these tooth movements.

INTERSTITIAL TISSUE. The loose connective tissue that passes between the principal fiber bundles consists of a fluid ground substance in which a number of different cellular elements are located. It also provides a path for blood vessels and nerves which thread their way between the fibers. The fluid ground substance helps cushion the vessels, nerves, and cellular elements against compression.

The fiber groups and the compressible nature of the fluid interstitial tissue collectively tend to dissipate forces placed on the tooth. All forces placed on the teeth are counteracted and these forces are translated into tension on the bone of the alveolus. Most of these forces are normally directed along the long axis of the tooth. Apparently these forces are first absorbed by the vascular bed and by hydraulic pressure release of fluid into the marrow spaces

of surrounding bone. Subsequently, the collagen fibers lengthen through an uncoiling mechanism. As the forces are released, fibers return to their original position. This characteristic of collagen fibers in combination with other features permits adaptation to a wide range of occlusal forces without damage to periodontal structures.

Functions of defense and tissue replacement and remodeling of the attachment apparatus are accomplished by the cellular elements within the interstitial connective tissue. Cells modified for formative functions provide new fibers, cementum, and alveolar bone of the socket. Fibroblasts are the most numerous cells in the interstitial spaces. These cells manufacture and maintain the collagen fibers of the principal fiber groups. Cementoblasts are cells modified for the apposition of cementum. New cementum is required to maintain the connection of the fibrous attachment apparatus at the tooth surface. Such a process is needed to allow for modification of tooth position and reattachment of new fibers to replace those lost through aging.

Alveolar bone is in a constant process of rearrangement because of the demands of stress placed upon it. The construction and removal of bone are accomplished by cells present in the periodontal ligament. Osteoblasts are the cells responsible for the formation of bone; osteoclasts are multinucleated cells that function in the resorption of the bone. Since all of these cells must be present in order for these functions to be operative, there are mesenchymal cells with multipotential powers present in the ligament. These primitive cells may then be modified into mature osteoblasts, cementoblasts, or fibroblasts in order to perform specific functions.

Other cellular elements are also present in the interstitial tissue. Among these are a multitude of cells available for defensive purposes since the periodontal ligament is subject to the ingress of toxic bacterial products from both the oral cavity and diseased pulpal tissue. Macrophages, lymphocytes, and wandering defense cells are present in order to destroy these bacterial products and nullify their toxic effects.

Epithelium plays a significant role in the formation of the tooth root. Clusters of epithelial cells, thought to be remnants from the embryonic development period, remain in the periodontal ligament after eruption (though the area is connective tissue). These are the *epithelial rests of Malassez*. These epithelial cells apparently are present as a connected latticework found in the interstitial tissue.

Occasionally calcified bodies are found in the interstitial spaces between periodontal fibers. These small items of cementum-like material are cementicles. These may be free in the connective tissue or attached to the root of the tooth. These cementicles probably have little significance clinically, but they may add to root roughness if exposed.

A particularly rich blood supply is found in the periodontal ligament. The arterial vessels are derived from three major sources. The primary vascular source is from branching vessels of the intra-alveolar arteries that pass through the interdental septum. Secondly, blood vessels entering the periapical area branch into the periodontal ligamemt. Finally, anastomoses are achieved with vessels from the gingiva. Studies have shown that the vascular bed is complex, containing extensive branching, glomeruli, and arteriovenous shunts. Veins and lymphatics generally follow the same routes as the arteries.

The sensory nervous supply serves three major purposes—pressure, pain, and proprioception. These responses are transmitted through special nerve and bulbs and free endings. The property that supplies information concerning spatial relations is termed proprioception. This particular property is well developed in the periodontal ligament. This enables a high degree of response on the part of teeth to the slightest pressure and aids in mastication.

The ability to determine small discrepancies between opposing teeth is an important feature attributable to the well-developed nerve supply.

Cementum

Cementum represents the tooth portion of the attachment apparatus. It corresponds in function to the alveolar bone which it also resembles in its structural composition. Cementum is slightly less hard than bone, being composed of 45 to 50% inorganic material and 50 to 55% organic matter and water.

The cementum covers all of the anatomic root of the tooth and is in direct apposition with the dentin. Although cementum is considerably softer than dentin, it is difficult to distinguish between dentin and cementum during scaling procedures.

In the region of the cementoenamel junction, different arrangements may occur between cementum and enamel. This cervical area of the root may have cementum making a blunt joint contact with the enamel, or the cementum may fail to contact the enamel leaving a gap. Most commonly, however, the cementum slightly overlaps the enamel. All of these designs may occur on different teeth or even on the same tooth. Such anatomic aberrations invite accumulation of bacteria and calculus deposition at the cementoenamel junction.

Considerable variation occurs in the width of the cementum. It is most narrow at the cementoenamel junction, but widens as it approaches the apex of the tooth. On some teeth the cementum is rather thick in this apical area. Often in the bifurcation and trifurcation areas of the tooth cementum is also thick.

TYPES OF CEMENTUM. Based on the presence or absence of cellular elements in the calcified connective tissue, two types of cementum can be determined. These are cellular cementum and acellular cementum. These two types differ also in their main anatomic location and morphologic construction.

Cellular cementum which occupies primarily the apical portion of the root strongly resembles bone. The cellular elements, cementocytes, occupy small spaces termed lacunae. These represent cementoblasts trapped during cementum formation. Connecting these lacunae are tiny channels called canaliculi, which provide for protoplasmic connection of the cementocytes. Since cementum lacks any blood vessels, these channels provide for nutrient exchange. In many lacunae located near dentin no cementocytes are present. This is presumed to be due to lack of nutrition from the surface in spite of the canaliculi. Therefore, cementocytes exist primarily in the more superficial layers.

The bulk of the cementum consists of collagen fibers embedded in a calcified matrix. The inorganic component is hydroxyapatite crystals. The collagen fibers are arranged, for the most part, parallel to the long axis of the tooth.

Layering of cementum is a conspicuous feature. These lamellae are distinguished by incremental lines. It is not unusual for acellular cementum to be laid down on preexisting cellular cementum or even for several layers of cellular and acellular cementum to be mixed.

A precemental layer of uncalcified substance and collagen fibers is found on the surface of the cementum. This layer, the cementoid, is continuously formed throughout the life of the tooth. External to the precementum, cementoblastic cells are located in the periodontal ligament.

The precementum or cementoid surface serves a most important protective function in that it apparently resists resorption. This is of considerabe importance because orthodontic movement depends on the fact that alveolar bone is more susceptible to resorption than cementum. Furthermore, the cementoid provides for the incorporation of Sharpey's fibers of the periodontal ligament, and this allows for repositioning of the tooth in response to demands placed on it, such as biting forces.

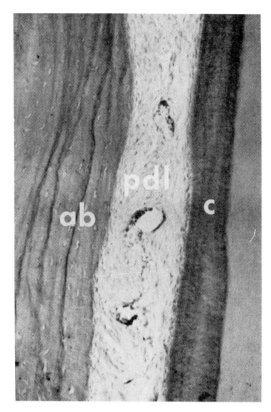

Figure 2–17. Cementum, Periodontal Ligament, and Alveolar Bone Proper. Sharpey's fibers are embedded in the cementum. This cementum is of the acellular type. (ab) alveolar bone, (c) cementum, (pdl) periodontal ligament.

Occupying the bulk of the coronal portion of the root is acellular cementum (Fig. 2–17). No cementocytes are located in this type of cementum, and often it is difficult to locate cementoblasts outside the cementum in histologic sections. Much of the original cementum formation adjacent to the dentin is of this acellular type. Growth lines are a prominent feature of acellular cementum. They may represent areas of fiber-free amorphous cementing substance. These areas alternate with broader zones containing coarse collagen fibers. Sometimes a fairly conspicuous layer of imperfectly formed cementum is located intermediate to the dentin.

It is important to note that apparently

there is little practical significance as to whether the root surface is comprised of cellular or acellular cementum. Both forms serve equally well as a base for precementum. The life of the tooth in its socket ultimately rests upon the vitality of the cementoid layer.

Apposition and Resorption. Apposition of new cementum is continuous throughout life. The amount of new cementum deposited is, however, generally not great. Cemental apposition occurs even on endodontically treated pulpless teeth. This continuous deposition is a logical arrangement to ensure an active attachment system with a capacity to be modified in response to functional demands.

In the apical region of the tooth, apposition of cellular cementum is a prominent feature which helps in forming the contour of the root apex, and, more importantly, allows for the tooth to remain in occlusal contact as wear occurs on the crown. This compensating mechanism may result in a rather heavy cemental deposit about the apex of some teeth.

New cemental growth occurs in areas of cementum or dentin resorption. Cemental apposition also takes place over root fractures. Hypercemental formation may be manifested in response to occlusal trauma or inflammation in the periapical region. Also, pressures on the tooth may sometimes result in bulges or spurs of cementum along the lateral surfaces of the tooth.

Numerous tiny microscopic areas of cemental resorption may exist. Sometimes these resorptive areas extend through the cementum and into dentin providing a potential place for bacterial accumulation and calculus formation when the crevice becomes deepened in these areas. It is believed that the resorption is carried out by modified cells with cementoclastic activity.

Although resorption and subsequent apposition of cementum may occur, this does not imply that remodeling takes place in cementum in the same manner as in bone. Bone, a vascular connective tissue, is constantly being reshaped. Cemental destruction and replacement occur only at the surface. As noted before, cementoid tissue seems to resist resorption.

Pressure obliquely applied to the tooth appears to markedly increase resorptive processes. This is particularly true when heavy lateral forces are sustained over long intervals. Thus massive cementum and dentin resorption may occur in some teeth undergoing orthodontic movement especially if tooth movement is attempted too rapidly.

Alveolar Process

The mandible and maxilla are composed of the basal bone and the alveolar processes. The alveolar processes represent the bony portion of the attachment apparatus. Working in harmony with the suspensory periodontal ligament and dental cementum the alveolar processes support the teeth in their sockets (alveoli). These flat bones of the jaws are derived via the intramembranous method of bone formation and are not unlike bone found elsewhere in the body in basic composition. The architectural arrangement of the alveolar process is modified, however, to serve its dental supportive function.

The alveolar processes consist of outer layers of dense compact bone termed the facial and lingual cortical plates. The crest of the bone interproximally between the roots of the teeth is also composed of the compact bone. Interdentally, these cortical plates are separated by a more spongy cancellous bone. Around the tooth the bone of the socket is modified as a perforated plate—the alveolar bone proper.

Structural variation in the arrangement of the bone occurs when mandible and maxilla are compared. Furthermore, area to area variation occurs in each arch. These differences are related to the position of tooth contact areas, the proximity of the tooth roots, and the faciolingual contour of the roots (Figs. 2–18 and 2–19).

Interproximal bone of the alveolar crest

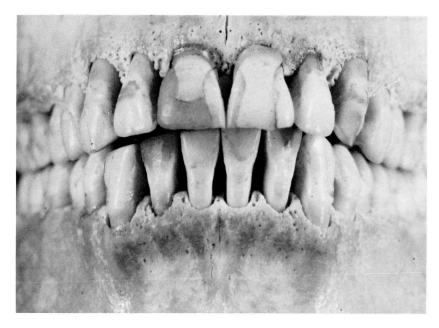

Figure 2–18. Anterior Osseous Morphology. In the anterior portion of the mouth the interproximal bone is pointed and the cortical plate is relatively thin. The small holes are openings for blood vessels. Compare with Figure 2–4.

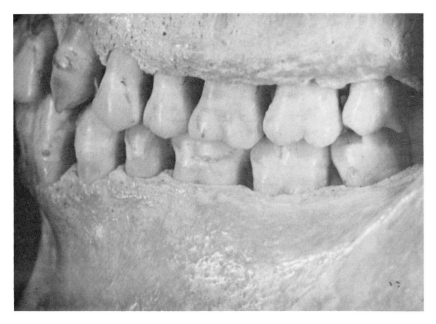

Figure 2–19. Posterior Osseous Morphology. In the posterior area of the mouth the cortical plate is thicker and the interproximal bone is more flattened. Compare with Figure 2–6.

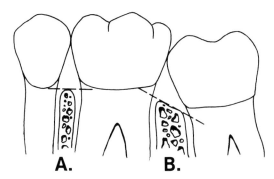

Figure 2–20. Contour of Alveolar Crest. Bone height interproximally is parallel to a line drawn between the cementoenamel junctions of two adjacent teeth. A. If teeth are evenly aligned, the contour is horizontal. B. If teeth are tilted or erupted to different heights, the contour is angular. (After Ritchie and Orban.)

is anatomically related to the cementoenamel junction of adjacent posterior teeth. When an imaginary line drawn between these is horizontal, then the crestal bone is flat. When a tooth is tipped, the bone then slants toward the more apically placed cementoenamel junction. This arrangement maintains sufficient space for healthy gingival fibers to exist between the bone and junctional epithelium (Fig. 2–20).

In the mandibular anterior region the fa-

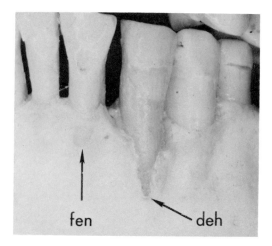

Figure 2–21. Dried Skull. In this specimen a thin plate of bone exists over the facial surface of roots of the teeth. (fen) fenestration, (deh) dehiscence.

cial cortical plate of bone is often thin. Roots of the teeth may perforate this thin plate. This is a fenestration or a window in the bone. At times a dip or cleft in the bone (dehiscence) may occur facially or lingually over the root of the tooth (Fig. 2–21). Interproximally in this area the bone assumes a pointed contour, and this arrangement is mimicked in the gingival tissue of this region since the interdental papillae are also pointed.

Posteriorly, the lower interproximal bony arrangement assumes a more rounded or flattened contour that may be related to the contact position and the relatively greater distance between the roots. In the bifurcation areas of mandibular molars the bone is more pointed, filling the interradicular space. This simulates the papillae form noted interproximally. In health the interproximal bone height is always positioned more coronally than on the facial or lingual aspect. This same pattern is seen in the gingival tissue, permitting a gentle rise and fall. The width of the facial cortical plate is fairly uniform. It is thinnest in the premolar region and thickest facial to the third molar. Lingually the bone is thicker in the premolar region and sometimes shows gross thickening in the form of mandibular tori.

The maxillary arch presents a somewhat different bony topography from that exhibited in the mandible. The facial cortical plate is thicker in the maxillary anterior region than in the mandible and fenestrations are less common. Between the central incisors a small cleft is sometimes noted. Facial to the maxillary canines, rather thick bony plates, the canine eminentias, are found.

The facial cortical plate of the maxilla is not as thick posteriorly as the mandible. Over the mesiofacial root of the first molar the bone often is extremely thin and dehiscences and fenestrations occur. The palatal cortical plate thickens as it proceeds posteriorly. Often small overgrowths of bone, exostoses, are located palatally in the region of the second molar. The relatively thin facial plate and the thickened palatal plate have clinical and therapeutic significance. Interproximally in the maxilla cancellous bone beneath the crest is more flattened posteriorly than anteriorly.

HISTOLOGIC ARRANGEMENT OF BONE. Bone is a connective tissue composed of fibers and cells residing in a calcified matrix. The organic and inorganic content are about equal such that bone is slightly harder than cementum. Unlike cementum, however, bone is penetrated by a blood vascular system that not only provides for nutrition, but also allows for easy reshaping of the bone.

Lining the outer aspects of the alveolar processes is a modified connective tissue, the periosteum. This is composed of two layers—an outer layer of dense collagenous fibers and an inner layer of connective tissue altered specifically for osseous deposition. Contained in this inner cambium layer are the cells, osteoblasts, responsible for bone formation. Also found here are osteoclastic cells capable of bone resorption. Just internal to the periosteum is a variable surface layer of noncalcified bone termed osteoid. Although the periosteum is tightly attached to the facial and lingual cortical plates, it can be surgically detached from the bone.

The cancellous portion of the bone is perforated by marrow cavities containing fat and a vascular bed. These inner cavities are lined by an endosteum similar to periosteum that is also capable of laying down or removing bone.

The facial and lingual cortical plates of the alveolar process are continuous with the basal bone of the mandible and maxilla. They consist of dense layers of compact bone. Compact bone consists of a calcified matrix of ground substance and fibers. Within this matrix are viable cells, osteocytes, which represent trapped osteoblasts. Residing in spaces in the bone called lacunae, these osteocytes are connected by cytoplasmic extension to one another. The canaliculi provide for exchange of fluid nutrients. Compact bone is made up of layers of this calcified, cell-containing matrix. Where these layers are concentrically formed around a small vessel, it is termed an haversian system. As many as twenty layers of bone may be formed in this manner though the number is usually less. Osteocytes are never far removed from a source of nutrition. Nearer the surface of the bone are more flattened periosteal lamellae. Irregular interstitial lamellae occupy spaces between haversian systems. Prominent cementing lines occur between the layers of compact bone indicating resting areas or places where resorption and apposition have occurred.

Bone is well supplied with vascular channels both from the periosteal side and from the inner marrow cavity side. These vessels, in Volkmann's canals, lead to haversian channels and from there fluid is passed on via the canaliculi.

Between the facial and lingual cortical plates of compact bone is the more spongy cancellous bone. In its composition and components cancellous bone is the same as compact bone, but architecturally it is arranged differently. Cancellous bone is made up of small beams of bone termed trabeculae which interlace to form the interproximal septa between adjacent teeth. These trabeculae are apparent as feathery radiopaque areas on the radiograph. The scaffolding constructed by the arrangement of these bars of bone lends a structural solidarity to the cancellous mass of bone and resists the stresses of occlusion (Fig. 2–22).

Located between the bone trabeculae are marrow cavities. This marrow is capable of production of blood cells in the young. As age increases, the nature of the marrow changes and becomes more fatty. Nevertheless, the marrow always provides pathways for vascular channels. Marrow spaces are lined by endosteum thus allowing for remodeling by osteoclasts and new bone apposition by osteoblasts.

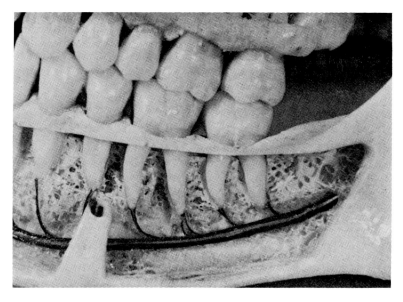

Figure 2–22. Dried Skull Specimen. In this view a portion of the facial cortical plate has been removed to show the underlying cancellous bone and vessels and nerves.

Alveolar Bone Proper. The bone comprising the wall of the alveolus is the alveolar bone proper. This cribriform plate is a layer of compact bone perforated by vascular and lymphatic channels. These perforations are continuous with the marrow spaces and aid in the hydraulic mechanism that partially absorbs occlusal forces on the tooth. The bone of the alveolus is modified to serve for the insertion of the Sharpey's fibers of the periodontal ligament. This type of bone has few conspicuous lamellae. This is largely due to lack of fibrils and increased amounts of cementing substance. This combination results in the alveolar bone proper being more radiopaque when seen on radiographs. This has resulted in the alveolar bone proper being termed the lamina dura in radiographs.

SUMMARY

The design of the oral tissue reflects an arrangement that merges form with function. In a state of health these tissues are mutually protective. When the oral structures are affected by disease, therapy is directed toward returning the tissues to their normal anatomic design insofar as possible. This restoration of form also aids in restoring the natural defensive mechanisms of the oral tissues.

BIBLIOGRAPHY

Ainamo, J. and Loe, H.: Anatomical characteristics of gingiva. A clinical and microscopic study of the free and attached gingiva, J. Periodontol., 37:5, 1966.

Arnim, S.S. and Hagerman, D.A.: The connective tissue fibers of the marginal gingiva, J. Am. Dent. Assoc., 47:271, 1953.

Bowers, G.M.: A study of the width of attached gingiva, J. Periodontol., 34:201, 1963.

Boyle, W.D., Jr., Via, W.F., Jr., and McFall, W.T., Jr.: Radiographic analysis of alveolar crest height and age, J. Periodontol., 44:236, 1973.

Cohn, S.A.: Transalveolar fibers in the human periodontium, Arch. Oral Biol., 20:257, 1975.

Coolidge, E.D.: The thickness of the human periodontal membrane, J. Am. Dent. Assoc., 24:1260, 1937.

Garguilo, A.W., Wentz, F.M. and Orban, B.: Dimensions and relations of the dentogingival junction in humans, J. Periodontol., 32:261, 1961.

Goldman, H.: The topography and role of the gingival fibers. J. Dent. Res., 30:331, 1951.

Henry, J.L. and Weinmann, J.P.: The pattern of resorption and repair of human cementum, J. Am. Dent. Assoc., 42:270, 1951.

Jones, J. and McFall, W.T., Jr.: A photometric study of the color of healthy gingiva, J. Periodontol., 48:21, 1977.

Kronfeld, R.: The biology of cementum, J. Am. Dent. Assoc., 25:1451, 1938.

Larato, D.C.: Alveolar plate fenestrations and dehiscences of the human skull, Oral Surg., 29:816, 1970.

Listgarten, M.A.: Electron microscopic study of the gingivo-dental junction of man, Am. J. Anat., 119:147, 1966.

McFall, W.T., Jr. and Kraus, B.S.: Histological studies of human prenatal oral mucous membranes, Periodontics, 1:20, 1963.

Mackler, S.D. and Crawford, J.J.: Plaque development and gingivitis in the primary dentition, J. Periodontol., 44:18, 1973.

Orban, B.: Clinical and histological study of the surface characteristics of the gingiva, Oral Surg., 1:827, 1948.

Orban, B. and Sicher, H.: The oral mucosa, J. Dent. Educ., 10:94, 1945 and 10:163, 1946.

Orban, B., et al.: Epithelial attachment (The at-tached epithelial cuff), J. Periodontol., 27:167, 1956.

Page, R.C. et al.: Collagen fiber bundles of the normal marginal gingiva, Arch. Oral Biol., 19:1039, 1974.

Ritchey, B. and Orban, B.: The crests of the interdental alveolar septa, J. Periodontol., 24:75, 1953.

Schroeder, H.E. and Listgarten, M.A.: Fine structure of the developing epithelial attachment of human teeth. Monographs in Developmental Biology, Vol. II, Basel, S. Karger, 1971.

Stern, I.: Electron microscopic observations of oral epithelium. I. Basal cells and basement membrane, Periodontics, 3:224, 1965.

Stern, I.B.: Current concepts of the dentogingival junction: The epithelial and connective tissue attachments to the tooth. J. Periodontol., 52:465, 1981.

Waerhaug, J.: Current concepts concerning gingiva anatomy. The dynamic epithelial cuff, Dent. Clin. North Am., Nov. 1960, p. 715.

Zander, H.A. and Hurzeler, B.: Continuous cementum apposition, J. Dent. Res., 37:1035, 1958.

Chapter | **3**

MICROBIOLOGY AND PATHOGENESIS OF INFLAMMATORY PERIODONTAL DISEASE

The complete etiology of inflammatory periodontal diseases is multifactorial and involves a complex set of local factors which relate to the extent and nature of irritants and systemic factors which determine the body's response to the irritants. The primary etiologic agent is bacterial dental plaque. Other factors are secondary and predispose to plaque accumulation or modify the individual's ability to protect against plaque's pathogenic effect.

Much recent research has been directed toward identifying specific bacteria in plaque that are periodontopathogens. It has become increasingly apparent that it is the quality of plaque, or bacterial types present, rather than the quantity of plaque that contributes most directly to the severity of periodontal diseases. From this aspect, inflammatory diseases that compromise periodontal support may be considered bacterial infections, not unlike other infections, but also exhibiting some unique characteristics. This chapter will concentrate on microbial factors in periodontal diseases, host defense mechanisms, and interrelationships that are potentially important in the pathogenesis of periodon-

tal diseases. Additional local and systemic factors will be discussed in Chapter 5.

DENTAL PLAQUE

Dental plaque has been defined as an adherent microbial film which cannot be removed by a strong water spray. This definition differentiates it from loosely adherent deposits such as food debris or materia alba. The outer layer of plaque, however, is always loosely adherent, and subgingivally, there is a distinct layer of loosely-bound plaque adjacent to the soft tissue wall. Consequently, a better definition of dental plaque would be bacterial aggregations that form on teeth and other hard surfaces in the oral cavity as well as in the protective environment of the gingival crevice.

Plaque Composition

Plaque is composed of a concentrated mass of cells, almost all bacterial, surrounded by an acellular matrix that imparts the cohesiveness to plaque. By weight these components constitute about 20% of plaque with the remainder being water.

Biochemically, the matrix is made up primarily of carbohydrates but also contains proteins and lipids. Bacterial synthesis of extracellular polysaccharides from dietary sugars constitutes the primary source of carbohydrate. Salivary glycoproteins may be degraded by some bacteria and constitute an additional source of carbohydrate and of protein. Other proteins in plaque matrix may be bacterial or salivary enzymes or immunoglobulins. The source for the lipid component of plaque matrix has not been well established. Lipids may be cell wall components from gram-negative bacteria or may originate from saliva. The most variable component of plaque matrix is carbohydrate. *Streptococcus mutans* in particular has the capacity to synthesize highly insoluble polysaccharides and contributes significantly to the formation of a thick cohesive supragingival plaque. These polysaccharides are polymers of glucose which are synthesized from sucrose through the action of the bacterial enzyme glucosyltransferase. The most stable glucose polymers are referred to as mutans and the ability of specific strains of *S. mutans* to produce this type of polymer relates directly to their cariogenic ability. Less stable glucose polymers, dextrans, and fructose polymers called levans, are also synthesized by *S. mutans* as well as by a number of other plaque bacteria.

If plaque is collected from several individuals and pooled to facilitate chemical analysis, the matrix makes up only about one third of the plaque dry weight with the remainder being almost entirely bacterial cells. These proportions vary on an individual basis. The matrix may increase to as much as 60% in the presence of a high sucrose diet where increased substrate for polylysaccharide synthesis is available. Levans are more prominent in the subgingival plaque matrix than are glucose polymers. Levans are not as stable as glucose polymers, but cohesiveness is not as critical for accumulation of subgingival plaque as it is for supragingival plaque. Major con-

tributors of levans in plaque are from the *Actinomyces* species, especially *A. viscosus* which is associated with gingivitis and root surface caries. Matrix components originating from saliva supragingivally are supplied by crevicular fluid subgingivally.

Plaque Distribution

The distribution of plaque is consistent with those areas that are least accessible to self-cleansing mechanisms in the oral cavity, proximal surfaces and cervical one-thirds of the clinical crowns of the teeth. Generally, there is more plaque on posterior teeth and on lingual surfaces of all teeth. Crowded or malaligned teeth also predispose to plaque accumulation. Distribution of plaque is often related to deficient oral hygiene habits and accordingly varies among individuals. The use of the Plaque Control Record as described in Chapter 6 involves the recording of plaque that is contiguous with the gingival margin and graphically illustrates specific areas where improved oral hygiene techniques are needed. Use of this record is helpful in educating patients in effective oral hygiene care for prevention of periodontal disease.

Stages of Plaque Formation

As many as 200 different bacterial species have been identified in plaque. There are probably many others not yet named or identified. The ability of a bacterial species to inhabit plaque is dependent upon a number of factors. Most important is the presence of a compatible surface to which bacterial cells may adhere. In the oral cavity this is a very selective process. Available surfaces include tooth surfaces, acquired pellicle, restorative materials, calculus, plaque matrix, other plaque bacteria and soft tissue surfaces. Additional determinants include the ability to overcome host defense capacity, the availability of nutrients for bacterial metabolism, and the presence of supportive atmospheric conditions. Based on respiratory needs, bacteria are categorized as: aerobes, requiring oxygen; anaerobes, unable to survive in oxygen; and facultative, adaptable to either environment. The set of growth requirements differs from species to species, but the variety of surfaces and conditions in the oral cavity provides favorable environments for a wide array of bacterial types. The complexity of oral microflora is especially increased with poor oral hygiene or through changes associated with oral diseases.

ACQUIRED PELLICLE. Within minutes of tooth cleansing, a film called the acquired pellicle is formed on the tooth surface. Supragingivally, this film is derived from saliva and exhibits a specific profile of salivary glycoproteins. This is a selective physicochemical process and does not just reflect a precipitation of saliva. The pellicle may afford some degree of protection of exposed tooth surfaces but also facilitates the initial attachment of plaque bacteria.

INITIAL BACTERIAL ADHERENCE. Within a few hours of pellicle deposition bacterial cells, again through specific interactions, adhere to the pellicle surface. Possible mechanisms for this adherence include the presence of bacterial cell wall appendages called *pili* or *fimbriae* or cell wall receptors called adhesins. Adherence is facilitated by the presence of cations such as free calcium ions in saliva that bridge the negative charges of tooth surface and bacterial cells.

Oral streptococci, primarily of the *Streptococcus mitior* and *Streptococcus sanguis* species are the first bacteria to adhere, at least in supragingival plaque. Much less is known regarding the initial stages of subgingival plaque formation. It is assumed that the pellicle is derived from serum components in crevicular fluid and that initial bacterial adherence is similar but may involve different bacterial species.

MICROBIAL CHANGES IN MATURING PLAQUE. In studies conducted in the 1960s, it was demonstrated that if plaque is permitted to accumulate on clean tooth surfaces with healthy adjacent gingiva, distribution of plaque bacteria progresses through three distinct stages (Fig. 3–1). Microscopic assessment of a patient's plaque sample can be a useful tool in oral hygiene education since the age of the plaque can be estimated according to bacterial types present. This assessment can be made based on shape, size and relative numbers of bacteria and does not require special slide preparation or staining if phase contrast or darkfield microscopy is used. In early plaque (1 to 2 days old), there is a predominance of Gram-positive cocci especially *S. mitior* and *S. sanguis*. Short aerobic gram-positive rods such as *Nocardia* species and Gram-negative aerobic cocci such as *Neisseria* species may also be present.

After 2 to 4 days of plaque accumulation, there is an increase in facultative filamentous bacteria such as *Actinomyces viscosus* and shortly thereafter an increase in *Fusobacteria* which are strict anaerobes. By 4 to 7 days the plaque mass appears to be a meshwork of these filamentous bacteria and fusiforms. Streptococci, which are facultative, still constitute a large proportion of the bacteria present but become less conspicuous because of their much smaller size. After 7 days, the appearance of motile forms, also anaerobes, begins to occur. These may be small gram-negative rods from the *Vibrio* class, larger flagellated rods such as *Selenomonas* species, and spirochetes. These bacteria do not predominate, except in deep actively-destructive periodontal pockets, but continue to increase in number as plaque continues to mature.

By 10 to 14 days of plaque accumulation, large numbers of these motile forms typify the final major morphologic change in plaque microbiology. This stage generally coincides with the appearance of clinical signs of gingivitis. Histological inflammatory changes begin after only 1 to 2 days of plaque accumulation, however. Subsequent microbial changes in plaque are dependent upon determinants mentioned previously.

Plaque forms more readily when the sal-

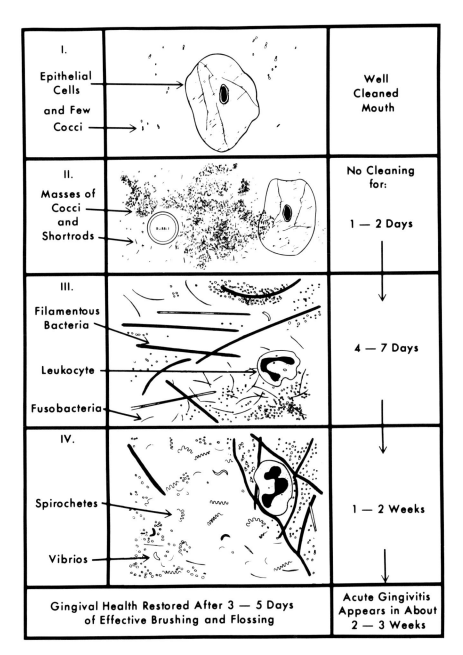

Figure 3–1. Bacterial Stages of Plaque Formation. Progressive changes in bacterial distribution in maturing supragingival plaque. (Courtesy of Dr. James Crawford, University of North Carolina School of Dentistry.)

ivary pH is slightly acidic and consequently tends to form faster during sleep when salivary flow is decreased. In general, as plaque matures there is an increase in the proportion of Gram-negative bacteria and in anaerobic species. In supragingival plaque, anaerobes occupy the inner portions of plaque and aerobes are found closer to the surface. Facultative bacteria are distributed evenly throughout the plaque mass.

Most of the information accumulated on the characterization of dental plaque has been derived from extensive studies of supragingival plaque. Less is known about these events for subgingival plaque. The mechanism by which subgingival plaque develops subsequently to supragingival plaque is not entirely clear. It may result either by apical extension of supragingival plaque or as discrete aggregations distant from supragingival plaque. Regardless, its initial accumulation is predisposed by inflammatory changes that occur at the gingival margin in response to supragingival plaque. That is, supragingival plaque contacting marginal gingiva at the opening of the crevice initiates an inflammatory tissue change such that bacteria may gain access into the crevice.

A sequence of plaque stages similar to that of supragingival plaque probably occurs in the development of subgingival plaque, but there are some key differences in the microbial distribution. The subgingival environment is more protective and more conducive to inhabitation by anaerobic bacteria. The pellicle, which is termed cuticle on subgingival surfaces, may contain the remains of the basal lamina from the epithelial attachment as well as material from crevicular fluid or from epithelial cell secretions. Leukocytes are usually seen in varying numbers in subgingival plaque. Many studies of subgingival plaque have focused on bacterial composition especially in association with different periodontal disease states. In general, subgingival microflora contains proportionately more an-

aerobes such as spirochetes and fusiforms and more Gram-negative bacteria such as *Bacteroides* species than are found in supramarginal plaque (Figs. 3–2 and 3–3). Streptococci are much less dominant and largely belong to the species *Streptococcus milleri, S. sanguis,* and *S. mitior.* Complex bacterial associations are more frequent, especially in periodontal pockets, than in supragingival plaque. Examples include the "corncob" association between cocci and filaments or the "test-tube brush" in which gram-negative rods attach to filaments at right angles and are usually limited to one end of the filament.

Subgingival plaque exhibits an adherent layer on the tooth surface composed primarily of gram-positive bacteria and a loosely adherent layer of Gram-negative bacteria and spirochetes adjacent to the crevicular wall.

Studies of the subgingival microflora have resulted in identification of a number of new species and even of new genera of bacteria. The periodontal pocket is apparently somewhat unique in supporting growth of many bacteria and further emphasizes the complexity of the oral environment.

Pathogenic Potential in Periodontal Disease

Most plaque bacteria are not generally described by microbiologists as pathogens. In fact, they may co-exist with the host indefinitely without causing overt infections. However, species of oral streptococci, *Bacteroides,* fusiforms, and spirochetes have been implicated in severe and life-threatening infections such as bacterial endocarditis, cellulitis, and brain abscess. These infections have usually involved transplantation of the bacteria from the oral cavity to another part of the body resulting from dental procedures, trauma, or extension of oral disease processes. In the area of the periodontium, most plaque bacteria do not possess the virulence factors which enable them to invade intact epithelium. Bacterial

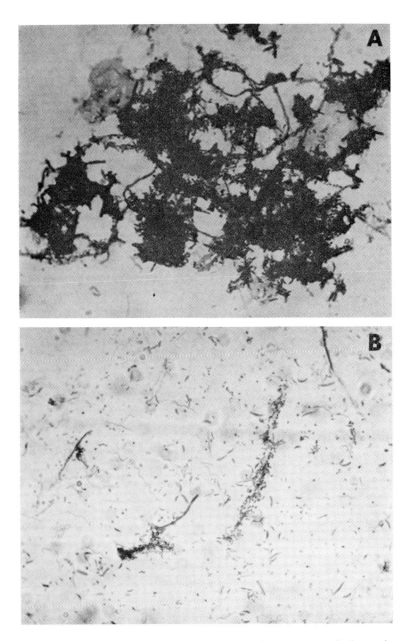

Figure 3–2. Bacterial (Dental) Plaque. A, Gram stain of supragingival plaque from a 46-year-old patient with chronic destructive periodontitis. Note the predominance of gram-positive (black) cocci and filaments and close cell-cell associations. B, Gram stain of subgingival plaque from same patient. Note the predominance of Gram-negative (gray) cocci, short rods. In contrast to A, subgingival plaque is more dispersed, but does contain some cell to cell interactions (cocci associated with long filamentous rods). (Courtesy of Dr. Dale Birdsell, University of Florida College of Dentistry.)

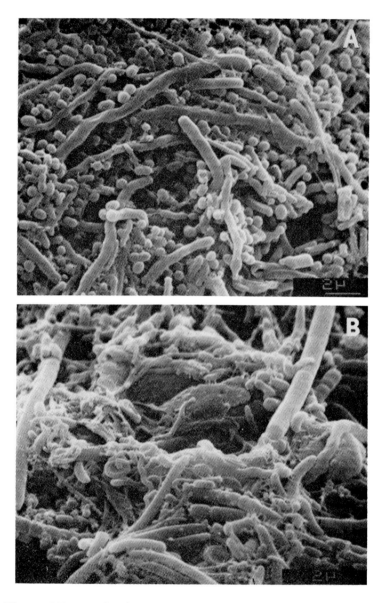

Figure 3–3. Electron Micrographs of Dental Plaque from the Same Specimen as in Figure 3–2. A, Supragingival. The scanning electron microscope reveals large numbers of cocci dispersed among long filamentous forms (× 6000). B, Subgingival. Long rod-shaped organisms are present together with fusiforms, spirochetes, and short rods. A few red blood cells are also evident (× 5600). (Courtesy of Dr. Werner Fischlschweiger, University of Florida College of Dentistry.)

Table 3–1. Some Products of Plaque Bacteria That are Potentially Damaging to Periodontal Tissues or Defense Components

Enzymes	Toxins
Collagenase	Endotoxin
Hyaluronidase	Leukotoxin
Chondroitin sulfatase	
Proteases	*Metabolic End-Products*
Phosphatase	
Aminopeptidase	Ammonia
Phosphoamidase	Hydrogen sulfide
Glycosidase	Indol
Fibrinolysin	Toxic amines
	Organic acids

invasion of periodontal tissues apparently can readily occur subsequent to tissue breakdown and established inflammatory changes.

A concentrated mass of bacteria, such as is seen in plaque, is an unusual occurrence in nature. Consequently, virulence factors that ordinarily have low pathogenic potential take on new significance. Potential pathogenic mechanisms of plaque bacteria involve bacterial products that may cause direct injury to periodontal tissues or defense components. These substances are probably responsible for at least the initial stages of tissue destruction in periodontal disease. Such products synthesized by plaque bacteria include enzymes, toxins, and waste products from bacterial metabolism (Table 3–1).

Enzymes produced by plaque bacteria include collagenase, hyaluronidase, and chondroitin sulfatase. These particular enzymes have the capacity to contribute to breakdown of collagen fibers and the ground substance in which the fibers are embedded. Other destructive enzymes such as proteases, have also been detected in plaque and may degrade immunoglobulins, transferrin, fibrinogen, and other body proteins important to defense or healing capacity. Waste products such as organic acids are irritating and potentially cytotoxic to body cells.

Endotoxins are lipopolysaccharide components of cell walls of gram-negative bacteria. As previously discussed, gram-negative bacteria are plentiful in mature dental plaque especially in periodontal pockets. Endotoxins can penetrate the crevice wall and have been implicated in bone resorption processes. They may also activate some host responses that have destructive potential. The participation of endotoxins in periodontal disease processes has been illustrated in tissue culture studies using extracted periodontally-involved teeth. When such teeth were placed in tissue culture with either epithelial cells or with gingival fibroblasts, the cells were killed or damaged. If endotoxin was chemically removed, a biologically acceptable environment was restored. Diseased cementum or calculus absorbs endotoxins and retains this substance in contact with the crevice wall indefinitely (Fig. 3–4). Endotoxins are primarily limited to superficial layers of cementum and therefore can be eliminated by scaling and root planing procedures.

Leukotoxin is produced by a bacterial species, *Actinobacillus actinomycetemcomitans,* which is associated with severely destructive periodontal diseases. Leukotoxin is cytotoxic for polymorphonuclear leukocytes (PMNs, neutrophils).

Although the participation of some of these bacterial products in periodontal destruction seems apparent, the relative importance of most of them is not clear. Since these substances are known to be produced by bacterial species in plaque, it is likely that they make at least a minor contribution to destructive processes.

Indirect bacterial effects are also potentially destructive. These relate primarily to the elicitation of inflammatory or immune responses which may result in tissue damage. All of these effects may occur in a sustained fashion due to the chronic plaque exposure that results when oral hygiene is inadequate. It is the chronicity of irritation and subsequent host response that often results in permanent damage. Host responses are described in greater detail later in this chapter. The point to be made here

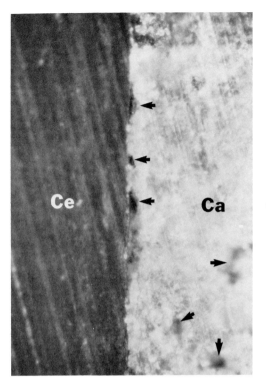

Figure 3-4. Endotoxin. Histologic section showing fluorescent-stained endotoxin (arrows) absorbed into calculus (Ca) and on surface of cementum (Ce) of an extracted periodontally-diseased tooth. (Courtesy of Dr. Heinz Topoll and Dr. David Simpson.)

is that bacterial cells, cell components, or cell products may function as antigens to elicit potentially immunopathologic responses or as chemotactic agents for polymorphonuclear leukocytes and other defense cells which in turn cause tissue destruction.

BACTERIAL SPECIFICITY IN PERIODONTAL DISEASE

In recent years, research has focused on attempts to identify specific bacterial species that are associated with disease processes in the periodontium. This avenue of research has been facilitated by the development of laboratory culture techniques that permit greater recovery of different types of bacteria from plaque, especialy an-

aerobes. These studies have led to growing recognition that the pathogenicity of plaque is related more to plaque quality than to plaque quantity. This is true especially for periodontitis where occurrence and severity appears to be dependent upon the presence of certain bacterial species. The identification of specific pathogens permits periodontal therapeutic approaches that are directed towards the elimination of those pathogens and not necessarily all of the bacteria in plaque.

Most research in this area has been conducted by identifying patients who exhibit various types and stages of periodontal diseases, and sampling of associated plaque. Microbial profiles that appear to be consistent with specific disease states have thus been determined. Establishment of this relationship does not necessarily elucidate a cause and effect relationship but does suggest participation in the disease process and provides a basis for additional investigation. Descriptions of bacterial flora that are associated with specific periodontal disease states are discussed next (Table 3-2).

Gingivitis

In the early stages of gingivitis (1 to 3 weeks), associated plaque is predominated by Gram-positive facultative microorganisms specially *Actinomyces* species such as *A. viscosus* and streptococci. *Actinomyces* species have been reported to constitute about 50% of bacteria present during this time. As gingivitis progresses to a more chronic or longstanding state, there is a shift to a more Gram-negative and more anaerobic microflora. *Veillonella* species and fusobacteria are typical of this disease state.

As described earlier in this chapter, all of these bacteria are typical of maturing plaque with minimal variation from person to person. Studies of experimental gingivitis demonstrate that virtually everyone will develop gingivitis if plaque is permitted to accumulate. The onset of gingivitis

Table 3–2. Predominant Bacterial Features Associated with Different Periodontal Disease States.

Periodontal Disease	Bacterial Features	Bacterial Species
Early Gingivitis	Increased quantities of Gram-positive, facultative flora in supragingival plaque	*Actinomyces* sp. *Streptococcus* sp.
Established Gingivitis	Increase in Gram-negative anaerobes and spirochetes, especially in subgingival plaque.	*Treponema* sp. *Veillonella* sp. *Fusobacteria* sp. *Bacteroides* sp.
Destructive Adult Periodontitis	Gram-positive flora attached to root surface Gram-negative anaerobes and spirochetes loosely-adherent adjacent to pocket epithelium	*Actinomyces* sp. *Streptococcus* sp. *Treponema* sp. *Bacteroides gingivalis* *Bacteroides intermedius* *Fusobacteria nucleatum* *Eikenella corrodens* *Wollinella recta*
Rapidly Progressive Periodontitis	Predominated by certain virulent species	*Bacteroides* sp. *Capnocytophaga* sp. *Actinobacillus actinomycetemcomitans*
Juvenile Periodontitis	Sparse plaque, few bacterial species that are consistently present	*Actinobacillus actinomycetemcomitans* *Capnocytophaga* sp.
Necrotizing Ulcerative Gingivitis	Zone of spirochetes invading tissue; Gram-negative bacteria predominating in supragingival plaque	*Treponema* sp. *Fusobacteria* sp. *Bacteroides intermedius*

is thus related to an increase in plaque quantity at the gingival margin with concomitant bacterial changes that consistently occur. It may be considered bacteriologically non-specific in comparison to other periodontal disease states.

Necrotizing Ulcerative Gingivitis

In the more unusual infection necrotizing ulcerative gingivitis (Fig. 3–5), microscopic evaluation of associated plaque reflects almost entirely a mixture of spirochetes and fusobacteria with spirochetes actually forming an invading zone in the affected gingival tissue. More recent studies have also documented the consistent presence of certain *Bacteroides* species as well. Several different species of spirochetes and fusobacteria that are present in mature plaque may be involved in necrotizing ulcerative gingivitis. Host defense mechanisms are apparently modified due to factors such as mental stress and poor eating and sleeping habits and the already-

present bacteria are permitted to overgrow resulting in the destructive lesions observed. The fusospirochetal combination involving the same or similar species has also been implicated in brain and lung abscesses. This indicates the level of their pathogenic potential that is normally controlled by homeostatic mechanisms in the oral cavity.

Periodontitis

The term periodontitis is applied when gingival inflammation progresses to involve pocket formation and destruction of underlying alveolar bone and periodontal ligament fibers. Although virtually everyone will develop gingivitis if plaque is retained, susceptibility to periodontitis exhibits extremes of individual variability. The differences in age of onset, rate of tissue destruction, severity, and clinical symptoms cannot be accounted for by presence and distribution of local factors alone. Systemic defensive factors play a

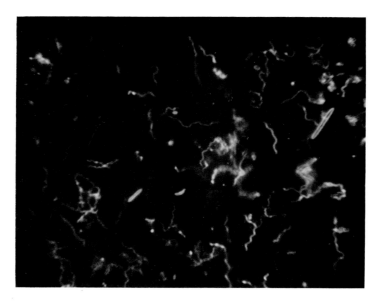

Figure 3–5. Microbiology of Necrotizing Ulcerative Gingivitis. Darkfield microscopic picture of the spirochetes and rodform microorganisms associated with this disease.

major role in determining susceptibility to periodontitis. These factors will be discussed later in this chapter. It is likely that deficiencies in the defense system relate to inability to control specific periodontal pathogens.

Most commonly, periodontitis occurs in adults with destruction becoming apparent after about age 30. Although the destructive changes appear to develop gradually over a long period of time, closer observations indicate that there are periods of disease activity occurring intermittently with periods of inactivity. Bacteria associated with adult periodontitis and especially with periods of disease activity have been characterized to include a limited number of species. More destructive forms of periodontitis involve different bacteria and will be discussed in the next section. Although microbial composition can be characterized, it is still not clear that a causal relationship exists between the bacteria present and the disease state. This information must be extrapolated from investigation of pathogenic mechanisms of isolated bacteria either using laboratory assays or animal study models in which to induce periodontal disease. Compared to the microflora associated with a healthy periodontium or with gingivitis, the bacteria in periodontal pockets consist of much greater proportions of Gram-negatives, anaerobes, and motile forms. Proportionate increases in motile rods and spirochetes observed with phase contrast or darkfield microscopy have been associated with increased disease activity. This type of microbial assessment may be useful in identifying active disease sites and monitoring results of periodontal therapy.

More detailed bacterial culture studies have revealed a predominance of Gram-negative anaerobic rods, in particular *Bacteroides gingivalis* and *Bacteroides intermedius. Eikenella corrodens, Fusobacterium nucleatum,* or *Wollinella recta* may also be present in large numbers. Numerous studies have demonstrated an increasing number of spirochetes in plaque as the severity of disease and pocket depth increases. In the spatial arrangement of bacteria in plaque, a consistent pattern is that the layer of plaque closest to a diseased root surface is predominately Gram-positive perhaps mediating attachment while the outer layer that is loosely attached is predominated by Gram-negative forms and spirochetes. The bacteria in the loosely bound layer would therefore be more likely to contribute to destruction of gingival and other periodontal tissues. The Gram-positive layer does not prevent the penetration of endotoxins which become absorbed into the underlying cementum. Other bacterial species frequently observed in periodontal pockets are *Vibrio sputorum* and *Selenomonas sputigena*. In a given individual the relative proportions of all of these various bacterial species is likely to vary, but in chronic destructive adult periodontitis, one or more is observed in large numbers.

Juvenile Periodontitis and Rapidly Progressive Periodontitis

The clinical characteristics and other features of these two unusually destructive diseases are described in Chapter 4. In juvenile periodontitis rapid and severe alveolar bone loss occurs usually around first molars and incisors in prepubertal or pubertal years. While rapidly progressive periodontitis may occur at any age, it most frequently is diagnosed in young adults who exhibit unusually rapid generalized bone loss. In both of these types of periodontitis, associated plaque contains an unusual bacterial flora.

As will be discussed in detail later, the polymorphonuclear leukocyte (PMN) is the most important defense cell in the initial response to a bacterial irritant. These cells are attracted to and move through the bloodstream to a site of irritation through a process called chemotaxis. Most bacterial cells produce chemotactic signals such that when they reach body tissues close to blood vessels, PMNs are mobilized into the area. A particular species of *Capnocytophaga, C. sputigena* is relatively inactive in promoting chemotaxis and thus depresses the host's ability to defend against it. This species is observed with frequency from patients with rapidly progressive periodontitis. *Capnocytophaga* species are also

isolated with high frequency from juvenile periodontitis but appear to be secondary to *Actinobacillus actinomycetemcomitans* as a pathogenic agent in this infection. *A. actinomycetemcomitans* is recovered from almost 100% of localized juvenile periodontitis (LJP) lesions. Its recovery from periodontally healthy individuals or in adult periodontitis is very low. *A. actinomycetemcomitans* is frequently found in healthy siblings and other family members of patients with juvenile periodontitis suggesting a genetic or environmental predisposition to its colonization in the oral cavity. Deficiencies in cellular defense mechanisms such as decreased chemotaxis of PMN's and depressed phagocytic ability that are common in LJP patients may in part account for the ability of *A. actinomycetemcomitans* to colonize. Additionally, these bacteria produce a number of factors that are capable of further inhibition of host defense mechanisms. These include leukotoxin which is toxic for PMNs, a PMN chemotaxis inhibiting factor, and a factor which can suppress some aspects of the immune system. These factors superimposed upon an already depressed defense ability may explain the rapidly severe periodontal destruction seen in juvenile periodontitis. The question of whether *A. actinomycetemcomitans* is a primary agent or an opportunist that contributes to the destructive process has not been fully answered. Nevertheless its consistent presence and pathogenic potential suggests that it is important in this periodontal disease. *A. actinomycetemcomitans* has also been implicated in severe periodontitis in insulin-dependent juvenile diabetic and in rapidly progressive periodontitis. Proportions and frequency in rapidly progressive periodontitis is not usually as dramatic as in juvenile periodontitis.

Fatal infections, such as bacterial endocarditis, caused by *A. actinomycetemcomitans* have been documented. Of special concern to the dental profession is the pathogenic potential coupled with a known resistance to penicillin. For patients who are suspected of harboring *A. actinomycetemcomitans* and who are at risk of developing bacterial endocarditis, supplemental precautions should be taken in planning an appropriate prophylactic antibiotic regimen with dental treatment. It is recommended that penicillin be supplemented with tetracycline to control the *A. actinomycetemcomitans* bacteria that may enter the bloodstream as a result of instrumentation (see Chapter 9).

DENTAL CALCULUS

A consequence of plaque accumulation on the teeth is that it may calcify and require professional intervention for removal. For most dental hygienists, calculus detection and removal occupies the greatest proportion of practice time and are complex skills that require years of experience to perfect. Even the most experienced clinician cannot assure complete removal of calculus in pockets greater than 4 mm, especially in furcation areas, without establishing direct access.

Although bacterial irritants from plaque are responsible for the inflammatory changes in periodontal disease, calculus usually forms and provides an increased surface area for plaque accumulation. It thus plays a major role in the maintenance and progression of the disease process. Calculus removal is an important preventive and therapeutic procedure but is not likely to be adequate if the patient does not practice good plaque control habits.

Classification of Dental Calculus

Dental calculus has traditionally been classified as supragingival and subgingival. Supragingival calculus is that which forms on clinical crowns of teeth while subgingival calculus forms on tooth surfaces within the gingival crevice. Supragingival calculus is found most commonly on surfaces opposite the duct openings of the major salivary glands, lingual surfaces of the mandibular anterior teeth opposite Wharton's duct openings from the submandibular salivary glands and on the facials of maxillary molars opposite Stenson's duct orifices from the parotid glands (Fig. 3–6). In many patients, supragingival calculus is found only in one or both of these areas. Some patients seem not to form supragingival calculus. Formation in other areas of the mouth is more highly dependent upon poor oral hygiene, tooth malalignment, malocclusion, and reduced mastication. It is not uncommon to find calculus on occlusal surfaces of teeth that do not have an opposing tooth in the opposite arch and thus do not participate in normal masticatory function. Very rarely does calculus form on occlusal surfaces of normally functioning teeth. Just as plaque forms on other hard surfaces besides teeth, calculus may also form on restorations and removable appliances.

Distribution of subgingival calculus does not exhibit such preferential localization and may be found anywhere in the mouth. It is most frequently present on proximal surfaces and more often on posterior teeth than on anterior teeth. Its relationship to oral hygiene and tooth malalignment is apparent in many patients.

Supragingival calculus is usually cream colored but may be stained by extrinsic factors such as coffee or tobacco. Initially it may be somewhat brittle and crumble easily especially if it forms rapidly. The density and tenacity of calculus tends to increase according to the length of time it has been present. Supragingival calculus usually follows the contours of the marginal or papillary gingiva. Subgingival calculus is often brown to black in color. Although not firmly established, this dark color probably reflects hemolyzed red blood cells from bleeding in the inflamed crevice. Bacterial pigments may also contribute to the color. The intensity of coloration as well as hardness and tenacity seem to increase with the age of the calculus. While supragingival calculus usually exhibits a smooth outer surface, subgingival deposits are most

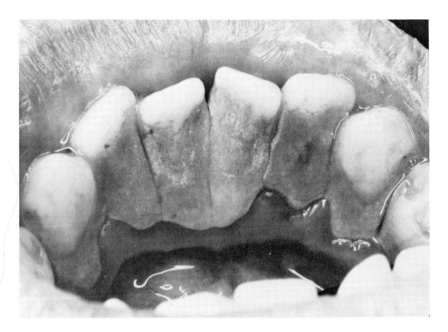

Figure 3–6. Calculus. Gross supragingival deposits on lingual of mandibular anterior teeth.

often irregular and rough-surfaced by comparison. Morphology may be described as nodular, ring-like, thin veneers, finger- or fern-like extensions or in islands or spots. The outer surface of calculus is almost always covered by a layer of unmineralized plaque. This is particularly deleterious in the gingival crevice where the soft tissues of the crevice wall continue to be irritated.

Composition of Calculus

Dental calculus is composed of 70 to 80% inorganic material although the degree of mineralization is somewhat dependent upon the age of the calculus. Inorganic components are primarily calcium and phosphorous forming crystals which are not unlike those in teeth and bone. Crystals formed early are brushite and octocalcium phosphate which are subsequently hydrolyzed to form hydroxyapatite and magnesium whitlockite crystals. Whitlockite is the more common form in subgingival calculus and in inner layers of supragingival calculus.

From 6 to 15% of calculus is organic constituents reflecting retention of plaque matrix material and of dead bacterial cells. Water constitutes the remaining 6 to 20% of calculus components.

Calculus Formation

Calculus formation involves the precipitation of calcium and phosphate into plaque. For supragingival calculus these ions are supplied from saliva and in subgingival calculus from serum by way of crevicular fluid. The exact mechanism by which this precipitation and crystal formation occurs has not been firmly established but several theories have been proposed. Central to all of the potential mechanisms is that an increase in pH results in Ca and P precipitation.

In the physicochemical theory, it is postulated that the increase in pH occurs as a function of salivary secretion. Secretion through the ducts occurs at a pressure greater than atmospheric pressure. As saliva is secreted, the pressure difference results in release of carbon dioxide from saliva and in an elevation of the salivary pH. Bacterial production of ammonia has also been suggested as an important mechanism in the pH increase.

The epitaxis theory of calculus formation places emphasis on the need for foci or "seeding" sites in plaque to provide the configuration whereby crystallization can occur. These foci may be provided by either matrix or bacterial components of plaque. Filamentous bacteria have in particular been associated with crystallization sites especially in developing supragingival calculus. The components of these various theories of calculus formation are not unrelated and it is likely that they are all involved to some extent.

Other factors such as salivary flow as well as viscosity and composition of saliva also influence calculus formation and in particular the rate of formation. Changes associated with age are apparently important since calculus is not usually seen in the prepubertal individual. All of these factors, not fully understood, account for the great individual variation in amount and rate of calculus formation in patients with poor plaque control.

Attachment of Calculus

Mechanisms of attachment of calculus to the tooth surface vary and were categorized a number of years ago into four different modes. These are: (1) by means of a secondary cuticle or pellicle interposed between calculus and tooth surface, (2) to microscopic irregularities in cementum where Sharpey's fibers were previously inserted, (3) mediated by penetration of bacteria into cementum, and (4) into areas of cemental resorption (Fig. 3–7). Obviously the nature of the underlying tooth surface would help determine the mode of attachment on any given area. The mode of attachment determines the tenacity of the deposit and consequently relates to the difficulty of calculus removal and ability of the hygienist to plane the surface to the desired smoothness.

HOST RESPONSES IN INFLAMMATORY PERIODONTAL DISEASES

Although bacteria and their products are recognized as essential and primary in the causation of inflammatory periodontal diseases, a variety of host responses may act together or individually to greatly influence the course of disease processes in a given individual. This might be in the form of deficiencies in certain defense mechanisms against bacteria or in the form of sustained inflammatory and immune responses that are destructive to localized tissue areas especially with the continued presence of a chronic irritant such as bacterial plaque. A number of these factors have been studied both in healthy and periodontally-diseased individuals. Although considerable information has been derived from those investigations, the exact role of specific responses in tissue destruction has yet to be fully elucidated. This section will discuss host defense mechanisms in terms of protective capacity and destructive potential. Finally, the sequence of cellular and tissue changes that occur in the progression of periodontal disease will be described.

PROTECTIVE MECHANISMS

The oral cavity and underlying supporting periodontal tissues are replete with mechanisms that have the potential to prevent infections, ameliorate the noxious effects of bacteria or their products, and to prevent the spreading of infection to other parts of the body.

Local Oral Factors

In addition to the mechanical barrier provided by an intact mucosa, salivary flow and crevicular fluid flow function to mechanically control or eliminate bacteria from the mouth. Normal masticatory function and self-cleansing mechanisms contribute to the maintenance of healthy tis-

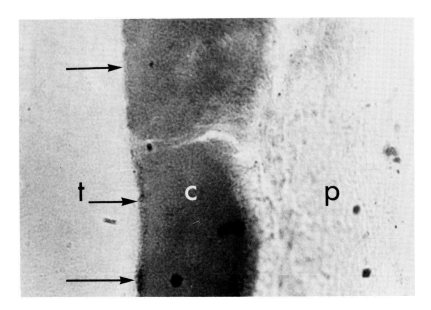

Figure 3–7.   Attachment of Calculus to Tooth.   The calculus (c) is in direct contact with the tooth (t) with projections extending into the tooth (arrows). Bacterial plaque (p) is on the surface of the calculus.

sues that have optimal resistance to infection.

Another mechanism of protection is provided by microbial balance in which indigenous microorganisms are able through several mechanisms to prevent the oral colonization of many potential pathogens. An example of the disruption of this important control mechanism is sometimes seen when antibiotic therapy selectively changes this balance and oral infections by resistant microorganisms such as *Candida albicans* results. A major concern in the development of antibacterial agents for plaque control is that an imbalance may be created and opportunistic infections could result.

In addition to mechanical and microbial defense factors, saliva contains several antibacterial components which play a significant role in the primary defense of the oral cavity. These substances include lysozyme, an enzyme that is bactericidal for some gram-positive bacteria and may damage other types of bacteria. Lactoperoxidase, another salivary enzyme, catalyzes the oxidation of salivary thiocyanate by bacterial hydrogen peroxide. The oxidation products from this reaction are bactericidal or bacteriostatic for some bacteria. Still another component lactoferrin can bind iron that is nutritionally required by some bacteria and thus prevent their survival in the oral environment. Antibodies from the IgA class of immunoglobulins are predominantly found in body secretions such as saliva. Although IgA antibodies to oral bacteria do not cause bacterial death, they can prevent bacterial adherence to oral surfaces, facilitate oral clearance, and neutralize some bacterial metabolic processes. This combination of antibacterial components in saliva constitute a major defense capacity in the oral cavity.

All of the above mechanisms function in the supragingival environment and, by exerting some control in this area, are important in the inhibition of the extension of plaque into the gingival crevice. When plaque causes irritation to the gingival or periodontal tissues, a set of responses mediated by systemic defense cells is initiated.

These responses are directed towards elimination of the irritant and prevention of spread of infection beyond the localized area. If the initial inflammatory response is ineffective in elimination of the irritant, inflammation progresses and additional defense cells particularly those from the immune system become involved.

The Inflammatory Response

Clinical alterations associated with periodontal inflammation are described in Chapter 4. These changes are related directly to underlying histologic events that begin within 24 hours of plaque accumulation. The sequence of events in the inflammatory response is directed towards elimination of the irritant, limiting destruction and initiation of healing. Consequently it is a very important defense mechanism.

Vascular Changes. Vascular alterations comprise the initial set of responses following the onset of an inflammatory challenge. There is an initial, but fleeting, vasoconstriction followed by a prolonged period of vasodilation. With vasodilation there is an increase in vascular permeability which results in movement of vascular fluid into the interstitial tissues. Blood viscosity is thereby increased and blood flow becomes sluggish. The increased heat and redness, typical inflammatory changes, result from the increased blood flow. Edema is a result of fluid accumulation in the surrounding tissue. Gingival inflammation most often progresses into a chronic state without going through an overt acute phase. Consequently the symptoms are usually subdued and may be difficult to detect. Some characteristic differences between acute and chronic inflammation are listed in Table 3–3. Of particular significance is that although reparative processes are occurring in chronic inflammation, the destructive potential from chronic irritation is likely to exceed the repair attempts and lead to permanent tissue damage in the periodontium.

Table 3–3. Comparison of General Features of Acute and Chronic Inflammation.

Acute	Chronic
Rapid onset	Gradual onset
Short duration	Longstanding duration
Pain	Little or no pain
Marked clinical symptoms	Subdued symptoms
Rapid tissue destruction with little repair	Tissue repair attempts along with destructive processes
Quick resolution if irritant is removed	Net destruction likely to result in irreversible damage

BIOCHEMICAL MEDIATORS. During the inflammatory response several biochemical substances are released or activated which are responsible for the observed increases in vascular permeability. Among these are histamine and serotonin which are released from degranulating mast cells during inflammation, kinins which originate from plasma or from connective tissue cells, and prostaglandins. Macrophages are a major source of prostaglandins found in gingival tissue.

CELLULAR CHANGES. Soon after the vascular alterations, circulating defense cells concentrate in the area of injury. The cells marginate along the inner wall of the blood vessel and then through a process called diapedesis, migrate between the endothelial cells of the vessel into the connective tissue. Bacterial chemotactic factors previously described, mediate this mobilization of defense cells. The major inflammatory cells involved in this response in the periodontium are the polymorphonuclear leukocyte (PMN), the first cell to respond, and the macrophage which is more prominent if inflammation is sustained.

Small numbers of PMNs are almost always found in the gingival area in healthy tissue. As dental plaque encroaches on the gingival tissues, greater numbers are attracted to and move to the area. The primary chemotactic factor that elicits this response is supplied by the bacterial cell itself. PMNs that move to the gingival area because of plaque irritation emigrate through the junctional epithelium and form a protective barrier in the gingival crevice and prevent or control plaque extension. The PMN is not mitotic and remains in tissue for only a short time before degranulating or being eliminated into the oral cavity.

The antibacterial capacity of the PMN rests in its ability to phagocytize or engulf bacterial cells and release destructive enzymes such as myeloperoxidase, lysozyme, and lactoferrin from intracellular granules causing bacterial death.

The critical role that the neutrophil or PMN plays in protecting the periodontium is most apparent in patients exhibiting PMN functional impairment who also exhibit severe periodontal breakdown. Impairments may be in the form of depressed chemotactic ability or depressed phagocytic ability. Conditions in which these changes are often observed include Chediak-Higashi syndrome, chronic granulomatous disease, insulin-controlled diabetes, and localized juvenile periodontitis. In patients with significantly decreased numbers of circulating PMNs as in agranulocytosis, neutropenia, or leukemia, the susceptibility to severe breakdown of oral tissues has been well documented.

As previously mentioned, *A. actinomycetemcomitans* is non-chemotactic for PMNs and may also be cytotoxic for these cells accounting in part for its virulence in periodontal disease.

The chemotaxis and phagocytosis activities of the PMN are additionally promoted or influenced by several mechanisms involving the immune system. Once immune responses begin subsequent to the inflammatory response, a number of additional chemotactic agents are activated. These will be described later in this chapter.

A second inflammatory cell of major importance in protecting the periodontium is the multifunctional macrophage. These cells, which differentiate from circulating monocytes when they reach tissue, appear later in the inflammatory response than

PMNs and are largely responsible for maintaining the response indefinitely as needed.

The macrophage, like the PMN, responds to chemotactic factors and is phagocytic. It is not an end cell and does replicate after it reaches the area of tissue injury. This cell participates in antigen recognition and processing for immune cells and thus is an important cellular component of the immune system. Its mobilization and activities are in turn strongly influenced by immune cells. The macrophage in addition to secreting antibacterial enzymes also synthesizes other enzymes such as collagenase and other proteases as well as prostaglandins which are important biochemical mediators of inflammation.

Recent investigations have shown that deficiencies in numbers and functions of macrophages are associated with increased periodontal disease. The extent of this influence has not been as well characterized as those involving PMN deficiencies.

Immune Mechanisms

As plaque irritation continues and the inflamed condition of periodontal tissues progresses into a more chronic state, the immune system is activated. The participation of immune cells is a reflection of the inability of the inflammatory cells just described to control the extension of plaque irritants and thus represents a second line of defense. The immune system has two major components, humoral immunity and cellular immunity (Fig. 3–8).

HUMORAL IMMUNITY. Humoral immunity is mediated by lymphocytes referred to as B-cells (bursa-derived cells) the primary function of which is the differentiation into plasma cells that synthesize antibodies in response to antigenic challenge by an irritant such as bacteria or bacterial components. There is evidence that antibody synthesis occurs locally in the gingival tissues in response to plaque antigens. Also, individuals exhibiting various periodontal

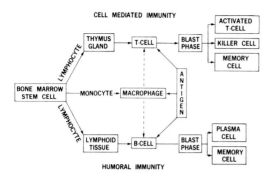

Figure 3–8. Immunologic Pathways. A series of cellular alterations results in the host acquiring immunity to antigenic substances.

disease states are shown to have circulating antibodies specific for bacterial pathogens involved in periodontal destruction. These findings, not observed in periodontally healthy individuals, indicate active participation of this type of immune response in periodontal defense.

There are five classes of immunoglobulins, the major ones in serum being IgG and IgM and in saliva, IgA. Antibodies that are present in the periodontal tissues are predominantly of the IgG and IgM classes and exert antibacterial effects in several different ways. Immune complexes of antibody and antigen are formed that may directly neutralize bacterial toxic effects or may activate the complement system (Fig. 3–9).

The complement system consists of at least 22 serum proteins that are activated

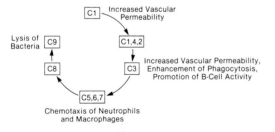

Figure 3–9. Complement System. Simplified scheme of sequential activation of the complement system and the functional activities related to periodontal disease. Activation may occur at C1 by antigen-antibody complexes or at C3 by endotoxins.

in a cascade fashion similar to that of blood clotting. Activation of complement is primarily induced by immune complexes but also may be induced directly by endotoxin. Each component of the complement system has a biological function such as chemotaxis of leukocytes, enhancement of phagocytosis (especially of gram-positive bacteria) and lysis of gram-negative bacterial cells. The complement system is very important in body defense and deficiencies may severely compromise resistance. B-cells which usually require interaction with T-cells and macrophages for activation also produce some biologically active substances called lymphokines. These are similar to those produced by T-cells and will be discussed next.

CELLULAR IMMUNITY. The T-cell or T-lymphocyte originates from bone marrow stem cells just as B-cells do but are then processed through the thymus gland and are destined to mediate cellular immunity. T-cells require the presence of macrophages for activation and like B-cells or plasma cells are responsive to specific antigenic stimulation. Some T-cells become "memory cells" and are probably responsible for maintaining the ability of the entire immune system to recognize and respond to antigens that the body has already been immunized against. Part of the function of T-cells rests in their ability to synthesize a set of substances referred to as lymphokines. Some of these are related to macrophage activities, such as macrophage chemotactic factor, macrophage inhibition factor (MIF) that prevents migration of macrophages out of an area of injury, and macrophage activating factor (MAF) that enhances the synthetic and proliferative functions of macrophages. Others include osteoclast activating factor (OAF) that results in bone resorption and lymphotoxin that is cytotoxic for fibroblasts. Given the destructive nature of the latter two, their protective function in the periodontium is not readily apparent.

Both cellular and humoral responses

occur at the same time, though one may be predominant depending upon the nature of the stimulus. Cellular immunity to plaque antigens like humoral immunity has been demonstrated in patients with periodontal disease.

POTENTIALLY DESTRUCTIVE MECHANISMS

Although the protective mechanisms just described are critical in maintaining the health of the periodontium and preventing extension of infection, they also have the potential for destruction of host tissues. It is likely that one or more of the host defense responses is responsible for much of the tissue destruction that occurs in periodontitis. Following are descriptions of potentially pathogenic host response mechanisms.

Inflammatory Cell Activities

While PMNs are important defense components, these cells contain a number of enzymes that can damage host tissue as well as destroy bacterial cells. These lysosomal enzymes gain limited access to periodontal tissues during the phagocytic process, but the primary exposure occurs when cell contents are released when the short-lived PMN dies. In the set of protective responses described, several chemotactic factors are generated that attract and maintain large numbers of PMN's at the site of irritation. While healing can occur with the removal of the irritant, continued replenishment of this cell population and subsequent enzyme release could result in net destruction without adequate healing. This likely occurs as plaque irritation continues indefinitely.

Similar chemotactic factors exist for the macrophage. The macrophage synthesizes and secretes collagenase, osteoclast activating factor, and prostaglandins. Prostaglandins are major mediators of inflammation and some have been shown to stimulate bone resorption. Concentrations of prostaglandins are higher in inflamed gingiva and even higher in periodontitis. Although other cells may synthesize prostaglandins, the macrophage is thought to be the major source in inflamed periodontal tissues. As with the PMN, the role of the macrophage in periodontal destruction relates to ongoing chemotaxis and stimulation due to continued plaque exposure.

Immunopathologic Mechanisms

Immunopathology, in the form of allergies or hypersensitivities, is known to participate in several disorders throughout the body. The potential for such participation in periodontal disease is clear given the immune responses that do occur in the periodontium.

ANTIBODY-MEDIATED RESPONSES. There are two pathologic responses mediated by antibodies that potentially contribute to destructive processes in the periodontium (Fig. 3–10). The first involves the activation of complement by antigen-antibody complexes (immune-complex response). As already discussed, complement components intensify the inflammatory response through chemotaxis of leukocytes and by increasing vascular permeability. If the immune complexes are deposited in gingival tissue, enzymes released from PMN's attracted to this area by the immune complex could cause tissue damage. There is also potential, though not demonstrated in the periodontium, that thrombosis of small blood vessels could result from this response and lead to localized tissue necrosis. Complement activation also can stimulate the production and release of prostaglandins by PMNs or macrophages which in turn can activate osteoclastic activity and bone resorption. It has been demonstrated in laboratory animals that hyperimmunization and subsequent antigenic challenge in the gingival crevice could result in periodontitis mediated by the complement system. Although not demonstrated to actually occur in the human disease, all components for this

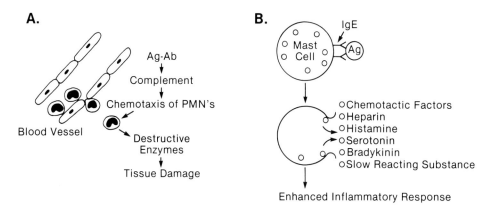

Figure 3–10. Antibody-Mediated Immunopathologic Reactions. A, Immune-complex reaction in which antigen-antibody complexes in tissue near blood vessels activate complement which attracts large numbers of polymorphonuclear leukocytes. B, Local anaphylaxis reaction in which antigen combines with IgE antibodies bound to mast cells causing release of substances that induce vascular changes.

pathologic response, including complement, are detectable in periodontitis states.

The second antibody-mediated immunopathologic response involves antibodies of the IgE class. IgE antibodies are not predominant in gingival tissue but have been detected and do exhibit specificity for plaque antigens. These antibodies are cytophilic and are attached in the gingival tissues to mast cells. When antigens react with the affixed IgE antibodies, the mast cells degranulate and release histamine, serotonin and other substances into the surrounding tissue. As mentioned earlier, these substances induce vascular changes, that, like complement intensify the inflammatory response. This response has been referred to as local anaphylaxis. Mast cells are present in gingival tissues and histamine levels are higher in inflamed gingiva than in normal gingiva and, therefore, this is a viable destructive mechanism.

The possibility of autoimmune reactions or production of antibodies against one's own tissues or cells has been investigated in periodontal disease, but there is no evidence that this response occurs.

CELL-MEDIATED RESPONSES. Lymphokines produced by T-lymphocytes have the capacity to contribute to tissue damage. In particular, the lymphokines that attract,

concentrate, and activate macrophages are potentialy destructive through the promotion of macrophage activities already described. Other lymphokines may increase vascular permeability, be cytotoxic for connective tissue cells, or stimulate bone resorption.

Either through lymphokine production or other mechanisms, T-lymphocytes from patients with periodontal disease have been demonstrated to be cytotoxic for epithelial cells and fibroblasts in tissue culture. This cytotoxicity either by sensitized lymphocytes or by non-specific action of so-called "killer T-cells" may contribute to tissue destruction in periodontal diseases.

It is clear from the preceding discussion of the potential destructiveness of host responses that they are interrelated. It has not been possible to identify a single mechanism as playing a major role. Furthermore, since their protective roles have been well established, it is difficult to determine the events that might precipitate progression to a destructive role.

HISTOPATHOLOGY OF INFLAMMATORY PERIODONTAL DISEASES

The sequence of histologic events in the initiation and progression of periodontal inflammation has been investigated in longitudinal studies of developing gingivitis and extrapolated from cross-sectional studies of different stages of periodontal disease.

The cellular and concomitant tissue histologic changes as gingivitis progresses to periodontitis have been well documented (Fig. 3–11). This progression begins with the initial lesion of gingivitis and extends to the advanced lesion of periodontitis. Observation of the sequence of changes that occurs in this progression has provided some of the information relative to the defense cells previously described. It should be emphasized that gingivitis does not always progress to periodontitis.

The Initial Lesion

Initial histologic changes are apparent after 1 to 4 days of plaque accumulation. These include vasodilation, increased migration of leukocytes (primarily PMNs, but also macrophages) from the blood vessels, some slight loss of collagen and the exudation of serum proteins from the blood vessels. These changes are limited to the area immediately subjacent to the junctional epithelium and are not accompanied by any clinical changes.

The Early Lesion

Features of what is termed the early lesion of gingivitis are apparent after 7 to 14 days of plaque accumulation. These include an accentuation of features of the initial lesion, an increase in the numbers of lymphocytes, cytopathic alterations in fibroblasts, further collagen loss and rete peg formation by junctional epithelium. Changes are still localized near the junctional epithelium and clinical signs of inflammation are apparent but may not be very dramatic. Some slight loss of tissue tone may be present due to collagen loss. Bleeding upon probing is indicative of these early inflammatory changes.

The Established Lesion

Changes that characterize the established lesion include progression of previous manifestations. Breakdown of collagen fibers now extends more laterally and apically. Epithelial rete pegs are more pronounced with junctional epithelium becoming detached from the tooth surface. This epithelial layer is now referred to as pocket epithelium and is often thin and exhibits ulcerated areas. With the extension of histologic inflammatory changes, clinical changes are readily apparent. A deepening of the gingival crevice and subgingival plaque deposition has now occurred. Mature plasma cells replace lymphocytes as the dominant defense cell and immunoglobulins may be detected in connective tissue. Lymphocytes, PMN's and macrophages are still present in the cellular infiltrate, however.

The changes to this point are restricted to the gingival tissue and do not involve alveolar bone loss. The progression and subsequent rate of periodontal destruction exhibits great individual variation. This is dependent in part upon the ability of protective mechanisms to inhibit further progression and in part upon the continued plaque exposure and virulence of plaque bacteria as previously discussed in this chapter. Although the established lesion state (chronic gingivitis) may exist indefinitely, this will progress into periodontitis in most individuals if plaque exposure continues.

The Advanced Lesion

This stage is characterized by the loss of alveolar bone. Inflammatory changes continue their extension laterally and apically and eventually affect periodontal ligament fibers and alveolar bone. The primary inflammatory pathway to underlying structures is along loose connective tissue around vascular channels into alveolar crestal bone (Figure 3–12). The loss of connective tissue fibers of the periodontal lig-

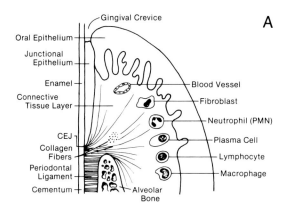

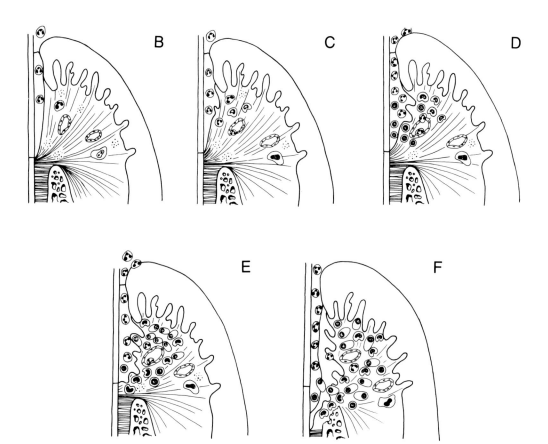

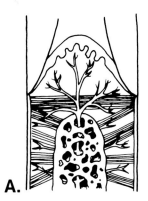 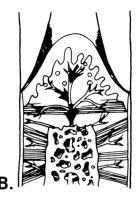 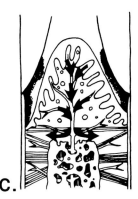

A.   B.   C.

Figure 3–12, A–C.   Pathway of Inflammation to Underlying Periodontal Structures.   A, Normal interdental area. B and C, Inflammation spreads along vascular channels; alveolar crestal bone resorbs; most coronal periodontal ligament fibers reestablish as transseptal fibers; transseptal fibers destroyed; junctional epithelium migrates apically and pocket is formed. (After Weinmann, J.P.: J. Periodontol. *12*:71, 1941.)

ament permits the apical extension of epithelium resulting in pocket formation. Although the existing gingival connective tissue attachment is destroyed in this process, it is usually reestablished more apically. This is particularly true of transseptal connective tissue fibers. These destructive processes that undermine periodontal support occur in most individuals in a cyclic fashion in which there are periods of remission when no destruction is occurring.

Clinically, pockets are detectable and vary considerably in location and topography depending upon the distribution of etiologic factors. The portions of cementum that no longer contain gingival or periodontal ligament fibers undergo changes. Cementoblasts, that are present in the periodontal ligament, are no longer available to maintain the integrity of this mineralized layer. The surface is usually rough because of previous fiber attachments and may become hypermineralized in some areas and cavitated in others. Because of the low inorganic content of cementum, it easily absorbs endotoxins and maintains an environment which is detrimental to periodontal tissues.

Figure 3–11, A–F.   Histopathology of Gingivitis and Periodontitis.   (After Page and Schroeder.) A, *Legend.* B, *Healthy Periodontium.* There are almost always a few defense cells, primarily PMNs, present in healthy gingiva. C, *The Initial Lesion of Gingivitis* (1–4 days). Characterized by an increase in numbers of PMN's and macrophages; slight loss of collagen fibers subjacent to junctional epithelium; beginning epithelial rete pig formation; vasculitis of blood vessels subjacent to junctional epithelium. D, *Early Lesion of Gingivitis.* (7–14 days). Characterized by continuing infiltration of PMNs and macrophages; influx of T-lymphocytes; extension of collagen loss and rete peg formation; presence of damaged fibroblasts. E, *Established Lesion of Chronic Gingivitis* (after 14 days and persisting indefinitely). Characterized by appearance and predominance of antibody-producing plasma cells; continuing replenishment of PMNs and macrophages; stabilization or decrease in numbers of T-lymphocytes; extension of collagen loss and rete peg formation; minimal or no bone loss or pocket formation. F, *Advanced Lesion of Periodontitis.* Characterized by continuing predominance of plasma cells; persistence of epithelial and connective tissue changes with some fibrosis at distant sites; extension of the lesion to alveolar bone and periodontal ligament with bone loss and pocket formation.

Gingival appearance varies considerably and some of the clinical inflammatory changes may have reverted to a level of normalcy in color and texture because of the ongoing repair attempts that are typical in longstanding chronic inflammation. Increased fibrosis or cyanosis may be present.

SUMMARY

Bacterial plaque is the primary agent in the etiology of inflammatory periodontal diseases although its effects may be modified by a number of additional local and systemic factors. Specific bacterial species in plaque have been identified in association with different types and stages of periodontal disease. The virulence of these species significantly influence periodontal destructiveness. The ability of bacteria to be destructive is related to bacterial products and to their ability to either withstand body defense mechanisms or to elicit destructive host responses. There are a number of protective mechanisms in the periodontium but when sustained by continued plaque irritation, they have the potential to destroy the tissues that are being protected.

BIBLIOGRAPHY

Allen, D.L. and Kerr, D.A.: Tissue response in the guinea pig to sterile and non-sterile calculus, J. Periodontol. 36:121, 1965.

Ebersole, J.L. et al.: Gingival crevicular fluid antibody to oral microorganisms. I. Method of collection and analysis of antibody, J. Periodont. Res. 19:124, 1984.

Jones, W.A. and O'Leary, T.J.: The effectiveness in in vivo root planing in removing bacterial endotoxin from the roots of periodontally involved teeth, J. Periodontol. 49:337, 1978.

Lehner, T.: Immunological aspects of dental caries and periodontal disease, Br. Med. Bull. 31:125, 1975.

Listgarten, M.A.: Electron microscopic observations on the bacterial flora of acute necrotizing ulcerative gingivitis, J. Periodontol. 36:328, 1965.

Listgarten, M.A.: Structure of the microbial flora associated with periodontal health and disease in man. J. Periodontol. 47:1, 1976.

Listgarten, M.A. and Ellegaard, B.: Electron microscopic evidence of a cellular attachment between junctional epithelium and dental calculus, J. Periodont. Res. 8:143, 1973.

Listgarten, M.A. and Hillden, L.: Relative distribution of bacteria at clinically healthy and periodontally diseased sites in humans, J. Clin. Periodontol. 5:115, 1978.

Listgarten, M.A. and Levin, S.: Positive correlation between the proportions of subgingival spirochetes and motile bacteria and susceptibility of human subjects to periodontal deterioration, J. Clin. Periodontol. 8:122, 1981.

Löe, H., Theilade, E. and Jensen, S.B.: Experimental gingivitis in man, J. Periodontol. 36:177, 1965.

Loesche, W.J. et al.: The bacteriology of acute necrotizing ulcerative gingivitis, J. Periodontol. 53:223, 1982.

Mandel, L.: Histochemical and biochemical aspects of calculus formation, J. Am. Soc. Periodontists 1:43, 1963.

Mashimo, P.A. et al.: The periodontal microflora of juvenile diabetics. Culture, immunofluorescence, and serum antibody studies, J. Periodontol. 54:420, 1983.

Nisengard, R.J.: The role of immunology in periodontal disease, J. Periodontol. 48:505, 1977.

Ohm, K., Albers, H.K., and Lisboa, B.P.: Measurement of eight prostaglandins in human gingival and periodontal disease using high pressure liquid chromatography and radioimmunoassay, J. Periodont. Res. 19:501, 1984.

Page, R.C. and Schroeder, H.E.: Pathogenesis of inflammatory periodontal disease, Lab. Invest. 33:235, 1976.

Page, R.C. and Schroeder, H.E.: Current status of the host response in chronic marginal periodontitis, J. Periodontol. 52:477, 1981.

Page, R.C. et al.: Rapidly progressive periodontitis, a distinct clinical condition, J. Periodontol. 54:197, 1983.

Page, R.C. et al.: Defective neutrophil and monocyte motility in patients with early onset periodontitis, Infect. Immun. 47:169, 1985.

Ritz, H.L.: Microbial population shifts in developing human dental plaque, Arch. Oral Biol. 12:1561, 1967.

Ritz, H.L.: Fluorescent antibody staining of Neisseria, Streptococcus, and Veillonella in frozen sections of human dental plaque, Arch. Oral Biol. 14:1073, 1969.

Ruzicka, F.: Structure of sub- and supragingival

dental calculus in human periodontitis. An electron microscopic study, J. Periodont. Res. 19:317, 1984.

Saglie, R. and Elbaz, J.J.: Bacterial penetration into the gingival tissue in periodontal disease, J. West. Soc. Periodont./Periodont. Abs. 31:85, 1983.

Savitt, E.D. and Socransky, S.S.: Distribution of certain subgingival microbial species in selected periodontal conditions, J. Periodont. Res. 19:111, 1984.

Slots, J.: Subgingival microflora and periodontal disease, J. Clin. Periodontol. 6:351, 1979.

Slots, J. and Dahlen, G.: Subgingival microorganisms and bacterial virulence factors in periodontitis, Scand. J. Dent. Res. 93:119, 1985.

Slots, J. and Genco, R.J.: Microbial pathogenicity, black-pigmented *Bacteroides* species, and *Actinobacillus actinomycetemcomitans* in human periodontal disease: virulence factors in colonization, survival, and tissue destruction, J. Dent. Res. 63:412, 1984.

Socransky, S.S. et al.: New concepts of destructive periodontal disease, J. Clin. Periodontol. 11:21, 1984.

Stambaugh, R.V. et al.: The limits of subgingival scaling. Int. J. Perio. and Rest. Dent. 1:30, 1981.

Tanner, A.C.R., Socransky, S.S. and Goodson, J.M.: Microbiota of periodontal pockets losing crestal alveolar bone, J. Periodont. Res. 19:279, 1984.

Theilade, E. *et al.:* Experimental gingivitis in man. II. A longitudinal clinical and bacteriological investigation, J. Periodont. Res. 1:1, 1966.

Van Dyke, T.E., Levine, M.J. and Genco, R.J.: Neutrophil function and oral disease, J. Oral Path. 14:95, 1985.

van Palenstein Helderman, W.H.: Microbial etiology of periodontal disease, J. Clin. Periodontol. 8:261, 1981.

Zambon, J.J.: *Actinobacillus actinomycetemcomitans* in human periodontal disease, J. Clin. Periodontol. 12:1, 1985.

Zander, H.A.: The attachment of calculus to root surfaces, J. Periodontol. 24:16, 1953.

CLASSIFICATION OF PERIODONTAL DISEASE

Periodontal disease is a broad term encompassing a number of pathologic alterations of the soft and hard supporting structures of teeth. These diseases and their prevention and treatment represent the essential reason for the profession of dental hygiene. Comprehension of the normal anatomy of the periodontium, the bodily defense mechanisms, the causative factors of disease, and the histopathologic changes in the tissues are essential to the hygienist's ability to successfully provide patient care. These have been presented in previous chapters. In the present chapter the clinical features manifested by pathologically affected tissue are provided.

Normal tissues are composed of cells, intercellular substances, and fluids that collectively provide a structural whole. In a state of health, all of the composite parts are carefully regulated and balanced. When changes in the environment occur, the basic harmony of the components is disturbed and a pathologic condition results. In subclinical instances subtle deviations occur that only can be ascertained through microscopic or laboratory analysis. More commonly, periodontal tissue response is manifested as clinically detectable alteration.

Basic pathologic mechanisms are common to various bodily tissue, and alterations occurring in tissues of the oral cavity are not unlike those found in other areas of the body. Tissue derangement is closely related to the nature of the contributory causes. Changes in clinical appearance of tissues due to pathoses is further modified by the anatomic arrangement of those tissues.

While the tissue response in the mouth to noxious influences resembles tissue response elsewhere in the body, there are unique problems with which oral tissues must contend. These are related to accessibility of the mouth to the external environment, the functions of oral structures, and the microbial flora of the mouth. Additionally, disease states originating in other regions of the body are often manifested in oral structures. Periodontal tissues comprise a distinctive soft tissue to tooth interface with resulting pathological aberrations demonstrated in no other body area.

PERIODONTAL DISEASES

Deviations of the gingival unit, the attachment apparatus, or both from health to a pathologic state are collectively termed periodontal disease. It is convenient to view these tissue changes as specific diseases and assign different names to each. This convenience in terminology is, however, somewhat misleading to the understanding of the pathologic process.

Great variation may exist in the clinical manifestation of periodontal pathoses in different individuals, though the etiology may be common. One individual may have relatively minor clinical changes in a periodontal disease state. Another person may demonstrate dramatic clinical alterations, yet both may have the same condition.

Not only do deviations occur among different people, there also may be variance within the same mouth from area to area, tooth to tooth, or on different surfaces of the same tooth. More than one periodontal disease or different stages of the same disease can occur in the periodontium on one individual. Thus the same mouth may demonstrate normality in some locations, slight alterations of the gingival unit in other areas, and areas of advanced destruction in other regions.

Protective Features

The periodontium is protected by the arrangement of the tissues, the vascular support mechanisms, and the cellular elements. Both epithelium and connective tissue components contribute to the defensive alignment. Epithelium of the keratinized masticatory mucosa serves as an effective barrier to irritants in much the same manner as the skin. The firm surface of the stratum corneum, constant shedding of epithelial cells, and the washing action of saliva all constitute defensive features of attached gingivae.

Crevicular epithelium and junctional epithelium, while lacking a keratinized surface, do desquamate cells constantly from superficial layers and replace them from basal strata. Junctional epithelium provides a pathway for defensive cells and fluids from connective tissue to battle microorganisms in the gingival crevice. In spite of these positive protective qualities, the epithelial lining of the gingival crevice provides the bacteria the opportunity to cause periodontal destruction.

Collagen fibers of the lamina propria and periodontal ligament provide support and binding to underlying hard tissues. Between these fiber groups are massed rich anastomoses of vascular channels and loose connective tissue. Protective and defensive cellular elements are available in these areas. Bone itself is protected indirectly by epithelial and directly by soft connective tissue and endothelial barriers. Alveolar bone is richly vascularized and capable of resorption and remodeling. Bone does not become necrotic in periodontal disease.

Fluids derived from blood serum are passed from connective tissue through junctional epithelium into the gingival crevice. This gingival crevicular exudate can carry antibodies, defensive cells, and systemically administered drugs into the crevice. Outward flow of crevicular fluid may aid in combating microbial flora. Though the amount of crevicular fluid is modest in healthy gingivae, it is markedly increased in disease conditions.

Destructive Factors

Aligned against the protective features of the periodontium discussed above and in Chapter 3 are a myriad of factors. The nature of the irritant and the response of the periodontal tissues combine to present the clinical signs representative of periodontal disease.

As previously stated, microorganisms are the principal causative agent of most periodontal diseases. The type of bacteria, the number of the organisms, and the virulence of the organisms strongly influence the nature of the tissue change. Clinical alteration is also influenced by the location of the organisms and the length of time the periodontal tissues are exposed to the microbial flora. This may be expressed as acute or chronic tissue changes.

Classification of Periodontal Diseases

Inflammation and the tissue changes in periodontal tissues have been previously detailed in Chapter 3. While the overwhelming majority of periodontal reactions are inflammatory in nature, other disease states also occur. These include changes in which the size, structure, or metabolism of the cells is altered. As a result of altered cellular metabolism tissue components may be over or under produced with detectable clinical manifestations. Specialized injury due to trauma associated with occlusion of the teeth also may affect the periodontium.

Many classifications of periodontal diseases have been developed over the years as more information on the nature and activity of tissue response has become available. During the 1950s an attempt was made to clarify the nomenclature and classification of periodontal disease. This classification has received further modification as the microbiologic and histopathologic features of disease conditions have evolved. Another factor that has influenced the classification system has been the desire for a standardized numerical system for computer use. This has resulted in development of broad general categorization of disease. All of these systems are, in a sense, artificial since several different diseases may be present in the same mouth at any given period in time. Classification, nevertheless, does provide for clarification of communication, and a simplified classification of periodontal disease states is presented below:

Inflammatory diseases
  Gingivitis
  Periodontitis
Atypical diseases
  Desquamative gingivitis
  Juvenile periodontitis
  Atrophy
Occlusal disturbances

Primary occlusal trauma
Secondary occlusal trauma

GINGIVITIS

Inflammation confined to the gingival tissues is termed gingivitis. In the United States it is the most common form of periodontal disease. Clinical signs of gingivitis range from the extremely subtle to the dramatic alteration of tissue. Both acute and chronic stages of the disease are recognized. The clinical signs of acute inflammation are swelling, redness, bleeding or exudation, and pain. All of these features are present in varying degrees in gingivitis with resultant change of gingival form and alteration of other normal characteristics (Fig. 4–1).

Any portion of the gingiva may be involved in gingivitis. Typically, the inflammatory process originates in the gingival crevice and proceeds through the initial, early, and established lesion stages in response to microbial activity. Clinical features are most apparent at the level of the established lesion. The inflammatory process may spread into marginal gingiva, the interdental papillae, or, in advanced stages, the attached gingiva. In gingivitis, however, no deeper involvement occurs and the attachment support of the tooth is not damaged.

Because no damage takes place in the attachment apparatus of the periodontal ligament tooth complex, any increase in crevicular depth is confined to the gingival unit. Gingival swelling due to inflammation may result in crevicular depth increase causing the presence of a false pocket or pseudopocket. When destruction of gingival connective fibers occurs a true gingival pocket is formed.

Certain forms of gingivitis are characterized by a sudden onset with an acute inflammatory response. In these acute states actual tissue degeneration and necrosis occur. Inflammatory changes also may be of a more chronic nature. With chronicity,

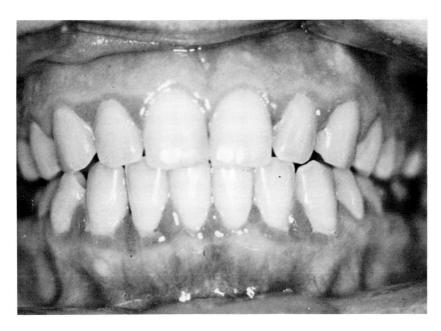

Figure 4–1. Acute Gingivitis. Marked color changes and poor gingival form are evident. (From McFall, W.T., Jr.: Tenn. State Dent. J., *45*:32, 1965.)

bodily resistance may be demonstrated by an increase in the number of tissue elements resulting in an overgrowth of the gingiva. Such an overgrowth is termed hyperplasia. Whether the gingival response is acute or chronic, if the causative factors are eliminated, there is a resolution of the inflammatory process.

Classification of Gingivitis

Inflammation is the underlying feature of all tissue changes in gingivitis (Fig. 4–2), but clinical alterations may take different forms. Many factors may modify the individual's response to tissue insult. The nature of the etiologic agent is a major factor in the determination of the tissue response. Certain microbial organisms cause more violent tissue response than others. The concept of bacterial specificity has been previously presented with regard to certain periodontal disease states. Local environmental and dental relations can create different tissue responses. Traumatic insult, as well as microbial attack, also may lead to variation in morphologic change. Host

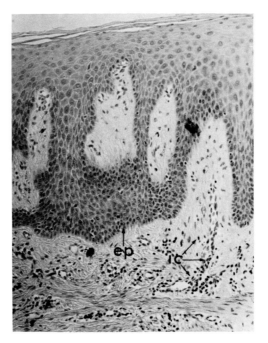

Figure 4–2. Gingivitis. This histologic section shows numerous inflammatory cells (ic) in the connective tissue and proliferation of the epithelial rete pegs (ep).

resistance factors, previous exposure to the organism, and degree of oral hygiene all contribute to a mixture of tissue reactions. The response of the host depends also on such factors as age, sex, general health status, and emotional state. A classification of gingivitis can be based on the type of gingival response to the multiple irritants and the nature of the individual in which they occur.

Gingivitis

Edematous gingivitis
Hyperplastic gingivitis
Necrotizing ulcerative gingivitis
Gingivitis associated with systemic states
    Gingivitis and puberty
    Gingivitis and pregnancy
    Hereditary gingival hyperplasia
    Phenytoin gingival enlargement
    Gingivitis and scurvy

Edematous Gingivitis

By far the most common inflammatory gingival response is gingivitis character-ized by edema (Fig. 4–3). When acute gingivitis occurs, the clinical manifestations are swelling, bleeding, redness, and soreness to pressure. Marginal gingival tissues become rolled and no longer present knife-edge contacts with teeth. Interdental papillae become swollen and bulbous. Gingival tone is lost and, with pressure, tissues feel spongy to the touch. Stippling is often diminished or lost. Gentle probing of the gingival crevice produces an instant bleeding response. Patients may complain of pain or of bleeding upon brushing.

These acute changes may involve only marginal gingivae and interdental papillae. The extent of the problem may be confined to single site, a group of teeth, or to a larger area. Variation in clinical signs may vary from area to area. Bleeding has been demonstrated to represent the earliest clinical sign, and clinical probing is an essential portion of the examination. The degree of redness and swelling may be of different intensity in various locations in the gingiva. Inflammation that spreads through the attached gingiva is a sign of more ad-

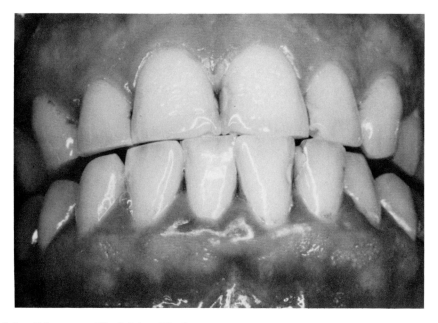

Figure 4–3. Edematous Gingivitis. The lower anterior gingival region demonstrates loss of contour and loss of stippling.

vancing disease. Plaque on teeth and gingiva is invariably present and calculus is not an uncommon feature.

Acute gingival reactions may take place in previously unaffected tissue or there may be an acute exacerbation of a chronic gingivitis. An acute state of gingivitis may subside and pass into a subacute or chronic form. The major feature of acute gingivitis is destruction exceeding repair with resultant clinical changes.

In the chronic form of edematous gingivitis the clinical signs are less intense than in the acute stages. Tissue tone may be firm, but marginal tissues are rolled. Stippling and the pinkish, normal color may be present. Pain is not a significant symptom with chronic edematous gingivitis. Bleeding from the gingival crevice generally does occur upon probing, but this bleeding is not intense and is somewhat delayed.

The more chronic forms of gingivitis represent an attempt by the body to balance destruction with repair in the presence of chronic irritants. Chronic gingivitis is time related and thus is a typical adult response. Large numbers of chronic inflammatory cells, particularly plasma cells, are spread throughout the lamina propria between reparative collagen fibers. Epithelial changes include proliferation with some interruption of integrity permitting the hemorrhage produced by probing.

Interesting trends are occurring concerning the presence of gingivitis. It appears that gingivitis is decreasing at all age levels. Gingivitis, as manifested by clinical signs, is not found to be significant during the primary dentition stage in spite of quantitatively large amounts of plaque. The highest degree of gingival inflammation occurs in teenage children. There also appears to be a gradual decrease in the prevalence of gingivitis in the elderly.

Hyperplastic Gingivitis

While swelling is a feature of all forms of gingivitis, in hyperplastic states proliferation of tissue is magnified with resultant gingival enlargement. The increase in size is, most commonly, due to an increase in the number of tissue elements, principally cells and fibers. This enlargement is the most prominent clinical sign of hyperplastic gingivitis.

Chronic irritation plays a significant role in gingival hyperplasia. Prosthetic appliances, orthodontic bands and appliances, faulty margins of restorations, improperly contoured fixed bridges, and mouth breathing habits all may contribute to hyperplastic responses. These hyperplasias also may take place in the absence of any detectable causation, and this is termed idiopathic gingival hyperplasia. Genetic traits also may influence this hyperplastic response. Because of the variance in etiologic agents, the hyperplastic response may be localized to a single area or more generalized. The area most conspicuously affected is the interdental papillae. Often the enlarged gingival papillae on the facial and lingual aspects can be separated from each other and the tooth with a blast of compressed air. Hyperplasia appears to occur more frequently in younger individuals.

Oral physiotherapy is frequently limited with gingival hyperplasia and plaque can accumulate with associated inflammatory tissue changes. The degree of this inflammation influences the clinical features. Gingival color may vary from pink to magenta, and stippling may or may not be present. Stippling also may be increased. Exaggeration of gingival form can take place. An increase in crevicular depth is noted due to gingival enlargement. For the most part, these deepened crevices are pseudopockets.

An increase in the number of collagen fibers in the gingival connective tissue is the major histologic feature. Epithelial cell proliferation also is present. The extent of round cell infiltration in the lamina propria is dependent upon the degree of inflammation, which also influences the amount of edematous fluid.

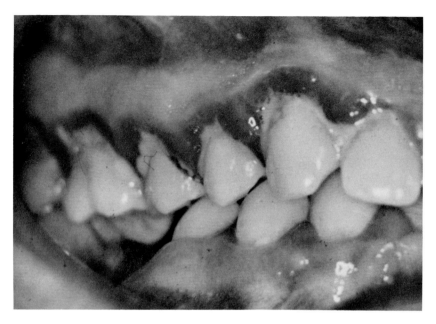

Figure 4–4. Necrotizing Ulcerative Gingivitis. The acute disease is responsible for edema, ulceration, and a pseudomembrane.

Necrotizing Ulcerative Gingivitis

This gingival disease is named on the basis of its most common clinical features: necrosis, ulceration, and inflammation of the gingiva (Figure. 4–4). The condition is also known as Vincent's infection because of its description by Vincent during the late nineteenth century. This disease was common during trench warfare of World War I and also has been termed "trench mouth." Because of its rapidity of onset, its destructive features, and the intensity of discomfort, patients afflicted with the condition usually seek professional care.

This disease condition appears to be seen less frequently than previously in this century. Though necrotizing ulcerative gingivitis was never as prevalent as other forms of gingivitis, it is becoming a relatively uncommon disease condition in the practice of general dentistry.

Necrotizing ulcerative gingivitis most commonly appears in an acute form, but some clinicians have described subacute or chronic stages of the disease. Since the condition has a tendency toward recurrence, the subacute stage may represent a recurrent form of necrotizing ulcerative gingivitis. Chronic stages are probably vestiges of the acute stage with permanently altered gingival form, such as loss of the tips of interdential papillae, due to initial severity. Various stages are distinguished by duration and severity.

Sudden onset, painful ulceration of interdental papillae, bleeding upon pressure, and foul taste and odor are the classic clinical manifestations of acute necrotizing gingivitis. In early stages, ulceration of the interdental col resulting in gingival papillary bleeding upon light probing may be the only clinical signs.

Erosion and necrosis of papillae are a major clinical feature of the severely acute stages of the disease. Extensive tissue destruction may cause the loss of the papillae resulting in a soft tissue crater (Fig. 4–5). A grayish pseudomembrane, composed of exfoliated cells and necrotic tissue debris, is sometimes present on the marginal gingiva. Marginal gingiva itself near ulcerated

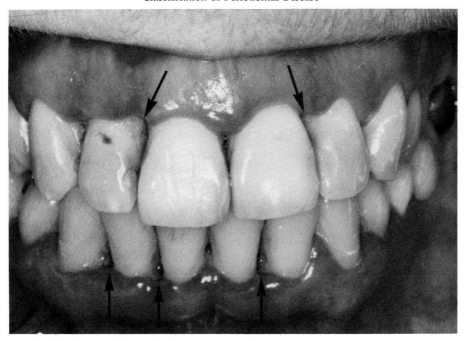

Figure 4–5. Necrotizing Ulcerative Gingivitis. The acute phase of this gingival disease has resulted in death and sloughing of portions of the interdental papillae. Arrows indicate interdental craters.

areas may appear fiercely red in color. Patients suffering from the condition most commonly report pain and foul taste as the major symptoms. Only in an advanced acute case is regional lymphadenopathy and a rise in temperature noted.

Acute necrotizing gingivitis is seldom found throughout the mouth. More commonly it is localized to several differentiated gingival areas with intervening areas of noninvolved gingiva. The disease is more commonly located in the periodontium of anterior teeth and facial areas are more usually affected than lingual ones. There is wide individual variation, and the disease may progress from one area to adjacent areas.

With chronicity, proliferation of some gingival areas may occur, while necrosis is present in other gingival areas. As a result, bizarre gingival contours with rolled margins, extensive interdental cratering, and loose flaps of tissue are presented. Gingival flaps associated with third molars are occasionally affected by the disease. In spite

of the destructive features observed in gingival tissues, extension of the disease into more apical tissues occurs rarely.

Diagnosis of necrotizing ulcerative gingivitis (NUG) is based upon the clinical changes noted previously. The disease is extremely rare in children. It is characteristically a disease of teenagers and young adults, most often occurring as the acute form (ANUG). Appearance of the disease in adults older than 30 is infrequent. Occasionally, the disease does occur in debilitated adults and may be superimposed upon preexisting periodontitis.

Necrotic epithelium with ulceration, debris, fibrin clots overlying a connective tissue infiltrated with polymorphonuclear leukocytes characterize the microscopic picture. A thin epithelium borders the ulcerated areas, and there is hyperemia of connective tissue.

Necrotizing ulcerative gingivitis has a complex causation. It is most certainly a bacterial caused condition, but other features also appear to sensitize an individual for the bacterial attack. Stress is one of those predisposing factors and it is not unusual for ANUG to occur in college students around the examination period or in military personnel undergoing training. Poor dietary habits, poor oral hygiene, lack of adequate rest. smoking, and overindulgence in alcohol all have been noted in individuals affected with this condition. It has been known for many years that there is a great increase in the number of spirochetes and fusiform bacilli in the mouths of patients with this disease. Formerly the spirochetes associated with this disease were thought to be *Borrelia vincentii*. Investigation with the electron microscope suggest that the majority of the spirochetes are of a different species. The favorable response of tissues to penicillin treatment confirms the spirochetal causation.

While most tissue changes in gingivitis are associated with microbial plaque and other local causative factors, systemic factors can and do modify tissue reactions. These systemic factors may include those of hormonal, nutritional, and hereditary origin. Gingival tissue alterations clinically represent variations of inflammatory responses.

GINGIVITIS AND PUBERTY. Pubescence is a period of enormous bodily change as the result of hormonal activity. In many young individuals just prior to puberty or during early puberty, a hyperplastic gingivitis is noted. This pubertal gingivitis is attributable in part to the hormonal alterations occurring throughout the body. Generally microbial flora growth is also present in the mouth.

While this type of gingivitis may subside spontaneously with increasing age, careful removal of irritants by health care providers is often needed. The young person must practice efficient oral hygiene to control the bacterial flora.

In pubertal gingivitis, gingival tissue overgrow, bleed easily, and may be reddish-blue in color. Sometimes these color changes may be quite dramatic involving marginal and attached gingiva (Fig. 4–6). Some pain may accompany these tissue alterations. More often the tissue changes are less severe. Orthodontic appliances, frequently worn by children during this age period, may contribute to the accumulation of plaque. Microscopic features include those normally associated with hyperplasia. There is thinning of gingival epithelium, sulcular ulceration, capillary edema, increase in tissue elements, and numerous inflammatory cells.

GINGIVITIS AND PREGNANCY. Approximately half of all pregnant women exhibit some clinically detectable gingival alteration. Local factors such as plaque are usually found, but endocrine disturbances appear to be the modifying influence (Fig. 4–7). The gingival inflammatory response during pregnancy appears to be the result of altered tissue metabolisms due to the hormonal influence. Even the attachment apparatus may be altered, and it has been noted that an increase in tooth mobility occurs during pregnancy.

The gingivitis of pregnancy ranges from mild to severe. Interdental papillae, particularly those between the anterior teeth, are primarily affected and demonstrate hyperplasia. Marginal gingiva exhibits redness, and both papillary and marginal tissues bleed with minimal irritation or trauma. Pain is not a dominant symptom, but slight discomfort is not unusual. Pregnancy gingivitis decreases with parturition.

Sometimes an exaggerated gingival reaction occurs in addition to the features of pregnancy gingivitis. A tumor-like mass may appear between teeth. These masses consist of hemorrhagic tissues termed pyogenic granulomas. Microscopic changes are manifested as capillary proliferations, intercellular edema and heavy inflammatory cell infiltrate beneath a thin epithelial cover.

These tumors, termed pregnancy granulomas, appear clinically as fiery red, pedunculated overgrowths of facial interdental papillae or, less frequently, lingual

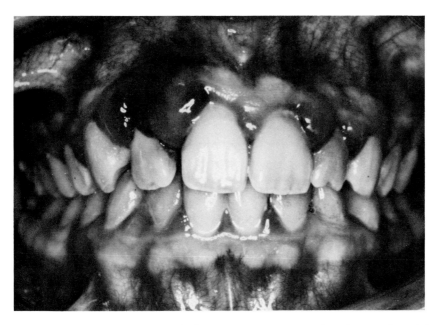

Figure 4–6. Gingivitis. These gingival alterations are associated with prepubertal hormonal changes in an 11-year-old girl.

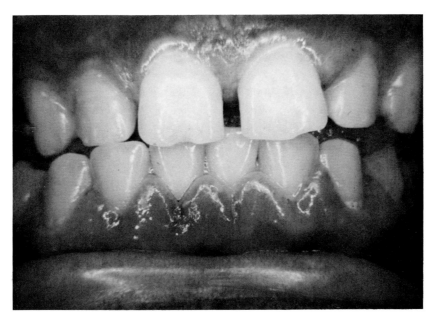

Figure 4–7. Gingivitis and Pregnancy. The gingival changes shown here are associated with pregnancy and local irritants.

papillae. They are most common during the second trimester of pregnancy. They are extremely fragile, bleed easily, and may require surgical removal. They tend to disappear following child delivery.

HEREDITARY GINGIVAL HYPERPLASIA. In certain families a type of gingival overgrowth occurs resulting in gross gingival changes. Apparently this is the result of certain inheritable tendencies. The condition may first appear with eruption of the teeth or may not appear until adolescence. Local causative factors may be lacking. Microscopic features are similar to those of other hyperplastic states except that the condition may have a greater number of collagen fibers. The condition seems more common in males, but such hyperplasia is uncommon. Diagnosis is based largely on family history.

PHENYTOIN GINGIVAL ENLARGEMENT. Dramatic overgrowth of gingival tissues are induced by diphenylhydantoin sodium, long marketed under the trade name Dilantin. This drug is used to control grand mal seizure of epilepsy. It is also widely used in other mental conditions. As such it is a valuable medication, but, unfortunately, some individuals taking the drug have severe tissue overgrowth. It is not a true hyperplasia. The exact mechanism of the reaction is not fully understood, but apparently certain fibroblasts are stimulated to produce a particularly dense form of collagen that causes the enlargement.

Gingival papillae are more affected by this drug than marginal tissues. There is great individual response to the drug, and, in severe cases, the gingival tissue may even obscure the teeth. Stippling may be present and the tissue may be pink and tough. In other instances, because of microbial flora, inflammation may be present with redness and bleeding (Fig. 4–8).

GINGIVITIS AND SCURVY. This is a most unusual gingival condition reflecting gingival alterations due to local bacterial irritants occurring in people with insufficient amounts of vitamin C. In the past, these gingival changes were part of the general bodily disease described as scurvy. With today's modern diet the disease is seldom seen. Ascorbic acid is so common in civilized society that the disease is extremely rare. The gingival changes in this condition are severe. Historically, the disease resulted in tooth loss due to progression into the attachment apparatus.

PERIODONTITIS

Periodontitis is an inflammatory disease that involves both the gingiva and the attachment apparatus of the teeth. The disease occurs predominanty, but not exclusively, in adults. Although periodontitis is probably the world's most common chronic inflammatory disease, the age of onset, the extent of destruction, and the prevalence varies among different populations in different nations. Asian nations have a higher prevalence than Western nations. Older terms for periodontitis included pyorrhea and periodontoclasia.

Periodontitis represents an extension of inflammatory changes associated with gingivitis into deeper supporting structures of the teeth. The disease is characterized by destruction of fibers of the periodontal ligament, apical migration of junctional epithelium, pocket formation, and loss of alveolar supporting bone. In advanced stages of periodontitis, tooth loss ultimately occurs because of lack of support. Periodontitis is the major cause of loss of teeth in adults.

In recent years, new data have caused a change in understanding of the progression of periodontitis. Formerly it was concluded that all patients with gingivitis, if left untreated, would eventually develop into periodontitis. Adult periodontitis does occur as a sequela of preexisting gingivitis, but probably many gingivitis cases do not progress to periodontitis. It now appears that periodontal disease progresses by recurrent acute episodes. Further, it appears that destruction with associated loss of at-

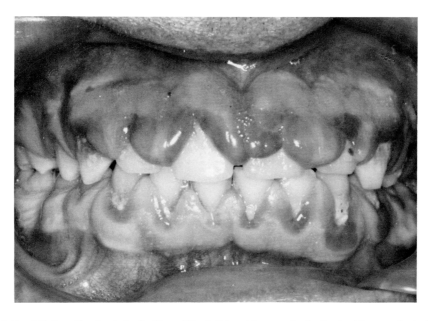

Figure 4–8. *Diphenylhydantoin Sodium Gingivitis.* The marked gingival hyperplasia is due to use of the drug diphenylhydantoin sodium.

tachment may occur at random sites around different teeth rather than as a generalized, progressive destruction. Some sites, in which active inflammation is taking place, may have never before demonstrated pocket formation. This concept of scattered sporadic activity in localized sites has been described as the "burst" concept of disease activity.

At sites of attachment loss, clinical changes are detectable in gingival tissues. These gingival alterations may be subtle or more dramatic. Acute gingival disturbances are manifested as swelling, erythema or cyanosis, loss of tissue form, and hemorrhage on provocation. These are the same features found in acute gingivitis, but there may be more purulent exudate. Inflammatory changes may spread to attached gingiva as well as continue in marginal and papillary tissue (Fig. 4–9). Both attachment loss and depth of probing increase beyond that found in gingivitis due to destruction of the attachment apparatus. These clinical features are consistent with the histopathologic changes described by

Page and Schroeder as the advanced lesion.

In other instances, the gingival changes in periodontitis reflect a continuation of chronic gingivitis with a gradual extension of inflammation with continued attempts by the body toward repair. Fibroblasts may produce increasing amounts of collagen fibers and defensive cells may be those associated with chronic inflammation and immunologic response. The clinical appearance is that of a thickened, toughened gingival tissue that may show stippling (Fig. 4–10). Probing of the pockets produces a slower bleeding response, and pain is not significant. Unfortunately, these clinical features and lack of symptoms mask a progressive loss of attachment and increasing bone destruction and diminished tooth support.

The key clinical feature of periodontitis is loss of attachment support of the teeth. This can be measured as attachment loss from a fixed reference point, or, more commonly, by an increase in separation of soft tissue from the tooth, a pocket. During the active destruction phase there is surface ul-

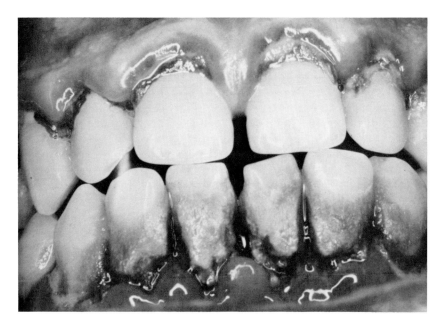

Figure 4–9. Periodontitis. Acute gingival inflammation, deep pockets, and drifting of teeth occur in this disease.

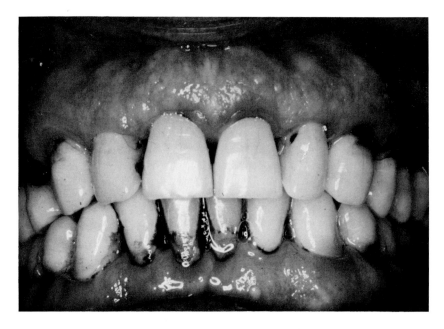

Figure 4–10. Chronic Periodontitis. The gingiva has become fibrotic in this chronic periodontitis. Deep pockets are present. (From McFall, W.T., Jr.: Tenn. State Dent. J. *45*:34, 1965.)

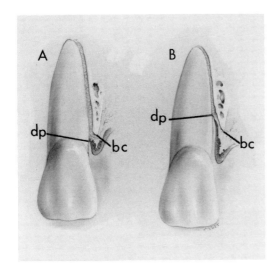

Figure 4–11. Pockets. A, A suprabony pocket, B, An intrabony defect with the base of the pocket apical to the bone crest. (bc) bone crest, (dp) depth of pocket.

ceration of the epithelium, bleeding and suppuration, fiber destruction, junctional epithelial migration apically, and resorption of alveolar bone. Pocket formation can occur with rapidity, but it is not continuously progressive. The presence of a pocket does not always indicate active inflammatory destruction. Apparently the degree of inflammation in a pocket is dependent upon the intensity of bacterial activity. Pockets may represent scars of previous destruction.

Unlike the pseudopocket or gingival pocket, due primarily to gingival swelling, the true periodontal pocket is a result of damage to the periodontal ligament and resorption of crestal supporting bone with apical migration of the junctional epithelial tissue. Periodontal pockets are classified as either suprabony or intrabony pockets. When the bottom of the pocket remains coronal to the alveolar bone level, a suprabony pocket is formed. An intrabony pocket occurs when the base of the pocket is apical to the remaining alveolar bone (Fig. 4–11).

Unless there is acute gingival changes or

abscess formation, pocket formation is usually painless, and suppuration may or may not be present. Radiographic evidence of bone loss is not a feature of early lesions of periodontitis. The only accurate determination of presence of periodontal pockets is through clinical examination with a periodontal probe.

As indicated in Chapter 3, microbial products are the primary cause of periodontal inflammation and pocket formation. As a result of these irritants connective tissue destruction first occurs beneath the base and sides of the gingival crevice. Dissolution of the collagen fiber barriers of gingival fibers and periodontal ligament allows the epithelial attachment to move apicalward. As the junctional epithelium proliferates apically, detachment of fibers takes place from cementum. A pocket is thus formed. A periodontal pocket is bordered on one side by exposed cementum and on the other by ulcerated epithelium (Fig. 4–12).

Deeper involvement of supporting tissues is the result of an extension of inflammation. This inflammatory infiltrate tends to follow the loose connective tissue adjacent to the vascular channels. Periodontal ligament fibers further apically are destroyed and alveolar bone is resorbed by osteoclastic activity. This osteoclastic bone removal is a portion of the bodily defense mechanism in response to the toxic effects of the inflammatory process. Bone does not become necrotic with periodontitis. While osteoclastic activity continues, there is also diminished osteoblastic activity. The result of increased resorption and minimal osteoblastic construction accounts for the pattern of bone loss.

Because periodontitis is most likely to occur in interproximal areas, the initial bone resorption takes place at the alveolar crest. Arterioles and venules pierce the alveolar crest in this interalveolar bone. Inflammatory exudate proceeds around the loose vascular connective surrounding these vessels. Seldom does the inflamma-

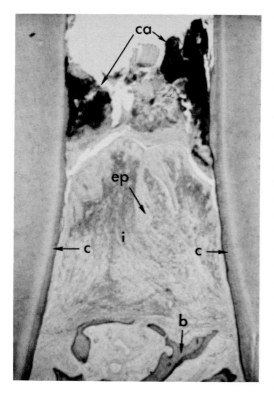

Figure 4–12. Periodontitis. Inflammation has spread through the interdental area. Destruction of many gingival fibers has occurred. (ca) calculus, (ep) epithelium, (i) inflammatory cells, (c) cementum, (b) bone.

tion spread directly through the periodontal ligament itself. Thus the osseous destruction most commonly happens where vascular channels pierce the crestal bone. This creates a cup-shaped resorptive area interproximally termed a crater. This type of bone loss is usually the earliest radiographic evidence of bone destruction.

Root cementum coronal to the bottom of the pocket becomes nonvital as the cementoblastic layer is lost. This exposed cementum provides increased areas for attachment of calculus and plaque. Toxic bacterial products are deposited on and in the structure of the root and on calculus. If the pocket continues to deepen, more and more fiber attachment is lost and greater root exposure occurs. With increased destruction of periodontal ligament alveolar

bone loss happens as a result of diminished function and spread of inflammation. The tooth so affected may become loosened or mobile. Teeth may drift or migrate with opening of interproximal dental contacts.

The most prominent radiographic feature in periodontitis is a gradual apical decrease in bone height. Early bone loss is expressed on radiographs as loss of crestal density and a scooped-out appearance of interproximal bone. Because changes in facial and lingual bone are unable to be seen on radiographs due to the image of the tooth, the interproximal area provides the best area for viewing osseous changes. Bone loss can also be radiographically evident in bifurcation and trifurcation areas, but these represent progressive stages of the disease process. The general pattern of bone loss in periodontitis is most commonly a stepladder-type of horizontal bone resorption (Fig. 4–13). Bone can assume rather unusual patterns of resorption that may not be radiographically evident.

Patterns of Periodontal Disease

Because of the variations in periodontal diseases, in recent times it has become necessary to create categories or patterns of the clinical stages of the disease. This convention has largely been brought about by the need to establish a uniform code of nomenclature that is computer compatible and can be used in reporting clinical conditions to third party insurance carriers. These codes, though somewhat artificial, are in wide general use in the United States, and the hygienist should understand their meaning. These are taken from the manual, *Current Procedural Terminology of Periodontics.*

(04500). Gingivitis. Inflammation of the gingiva characterized clinically by gingival hyperplasia, edema, retractability, gingival pockets and no bone loss represent the gingivitis code.

(04600). Early Periodontitis. This is represented as progression of gingival inflammation into the alveolar bone crest and

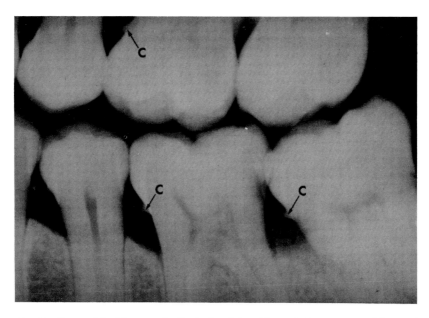

Figure 4–13. Radiographic Changes In Periodontitis. There is interproximal bone destruction, and calculus (c) is evident on the teeth.

early bone loss resulting in moderate pocket formation.

(04700). Moderate Periodontitis. A more advanced state than early periodontitis, this is characterized as increased destruction of periodontal structures associated with moderate to deep pockets, moderate to severe bone loss and tooth mobility.

(04800). Advanced Periodontitis. This pattern is represented by further progression of periodontitis with severe destruction of the periodontal structures with increased tooth mobility.

(04900). Refractory Progressive Periodontitis. This is a condition of continued destruction in spite of clinical treatment.

Progression of Periodontitis

As discussed above, most inflammatory periodontitis is preceded by gingivitis, but the hygienist should understand that the concept of continuing progression from early periodontitis to more advanced states is undergoing critical reexamination. It is clear that periodontal destruction progresses at different rates in different pa-

tients and at different sites in the same individual.

Gingivitis may or may not progress to early periodontitis; early periodontitis may or may not progress to moderate periodontitis, and moderate periodontitis may or may not progress to advanced periodontitis. Indeed, the number of individuals with advanced periodontitis is small when compared with the whole population. Even in those individuals with advanced destruction not all teeth may be similarly involved.

Though rates of progression vary, the predominant progressive pattern is slow involving months and years. Although there have been reports of rapid destruction known as rapidly progressive periodontitis, it should be emphasized that this is uncommon. Even if the rates of progression are slow, the results of periodontitis are sure—loss of attachment and tooth support.

All of the above characterize a widespread inflammatory disease affecting an enormous number of people on a worldwide basis. Each individual affected by the disease must be treated on an individual basis. Prevention and treatment of these diseases are of paramount import and will be discussed in future chapters.

ATYPICAL DISEASES

Inflammation is a characteristic of all periodontal diseases. Certain conditions affecting the periodontium have other histopathoses that are the major cause of the clinical changes. These conditions may be confined in the superficial soft tissues or deeper periodontal structures.

Desquamative Gingivitis

Dystrophic diseases refer to pathologic conditions in which cells undergo certain metabolic changes leading to cellular atrophy or cellular death. These types of cellular modifications are rare in periodontal tissues when compared with inflammatory alterations. A disease that affects the gingival tissues in this manner is termed desquamative gingivitis.

The most prominent clinical feature in this rare disease is the presence of areas of gingiva from which the epithelium has been lost (desquamated). These areas may be scattered among areas of normal appearing gingiva. Large amounts of marginal, interdental papillae, and attached gingiva may become involved (Fig. 4–14).

While no specific etiology for this condition has been determined, some evidence points to hormonal or nutritional disturbances in the causation. There are similarities between desquamative gingivitis and some dermatologic disorders that affect oral structures, notably benign mucous membrane pemphigoid (BMMP). Females who have completed menopause appears to be the group most commonly afflicted with this condition, but the disease has been found in older males. Other periodontal inflammatory disease states may be present as well.

When epithelium is desquamated, underlying connective tissue is exposed as a raw red wound. In some cases the epithelium is not completely lost and vesicles and ulcerations are sometimes present. When gingiva is scraped vigorously, the epithelium is peeled off in some cases.

Denuded connective tissue becomes secondarily infected by bacteria. This inflammatory process accounts for the gingivitis portion of the name desquamative gingivitis. With exposure of connective tissue, pain and burning sensations are experienced by the patient.

Microscopic features include a thinning or an absence of epithelium with few rete pegs present. Edema and disruption of cellular layers of epithelium may be found. The basement membrane is atrophic. Connective tissues are disorganized with fiber degeneration and inflammatory cell infiltration.

Juvenile Periodontitis

A disease of much more serious tooth threatening consequences is juvenile periodontitis. This is an atypical disease of the periodontium involving cementum, periodontal ligament, and alveolar bone. Primarily a disease of adolescence, it was formerly termed periodontosis.

Although juvenile forms of periodontitis affect only a small number of individuals in comparison with other forms of periodontitis, the rapidly destructive nature of the disease and the youthful age of onset make it significant. In recent years a great amount of research has been done on this disease and underlying causation and methods of treatment are now better understood.

One of the interesting clinical features of the disease is that gingival inflammation is not prominent in early stages. There may be no overt change in gingival color, texture, or form. Deep pocket formation, determined by probing, is the earliest clinical indication of the disease. Radiographic evidence of extensive bone loss is another diagnostic indicator. Occasionally, the individuals with this condition may note

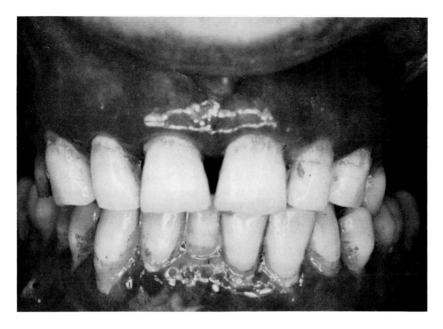

Figure 4–14. Desquamative Gingivitis.   Epithelium has been lost in most areas of the gingivae.

drifting or extrusion of their teeth. Pain is not a significant finding.

Two forms of juvenile periodontitis are most commonly reported. In the classical form of the disease, deepened pockets and rapid bone loss are associated with first permanent molars and permanent incisors exclusively. In the other form, there is a more generalized pattern of bone loss affecting many teeth. This generalized pattern may be related to systemic conditions, may be adult periodontitis superimposed on juvenile periodontitis, or may represent a rapidly progressive form of the disease. When bone loss and pocket formation are associated with a single dental unit, these lesions are commonly excluded from the classification of juvenile periodontitis.

Diagnostic clues relative to juvenile periodontitis rest with the young age of the patient, the depth of the periodontal pockets, the predilection for incisor and molar teeth, and the radiographic image of angular patterns of bone loss. Roentgenographic pictures are of some value in diagnosis in that extensive bone loss is unusual in young individuals. A steep ver-

tical type of bone resorption occurs on proximal surfaces of affected teeth (Fig. 4–15). This may involve both mesial and distal surfaces of the teeth, particularly in regard to first molars. Both arches may be affected and bilateral bone loss patterns are not uncommon. In other instances only one proximal root surface may present such an angular defect. Angular patterns of bone loss are not, however, confined to juvenile periodontitis.

Histopathologic findings in juvenile periodontitis are characterized by dissolution of periodontal ligament fibers and resorption of alveolar bone. Gingival inflammation is a variable feature, but most aspects of periodontitis, including an inflammatory infiltrate, are present. The etiology of this disease is discussed in Chapters 3 and 5.

Loss of teeth in this condition is accounted for by the combination of tooth migration, deep pocket formation, alveolar bone loss, and occlusal forces on teeth whose support has been weakened. The early age of onset also means that affected teeth are at risk longer to microbial attack. Some adults may maintain affected teeth

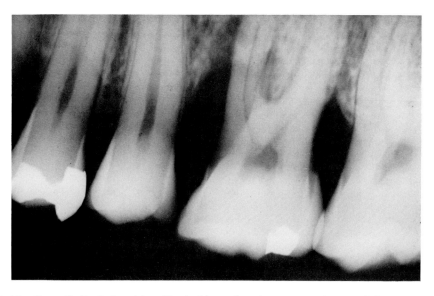

Figure 4–15. Juvenile Periodontitis. Vertical bone loss has occurred around the first molar in a 19-year-old girl.

for some time, thus sometimes presenting a diagnostic quandary.

PERIODONTAL ATROPHY

Atrophy refers to a condition of gradual wasting away of cells or tissues with a resultant diminution in size. In the periodontium this may be expressed as gingival recession with exposure of the root. Also, atrophy of disuse may take place in the periodontium surrounding a tooth with diminished function or lack of function.

GINGIVAL ATROPHY. Gingival recession is a common clinical feature in older individuals. With the longer life expectancy and greater number of individuals reaching advanced ages, it can be anticipated that gingival recession will be a more frequent clinical finding in the future. This gingival atrophy is often accompanied by concomitant resorption of alveolar bone without pocket formation. As the gingival tissues recede apically, cementum is exposed, and this cementum may then be subject to abrasion or caries. Gingival inflammation is a variable feature.

Sometimes a vertical groove occurs in the gingiva through the free gingiva over the middle of a prominent root. Such a condition is termed a Stillman's cleft. In other instances recession may result in prominent rolls of gingiva. These configurations are referred to as McCall's festoons. Neither of these terms are in common usage.

The concept of gingival atrophy or physiologic recession is open to some question. So many etiologic factors may contribute to gingival recession that pure recessional atrophy probably seldom takes place. Teeth, particularly mandibular teeth, may erupt in a facial position too close to the mucogingival junction, and the teeth may never have much attached gingival tissue. Other factors include frenulum attachment, faulty toothbrushing methods, rotation of teeth, orthodontics, and calculus.

Gingival recession may also be found in children, particularly in facial areas. This may be due to an eruptive phenomenon, trauma, faulty brushing, pernicious habits, and frenulum tension. Preventive grafting surgical procedures are available to deal with these recessional problems.

DISUSE ATROPHY. Some exercise is required to keep any bodily organ functioning in health. This stimulus for the teeth and periodontium is provided by a functioning occlusion. If a tooth loses its functional stimulus, as in the case of a tooth without an antagonist, then disuse atrophy of the periodontium can take place.

The fibers of the periodontal ligament, lacking usage, are diminished in number. Remaining fibers become irregularly arranged and the width of the periodontal ligament is decreased. Sometimes the thickness of adjacent cortical bone is reduced and marrow spaces in cancellous bone are enlarged. Radiographic findings may include a narrowed periodontal ligament space.

Disuse atrophy is probably never complete in the periodontium. Action of the tongue and cheeks and passage of food continue to supply some stimulus to the periodontium. If a tooth so affected is subsequently returned to function, a return to normality gradually ensues.

OCCLUSAL TRAUMA

Trauma implies an injury of tissue. Such an injury may be produced by forceful occlusion of teeth with one another. This mechanism of occlusal trauma and the influence of untoward occlusal forces is discussed in Chapter 5.

As noted previously, a certain amount of activity of the teeth is required to maintain integrity of the periodontium. Even fairly heavy forces, if intermittently applied, are well tolerated by compensatory thickening of periodontal ligament fibers and construction of additional bone in the socket walls.

When occlusal forces exceed physiologic limits and produce damage in an otherwise healthy periodontium, this is *primary occlusal trauma*. All changes are confined to the attachment apparatus and there are no inflammatory features. The gingival crevice is not deepened and there is no pocket formation. Clinically, an increased tooth mobility, coronal facets, and food impaction

may be noted. The patient may experience soreness or discomfort and may avoid the tooth during mastication. A similar type of trauma to the attachment apparatus occurs with orthodontic tooth movement.

Histopathologic alterations of the attachment apparatus are dependent upon the magnitude, duration, and direction of the occlusal forces on the tooth. When forces are in the direction of the long axis of the tooth, the fiber arrangement is well designed to resist this stress and the major response to the force is a thickening of the alveolar bone proper. Most forces, such as those generated in grinding habits, are directed in a faciolingual manner resulting in tension and compression of the periodontal ligament. Periodontal fibers are stretched on the side from which the pressure is applied and cemental tearing can occur. Tension is transferred to adjacent bone. On the side opposite to that from which pressure is applied, compression of fibers and vessel occurs and bone resorption may occur. With continued strong force crushing necrosis of the ligament and extensive bone resorption takes place.

On radiographs these changes are manifested by an uneven widening of the periodontal space, increased density and thickening of the lamina dura and root resorption. Since there are repair attempts by the body for response to these forces there may be hypercementosis at the apices of roots. Bone may compensate with additional construction.

When tooth support is seriously diminished by inflammatory periodontal destruction, even normal occlusal forces may produce injury. The lesion produced in the attachment apparatus is known as *secondary occlusal trauma*. Occlusal forces thus become a secondary factor, which can alter the rate or extent of damage. Pathways of inflammation may be modified with occlusal forces resulting in inflammatory infiltrate proceeding through the periodontal ligament itself.

Clinical features of secondary occlusal

trauma are the same as those seen in periodontitis. Mobility may be marked. Radiographic features are those of advanced periodontitis, and there may be angular bone defects.

Experimental evidence has repeatedly demonstrated that excessive occlusal forces will not initiate gingival inflammation or produce periodontal pockets. In order to initiate inflammatory changes microbial factors must be present.

PERIODONTAL ABSCESS

The periodontal or lateral abscess represents a localized inflammation of the purulent type in the attachment apparatus. They should be differentiated from the occasional gingival abscess, caused by foreign bodies, which is confined to marginal tissues. Gingival abscesses do not usually destroy deeper supporting tissues.

A periodontal abscess is usually associated with a preexistent periodontal pocket. A collection of neutrophils is assembled to combat microbial irritants in the pocket. As long as drainage is possible through the orifice of the pocket, no abscess occurs. If the opening of the pocket becomes obstructed, or in deep pockets where drainage is inhibited then the neutrophils die and pus is formed. As pus continues to form it seeks escape. This is achieved by destruction of cortical bone and penetration through overlying soft tissue.

Clinically, the acute periodontal abscess appears as a pronounced swelling (Fig. 4–16). The gingiva is edematous and reddened. Periodontal exudate can usually be expressed from the gingival opening of the pocket by probing. In some instances the abscess may "point" or come to a head in the soft tissue. The patient may report pain, tooth looseness or soreness, regional lymph node swelling, and, in some cases, fever. Symptoms vary with size and location of the abscess.

Chronic abscesses are less common but do occur, usually with a patent fistula.

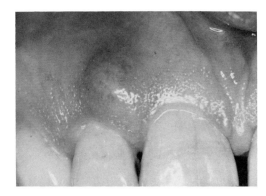

Figure 4–16. Periodontal Abscess. An acute periodontal abscess has formed in association with a deep pocket on the facial of the lateral incisor.

These tracts occasionally ooze exudate and may become reinfected. Chronic periodontal abscesses are often surprisingly symptomless.

Radiographic findings associated with a periodontal abscess are often scant. In the early phases of an acute lesion they are totally lacking. With chronicity, a radiolucent area may appear lateral to the surface of the root.

Certain clinical conditions lend themselves to this pathologic process. Narrow, deep intrabony pockets can become blocked and are prone to abscess formation. Bifurcation and trifurcation areas are also common sites for abscess formation. In persistent deep pockets recurrent abscess formation may occur with each attack further weakening tooth support.

Foreign bodies in the form of impacted food, dental materials, and toothbrush bristles have been implicated in periodontal abscess formation. More frequently the lesion occurs in association with calculus deposits. A relativey high incidence of periodontal abscesses have been noted in patients with diabetes.

HERPETIC STOMATITIS

Acute herpetic gingivostomatitis is not strictly a periodontal disease, but it does effect periodontal tissue. It is included here because of its occurrence in gingival tissue and of the confusion of this condition with other inflammatory gingival disturbances.

Herpes simplex virus is responsible for herpetic gingivostomatitis. This disease occurs in both sexes and appears most commonly in infants and children. The lesions of this disease occurs primarily as small vesicles on any part of the oral mucosa. These vesicles soon rupture and painful, small, yellow-rimmed ulcers form. Areas may be secondarily infected by bacteria.

There may be diffuse inflammation of the gingiva with variable degrees of swelling and bleeding (Fig. 4–17). Sometimes there is widespread gingival erythema with minimal vesicle formation and ulceration. The disease can be quite painful and debilitating but it is self-limiting, and the disease runs its course in 1 to 2 weeks.

In the adult, recurrent herpetic lesions are common and occur almost exclusively extraorally, primarily on the lips. Secondary herpes appear as a painful vesicle that erupts into an ulcer. A clot covers the ulcer and the wound heals in approximately a week and a half without residual scarring. During the ulcer stage the herpes virus is transmissible to other individuals.

SUMMARY

In this chapter the clinical and histopathologic features of the major diseases affecting the periodontium have been described. These diseases are primariy inflammatory in nature, but there may be other changes as well. Atypical conditions and traumatic injuries are also part of periodontal diseases. Pathologic alterations disrupt the normal integrity of periodontal tissues. In Chapter 3 and the present chapter the mechanisms of these changes and the clinical manifestations have been presented. These pathologic features are primarily the result of local irritants but may be modified by systemic states. In the next chapter these causative relations to periodontal disease are discussed. A classifica-

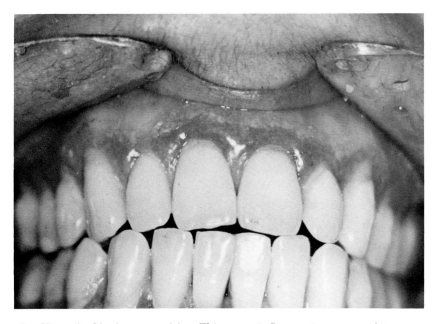

Figure 4–17. Herpetic Gingivostomatitis. This acute inflammation occurred in a young father who contracted it from his baby.

tion of periodontal disease based on these manfestations is presented.

BIBLIOGRAPHY

Chilton, N.W. and Miller, M.F.: Epidemiology: A position paper and review of the literature, International Conference on Research in the Biology of Oral Disease, Chicago, 1977, p. 135.

Cohen, D.W., Shapiro, J., Friedman, L., Kyle, G.C. and Franklin, S.: A longitudinal investigation of the periodontal changes during pregnancy and fifteen months post-partum, J. Periodontol., 42:633, 1971.

Cox, M.O., Crawford, J.J., Lundblad, R.L. and McFall, W.T., Jr.: Oral leukocytes and gingivitis in the primary dentition. J. Periodont. Res., 9:23, 1974.

Douglas, C.F., Gillings, D., Sollecito, W. and Gammon, M.: National trends in the prevalence and severity of the periodontal diseases, J. Am. Dent. Assoc., 107:403, 1983.

Goodman, S.F., Derdivanis, J. and Hornbuckle, C.: Current Procedural Terminology for Periodontics, Chicago, The American Academy of Periodontology, 1977.

Greenstein, G.: The role of bleeding upon probing in the diagnosis of periodontal disease. A literature review, J. Periodontol., 55:684, 1984.

Hassell, T.W., Page, R.C. and Lindhe, J.: Histologic evidence for impaired growth control in diphenylhydantoin gingival overgrowth in man, Arch. Oral. Biol. 23:381, 1978.

Listgarten, M.A.: Electron microscopic observations on the bacterial flora of acute necrotizing ulcerative gingivitis, J. Periodontol., 36:328, 1965.

Loe, H. and Silness, J.: Periodontal disease in pregnancy, Acta Odont. Scand., 21:533, 1963.

Lyon, H., Bernier, J., and Goldman, H.M.: Report of the Nomenclature and Classification Committee, J. Periodontol., 30:74, 1959.

Mackler, S.B. and Crawford, J.J.: Plaque development and gingivitis in the primary dentition, J. Periodontol., 44:18, 1973.

Matsson, L. and Goldberg, P.: Gingival inflammatory reaction in children at different ages, J. Clin. Periodontol., 12:98, 1985.

Newman, M.G. and Socransky, S.S.: Predominant cultivable microbiota in periodontosis. J. Periodont. Res., 12:120, 1977.

Page, R.C. and Schroeder, H.E.: Periodontal Disease, in Schluger, S., Yuodelis, R.A. and Page, R.C. (Eds.), Philadelphia, Lea & Febiger, Chapter 7, pp. 168, 1977.

Page, R.C. et al.: Rapidly progressive periodontitis, J. Periodontol., 54:197, 1983.

Schluger, S.: Osseous resection—a basic principle in periodontal surgery, Oral Surg., 2:316, 1949.

Slots, J., Reynolds, H.S. and Genco, J.R.: Actinobacillus actinomycetemcomitans in human periodontal disease, Infection and Immunity, 29:1013, 1980.

Socransky, S.S., Haffajee, A.D., Goodson, J. and Lindhe, J.: Changing concepts of destructive periodontal disease, J. Clin. Periodontol., 11:21, 1984.

Waerhaug, J.: Pathogenesis of pocket formation in traumatic occlusion, J. Periodontol., 26:107, 1955.

Weinmann, J.P.: Progress of gingival inflammation in the supporting structures of the tooth, J. Periodontol., 12:71, 1941.

Wentz, F.M., Jarabak, J. and Orban, B.: Experimental occlusal trauma imitating cuspal interference, J. Periodontol., 29:117, 1958.

CONTRIBUTING FACTORS IN THE ETIOLOGY OF THE PERIODONTAL DISEASES

Overwhelming evidence supports the contention that the primary etiology of the periodontal diseases is microbiologic in nature. The high majority of periodontal problems encountered by the dental hygienist on a daily basis is inflammatory in nature caused by tissue response to irritants produced by oral microorganisms, usually organized as dental plaque. The plaque is usually attached directly to the tooth surface, to dental calculus, to dental restorations or to irregularities of the tooth surface. Many of the preventive procedures employed by the dental team for the patient are directed towards the inhibition of or removal of dental plaque. The role of dental plaque and dental calculus in periodontal diseases has been discussed in previous chapters.

There are, however, other factors of a local or systemic nature which may predispose the patient to be more susceptible to developing periodontal disease. Local conditions in the mouth may promote plaque and calculus formation. Irritants other than microorganisms may elicit the inflammatory response in the periodon-

tium. The inflammatory response of a patient may be modified or influenced by various systemic diseases or factors. This chapter will be concerned with those factors which may contribute in the etiology of periodontal disease for any one given patient.

LOCAL FACTORS OTHER THAN PLAQUE AND CALCULUS

STAINS. Stains are not as important as bacterial plaque and dental calculus in the causation of periodontal disease. The complete removal of stains, however, is important for several reasons. The hygienist cannot be sure that all plaque and calculus have been removed unless the teeth are clean of all extraneous material. Stains produce irregularities on the teeth that may promote plaque or calculus formation. A patient's hygiene cannot be evaluated at a subsequent appointment unless it is known that the teeth were clean at the time they received oral physiotherapy instructions. The patient with scrupulously clean teeth is more highly motivated to keep

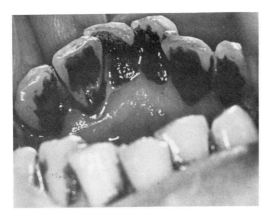

Figure 5–1. Stain. Heavy deposits of tobacco stain on the lingual of the mandibular anterior teeth.

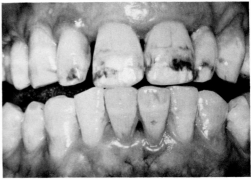

Figure 5–2. Dental Fluorosis. Mottled, brownish-opaque discoloration of teeth due to incorporation of excessive amounts of fluoride during the development of the teeth. (Courtesy Dr. Richard Courtney.)

them that way. Stains may be noticeable and create a cosmetic problem for the patient. Patients will not gain confidence in the hygienist unless they are assured that she has done a thorough dental prophylaxis for them.

Extrinsic stains form on the teeth from the use of tobacco, coffee, tea, certain drugs, and certain food (Fig. 5–1). Chromogenic microorganisms may also produce discoloration on the surfaces of the teeth. A study suggests that black stain is produced by certain microorganisms that cause a reaction to occur in the saliva between hydrogen sulfide and iron, resulting in the formation of ferrous sulfide. Perhaps other stains are produced in a similar manner. These vary in color and may be orange, red, green, brown, or black. Microbial stains are seen usually on the teeth of children. Extrinsic stains are removable by adequate scaling or polishing procedures.

Intrinsic stains are present within the substance of the tooth and cannot be removed by scaling or polishing. If a patient has ingested excessive quantities of fluoride during the formative stages of the teeth, the teeth will be mottled with a brownish-opaque discoloration (Fig. 5–2). This condition is referred to as dental fluorosis. Frequently, there are localized lines of brown stain around silicate cement res-

torations resulting from the fluoride content of the cement.

Teeth which have been exposed to an excessive amount of tetracycline drugs during the period of formation may be intrinsically stained as a result of the antibiotic. The color of the stain varies and may be yellow, brown, or orange.

Teeth which have been treated for caries arrestment or hypersensitivity by topical application of silver nitrate may exhibit a grayish-black discoloration. This change is usually seen around amalgam restoration and gives the appearance that the source of the stain is below the surface of the tooth. The crowns of teeth in which the pulp has degenerated present a grayish discoloration with loss of translucency.

ANATOMIC CONSIDERATIONS. Ideal alignment and relation of the teeth promote the physiologic as well as anatomic configuration of the gingivae, attachment apparatus and alveolar bone. Deviations from these ideal relations are caused by irregularities in the eruptive sequence of the teeth, premature loss of the primary teeth, loss of permanent teeth without appropriate space maintenance, non-compatibility of teeth size or tooth and jaw size, or anomalies of the size or shape of the teeth.

Any alteration in the ideal alignment and

relation of the teeth can lead to conditions which promote plaque and calculus formation. Open interdental contacts and marginal ridge discrepancies result in food impaction which irritates the interdental papillae. Crowding of teeth and other forms of malocclusion make oral physiotherapy procedures more difficult for the patient and create clinical challenges for the hygienist when performing preventive and therapeutic procedures.

As is true of most tissues and organs, with the gingivae there is a direct relation between anatomic form and function. The form of the gingivae as well as the supporting bone is determined primarily by the form and alignment of the associated teeth. If the teeth are normal in size and shape and are in proper position and alignment, the related periodontium will tend to be of ideal form (unless periodontal disease is or has been present). If, for example, a tooth is malaligned in a facial direction, the facially attached gingival and alveolar bone will be receded and thin. When a tooth is lost, a major portion of the associated alveolar bone eventually will resorb. When a tooth drifts into an adjacent space created by the extraction of teeth, bone will resorb on the side of the tooth in the direction it leans. Intrabony pockets occur most frequently when the interproximal distance between adjacent tooth roots is greater than 2 mm. Every attempt needs to be made by the dental team to promote retention of the integrity of the dental arches as well as the physiologic arrangement of the dental units.

FOOD IMPACTION AND RETENTION. The impaction of food between the teeth may result in physical injury to the interproximal gingival tissues. If the food particles are allowed to remain in the mouth and to degenerate, chemical substances are produced that are irritants to the gingival tissues and that favor the overgrowth of microorganisms. The breakdown products of certain foods are also thought to be important in the etiology of dental caries.

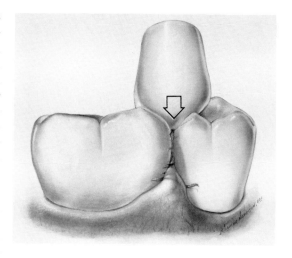

Figure 5–3. Plunger Cusp. Maxillary premolar cusp has forced fibrous food through the interdental contact area of the mandibular teeth (lingual view).

Chronic areas of food impaction are naturally more significant in the production of gingival inflammation than are areas where food is only occasionally retained.

The integrity of the dental arch plays an important part in protection from food impaction. If there is a contiguous arrangement of teeth with firm interdental contacts, there is less likelihood of food impaction than if there are missing teeth or weak interdental contacts. The cusp of a tooth which fits tightly into the occlusal embrasure formed by the marginal ridges of two opposing teeth may force food through the interdental contact area into the gingival embrasure. Such a cusp is called a plunger cusp (Fig. 5–3). This mechanism of food impaction is more likely to occur if there is a weak or poorly placed interdental contact. Vertical food impaction occurs when food is forced between the interdental contacts. Horizontal food impaction may occur in open gingival embrasures from tongue or cheek activity while eating.

Malaligned teeth due to developmental patterns of eruption or due to migration following dental extractions create discrep-

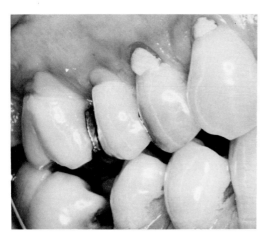

Figure 5–4. Gingival Recession and Cervical Abrasion. Horizontal scrubbing with a toothbrush has resulted in these defects. Two of the abraded areas have been repaired with poorly contoured restorations.

ancies in the dental arch that favor food impaction and retention. Adjacent marginal ridges at different occlusal heights also promote food impaction.

Fibrous foods such as meat are usually more readily impacted than other foods. Nondetergent or soft foods are of the type more likely to be retained around the necks of the teeth. Coarse, detergent foods may aid in the removal of soft debris and bacterial plaque from the surfaces of the teeth.

Inadequate Oral Physiotherapy

In essence, all of the potent sources of local irritation can be related to oral physiotherapy. The degree of development of bacterial plaque, dental calculus, and food deposits is inversely proportionate to the effectiveness of the patient's oral hygiene procedures as well as to the dental and hygienist service which the patient receives. Occasionally a patient is seen who has practiced a good brushing and home care regimen, but who has developed a serious periodontal problem. This is certainly the exceptional situation, however.

Inadequate oral physiotherapy has a twofold deleterious effect on the periodon-

tal tissues. Faulty or ineffective techniques result in the formation of plaque and calculus on the teeth. The other deleterious effect is insufficient gingival stimulation, which results in a decrease of gingival tone, a decrease in surface keratinization, and a decrease in blood circulation through the tissues. Lack of adequate tone, keratinization, and circulation reduce the general resistance of the gingival tissues to combat the irritating effects of harmful substances. Too vigorous brushing, however, especially with a hard toothbrush in a horizontal manner, may result in gingival recession and cervical abrasion (Fig. 5–4). These conditions are most likely to occur around teeth which are prominent in the dental arch.

Proper brushing procedures may aid in the expression of tissue fluid through the gingival crevice, helping to keep the crevice free of irritating substances. The many reasons why a patient may not be accomplishing good daily oral hygiene procedures are discussed in Chapter 8.

Nonphysiologic or Inadequate Dental Treatment

The lack of dental treatment or the placement of nonphysiologic dental restorations may actually initiate or promote the development of periodontal disease.

LACK OF DENTAL TREATMENT. Dental caries can result in the loss of interdental contacts, thereby promoting the impaction and retention of food debris between the teeth (Fig. 5–5). Bacterial plaque forms readily around the rough margins of carious lesions. The carious area itself is contaminated with a heavy accumulation of microorganisms and may hold these in close association with the gingival tissues. If the tooth is sensitive because of caries, the patient will avoid it while eating, brushing, and rinsing. This favors the build up of plaque and calculus in that area.

Dental extractions without replacement often result in the drifting mesially, dis-

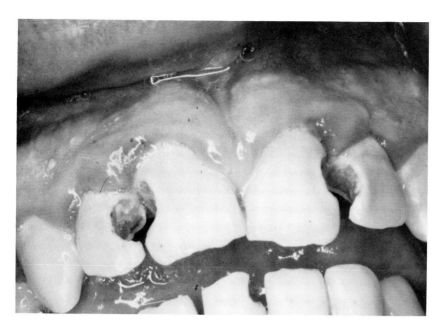

Figure 5–5. Caries and Periodontal Disease. The loss of interproximal contacts due to carious lesions has resulted in an exaggeration of gingivitis between the central and lateral incisors.

tally, or occlusally of the adjacent or opposing teeth. This results in the tilting of teeth, the opening up of interdental contacts, and the development of discrepancies in the level of adjacent marginal ridges. All of these create situations which may lead to food impaction and retention and frequently make oral physiotherapy procedures more difficult. The loss of teeth on one side of the mouth may influence the patient to perform most of the masticatory activity on the more efficient side. This can lead to an increasing formation of plaque on the unused side.

Patients who need orthodontic treatment frequently have teeth so malaligned as to favor foot retention and to interfere with adequate oral hygiene.

NONPHYSIOLOGIC DENTAL TREATMENT. Overhanging gingival margins of dental restorations are encountered too frequently. These are usually produced by the lack of or incorrect use of matrix bands when amalgam restorations are placed (Fig. 5–6). If an explorer tine is run under the overhang, a white material consisting

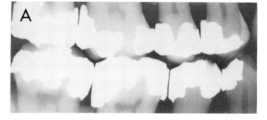

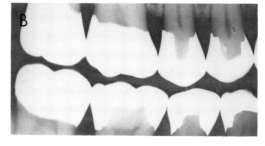

Figure 5–6. Replacement of Nonphysiologic Restorations. A, Restorations with gingival overhanging margins, improper contours, and faulty and open interdental contacts. B, Same teeth with physiologic restorations. (Courtesy Dr. W.D. Strickland, UNC School of Dentistry.)

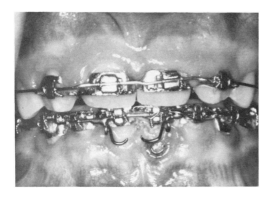

Figure 5–7. Hyperplastic Gingivitis. Enlargement of the gingivae resulting from chronic irritation due to orthodontic appliances and inadequate oral physiotherapy.

almost entirely of microorganisms adheres to the instrument. While the overhanging restorative material may produce mechanical injury to the crevicular tissues, it is most likely that the retention of bacterial plaque in this area is more significant in the incitement of gingival inflammation. This form of irritation is located where it can do the greatest amount of injury, that is, close to the epithelial attachment. In a controlled study, interproximal bone loss was greater around teeth with overhangs (Jeffcoat, 1980.)

Open or weak contacts, marginal ridge discrepancies, or nonphysiologic contours of restorations may lead to food impaction and food retention. These are problems which can usually be corrected only by replacement of the restoration. It is important, however, that the hygienist recognize the source of these problems and not expect scaling and home care procedure alone to correct the periodontal pathologic condition which may be present.

The clasping action of conventional partial dentures may create excessive forces on the abutment teeth, resulting in looseness of the teeth. This may exaggerate the rate of loss of supporting bone around the teeth, especially in the presence of periodontal disease. The mobility of the tooth may lead to food impaction and sensitivity.

Fixed bridge pontics often create situations favoring food retention and demanding special oral physiotherapy procedures. This is especially true in situations where the pontics have not been contoured to deflect food or in situations where there has been encroachment of the interdental area because the pontics are too bulky.

Orthodontic appliances are notorious in producing conditions which interfere with adequate oral hygiene. The complex of bands, brackets, and wires greatly enhances the accumulation of food debris and bacterial plaque. They interfere with brushing and gingival massage. The bands themselves, which usually extend subgingivally, may provide mechanical irritation to the crevicular tissues. The reaction in many young patients to the irritation is one of hyperplasia of the gingival tissues (Fig. 5–7). This overgrowth of tissue results in an increase in depth of the gingival crevice and a thickening of the marginal gingiva. These gingival changes increase the difficulty of maintaining good oral physiotherapy. The practice of directly attaching brackets to teeth, thus eliminating the bands, has made the orthodontic appliance somewhat more hygienic.

Factors in Common of Most Local Irritating Factors

The local factors previously discussed are those most frequently encountered clinically and those most significant in the etiology of periodontal disease. These factors have several commonalities that may be considered. They all promote the accumulation or overgrowth locally of oral microorganisms. They all interfere with oral hygiene or are the result of inadequate oral physiotherapy. Many of them provide at least some degree of mechanical irritation. These irritants are present continuously or recur at frequent intervals. The resistance of the periodontal tissues to injury is high, but the chronic nature of these irritating agents eventually results in pathologic changes.

Disease occurs at the cellular and subcellular levels. All of the local factors create a situation which permits chemical irritants to exist in concentrations sufficient to damage the cells and to interfere with the functions of cells. These cellular alterations in the gingival tissues when extensive enough and severe enough are seen clinically as periodontal disease.

Role of Dental Occlusion in the Etiology of Periodontal Disease

In the broadest sense, dental occlusion is the relationship of the mandibular teeth to the maxillary teeth in all the various positions and movements of the mandible. The physiology of mandibular positions and movements is highly complex and is ultimately controlled by the central nervous system through the nerves and muscles that are responsible for mandibular activity.

The stomatognathic system normally contributes to the performance of the functions of mastication, deglutition, and speech. The role of the opposing dental arches in these activities is referred to as functional dental occlusion. When the teeth are brought into contact to perform such activities as habitual grinding (bruxism) or clenching or to perform tasks which are not part of their normal function, it is referred to as dysfunctional dental occlusion.

If damage occurs to the periodontal tissues as a result of functional or dysfunctional occlusion, the injury is termed occlusal trauma (traumatic occlusion). A diagnosis of occlusal trauma can be made only if an injury to the periodontium related to the occlusion can be demonstrated. Unlike the injury of gingivitis or periodontitis, which begins in the gingival tissue, the lesion of occlusal trauma begins in the periodontal ligament and involves the cementum and alveolar bone. Clinically, mobility of teeth, sensitivity to pressure, migration of teeth, and an increased or uneven width of the periodontal ligament

space as seen on the radiograph (Fig. 5–8) are the most important indications of occlusal trauma.

It is generally believed that occlusal trauma is not a primary factor in the etiology of periodontal disease. That is to say, local irritants must be present to cause inflammation and pocket formation. Clinically, occlusal trauma appears to promote or aggravate the existing periodontal tissue destruction. In many cases it is dysfunctional rather than functional occlusal patterns which are significant in the etiology of periodontal disease.

The forces of occlusion which are applied to the teeth are utimately absorbed by the periodontal ligament and attached bone. Occlusion may complicate the periodontal problem by either placing excessive forces on the periodontium or by resulting in an insufficient amount of stimulation to the supporting structures of the teeth.

There are several possibilities by which too much pressure may be applied to the periodontium. If two opposing teeth contact prior to the full meeting of all the teeth on closing, excessive stress may be placed on the periodontium of those two teeth. Such teeth are said to be in premature contact. Likewise, if only one or a few teeth in each arch are contacting in the various sliding movements of the mandible, they will carry a disproportionate amount of occlusal force. If opposing teeth on the nonfunctioning side are contacting more forcefully than teeth on the functioning side, the nonfunctioning teeth will carry an excessive amount of force. All of these situations are accentuated if the occlusal contacts occur on incline planes rather than on flat surfaces.

If heavy occlusal forces are placed on the teeth, it is desirable that they be applied in a vertical direction so that the maximum number of periodontal fibers are utilized for dispensation of the force over a wide area of supporting bone. The dispensation of a force applied to the tooth in a vertical direction is illustrated in Figure 5–9A. Fig-

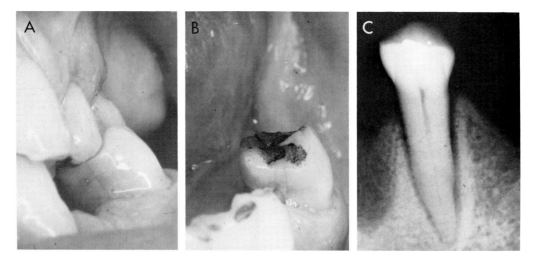

Figure 5–8. Occlusal Trauma.   A, Occlusal relationship of mandibular premolar. The tooth is in a crossbite relationship and is unsupported since both adjacent teeth are missing. B, The articulating paper markings on the occlusal surface indicate the excessive amount of occlusal contact. C, Radiograph showing increased width of periodontal space and lamina dura. Since there is no periodontitis or pocket formation, this is primary occlusal trauma.

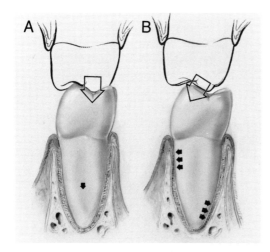

Figure 5–9.   Influence of Direction of Occlusal Forces on Periodontal Ligament.   Large arrows indicate the direction of the occlusal force. A, Favorable situation. The force is parallel to the long axis of the tooth. Most periodontal fibers are active in resisting the applied force. B, Unfavorable situation. The force is applied at an angle to the long axis. The fibers indicated by the small arrows are crushed due to the displacement of the tooth in the alveolus and therefore do not help support it.

ure 5–9B shows the unfavorable distribution of stress when the force is applied to an incline plane of the tooth. Notice the amount of periodontal ligament utilized in each situation.

Another manner by which excessive force may be placed on the periodontium is by too frequent contact on the teeth. It is doubtful that normal functional use of the teeth alone would ever result in this type of abuse if the teeth have adequate periodontal support. However, dysfunctional habits such as bruxism and clenching or chewing on pipe stems or pencils may result in damage to the periodontium. This same problem may develop in beauticians who open hair pins with their teeth, tailors who bite thread with their teeth, or carpenters who hold tacks between their teeth. While these or other occupational or avocational habits may not be significant in the population in general, they may be extremely important in the overall dental treatment of any one patient.

The significance of occlusal trauma in the prognosis of a patient's periodontal condition increases considerably as the degree of periodontal destruction increases. When there is a normal level of alveolar bone and periodontal ligament supporting a tooth, excessive force may be absorbed without any appreciable damage resulting. When, however, periodontal support has been lost, the remaining periodontium may no longer be able to withstand the excessive force. A tooth may lose so much support from periodontitis that even normal use may result in injury to the periodontium. Such a condition is called secondary occlusal trauma.

Poorly fitting or improperly designed partial dentures may produce unfavorable stresses which result in the production of occlusal trauma of the abutment teeth. Dental restoration left heavy in occlusion may result in damage to the attachment apparatus of the involved or opposing teeth.

Insufficient function of the teeth and periodontium may create a situation that is not conducive to the maintenance of health. The gingiva, periodontal ligament, and alveolar bone maintain an optimal degree of structural design and density when they receive a proper amount of stimulation. The alveolar bone atrophies around teeth that are not in function because the opposing teeth have been extracted and not replaced. The principal fiber groups of the periodontal ligament become poorly arranged and begin to disappear. The gingivae lose part of the normal texture, tone, and keratinization.

Frequently patients stop eating on the side where teeth have been extracted. In addition to the decrease in masticatory stimulation to the periodontium, plaque begins to form on the teeth. This is because part of the cleansing mechanism provided for the passage of food over the surfaces of the teeth is lost. Other situations such as dental sensitivity from caries, a faulty restoration, or occlusal trauma may result in unilateral mastication. The formation of plaque and calculus on the side not used

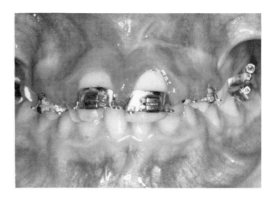

Figure 5–10. Mouth Breathing. Gingival changes of redness, swelling, and loss of stippling in the maxillary area. The malocclusion, especially in the anterior area, predisposes the patient to this condition.

for mastication leads to gingivitis and periodontitis.

Mouth Breathing

Because of difficulty in nasal breathing due to nasal obstruction, abnormal nasal development, enlarged adenoids, or malocclusion, some patients perform a large portion of inspiration through the oral cavity. In such individuals, mouth breathing may be a complicating factor in the etiology of their periodontal problems.

The mechanism by which mouth breathing irritates the gingivae is not known. It may be that excessive drying or the continuous wetting and drying of the tissue results in an alteration of the metabolism of the cells. It is the area of the gingiva which is exposed to the air that is affected. These areas are usually the labial and palatal gingivae of the maxillary anterior region. The response of the gingival tissue to mouth breathing is one of hyperplastic gingivitis (Fig. 5–10). The involved gingivae are increased in bulk, are usually red in color, and frequently demonstrate an increased bleeding tendency.

Having the patient cover the area with a lubricating agent such as petroleum jelly before retiring usually helps the condition. Of course, correction of the basic cause of the mouth breathing is the ideal treatment.

SYSTEMIC FACTORS

All parts of the body are interrelated anatomically and functionally. Any generalized disease, nutritional deficiency, endocrine dysfunction, or physiologic disorder could affect the development or metabolism of cells anywhere in the organism. The general resistance of the organism to any etiologic agent is influenced by general body health as well as by local health and integrity of tissues.

While it must be assumed that general health affects a patient's resistance to the development of periodontal disease, no specific systemic disease has been shown to produce gingival inflammation or periodontal pocket formation in the absence of local irritating factors. Periodontal disease can be successfully treated in patients with various generalized disease states. On the other hand, no specific system disease is cured by the treatment of periodontal disease. Periodontal disease is treated to preserve the teeth and their supporting structures in health, function, and comfort, not to cure other medical problems which the patient may have. However, through better digestion and nutrition, a patient's general health may be improved. This is beneficial, but admittedly, an indirect result of periodontal therapy. General body health may be improved by the elimination of any area of infection or inflammation, including those of the teeth and periodontium.

There are certain systemic factors which may modify a patient's response to local irritation. It is within the framework of this general concept of the modification of response that systemic factors are discussed in this chapter. Occasionally patients are seen clinically with advanced periodontal bone loss and little in the way of quantitative local irrational factors. It is in such patients that systemic factors have been suspected as being significant in the etiology of their periodontal condition. However, no specific factor has been identified

in these patients to explain the cause of the periodontal disease.

Age and Sex

Epidemiologically, it has been shown that the prevalence and severity of periodontal disease increase with age. Most investigators agree that the majority of children examined have some degree of gingivitis. Periodontitis generally appears first during the third decade of life. The percentage of people with periodontitis and the degree of periodontal involvement increase in the middle and older age groups. This would be expected since obviously the older age groups have been exposed to local irritants for a longer period of time than the younger groups. As has been mentioned previously, necrotizing ulcerative gingivitis occurs almost entirely in the 18 to 30 year age group.

Periodontal disease has a somewhat higher incidence in the male than in the female, probably due to better oral hygiene practices of the female. Juvenile periodontitis, however, is reported to be more frequent in the young female.

Hormonal Status

Gingivitis and periodontitis have been noticed clinically to be more severe in some patients during periods of hormonal change or imbalance. In the prepubertal, pregnant, and postmenopausal patients an exaggerated inflammatory response to local irritation may be evident. Teeth may become more mobile during pregnancy. Hormonal status in general does have an influence on the inflammatory response. Patients need adequate periodontal care by the hygienist and meticulous home care during these periods of life.

Diabetes mellitus is a chronic disease of carbohydrate metabolism initiated by a disturbance in the action of insulin. Insulin is a hormone produced by certain cells in the pancreas. The patient with uncontrolled diabetes is more susceptible to infection than the nondiabetic patient. These people develop periodontal abscesses and "dry-sockets" following dental extractions more readily than most other patients. Periodontal surgical wounds usually heal at a slow rate. It is more difficult to maintain gingival health in these patients, assumably because of the generalized lower tissue tolerance to irritation. The juvenile diabetic is more likely to have a complicated periodontal problem than the individual who develops diabetes mellitus late in life.

Corticosteroid derivatives are used in the treatment of a wide range of systemic diseases including rheumatoid arthritis, allergy, and pemphigus. These hormones depress the natural defensive mechanisms including inflammation. The depression of the inflammatory response may have a deleterious effect on the progress of periodontal disease. Any stressful situation especially of a chronic nature may result in an alteration of the production of corticosteroids from the adrenal glands. Some of these hormones promote inflammation and some are antagonistic to it. Rather dramatic changes in the periodontal tissues have been produced in experimental animals which were placed under stressful situations which affect the normal production of corticosteroids.

Nutritional Status

Nutritional deficiencies result in disease because the organism is deprived of elements which are essential for optimal health. As with other systemic diseases all body cells may be adversely affected by the deficiency of an essential nutrient. The cells of the periodontium are no exception. However, nutritional deficiencies alone are not known to cause periodontal disease.

Most of the investigations have been done by inducing a deprivation state of a single or a group of related nutrients in laboratory animals. In general there is decreased formation of periodontal ligament and decreased osteoblastic and cementoblastic activity in these animals. These changes are more severe in young animals

than in mature animals. It is most unusual to see a patient whose diet is totally lacking in a single or group of related nutrients (deprivation state). Hence, one cannot directly apply the information gained from these experimental laboratory studies to clinical situations.

Vitamin deficiencies are probably given more significance in the etiology of periodontal disease from a clinical standpoint than the other nutritional substances. Vitamins are essential for life and their importance in health should not be underestimated. Their role in the etiology of peridontal disease may be overemphasized in some dental practices.

It was reported centuries ago that sailors with scurvy developed serious periodontal problems with bleeding gums and loosening and exfoliation of the teeth. Ascorbic acid (vitamin C) plays an important role in the normal functions of fibroblasts, osteoblasts, and odontoblasts. Wound healing is greatly reduced in animals with scurvy. However, it has been shown that monkeys with scurvy did not develop periodontal pockets if good oral hygiene was carried out (Waerhaug, 1958). Likewise, it has been shown clinically that good oral hygiene counteracted the harmful results of scurvy on the periodontium of the human (Crandon, Lund, and Dill, 1940).

Following World War II an unusual gingival disorder named *gingivosis* was described in a group of Italian children (Schour and Massler, 1947). It was suspected that poor dietary regimen necessitated by wartime conditions may have caused this disease. Because of the response of the children to vitamin therapy, it was concluded that the primary etiology of this disease was probably a deficiency of the B-complex vitamins.

For the majority of periodontal patients it is unlikely that vitamin deficiencies are significant in the etiology of periodontal disease. There is no rationale to justify specific or multivitamin therapy for the treatment of periodontal disease unless a vitamin deficiency state is present. In such a case, the patient should be under the care of a qualified health professional.

Protein is extremely necessary in the nutritional requirements of man. Cells must receive all of the essential amino acids in order to reproduce themselves and to replenish the body stores of worn out and used up biochemicals. Much periodontal tissue is synthesized and maintained from protein. Protein synthesis by defense cells is essential in order to maintain their functions. Antibodies which are important in the body defense mechanism are protein in nature.

Experimental animals on protein deprivation diets demonstrate degeneration of connective tissue including that of the periodontal tissues. There is diminished alveolar bone and cementum formation. Several investigations have shown that periodontal disease develops more severely in protein-deprived animals when local irritating agents are present.

Carbohydrates may directly or indirectly play a role in the etiology of periodontal disease. Directly they may aid in the production of bacterial plaque since they are readily retained around the teeth. Carbohydrates may serve as a nutritional source for microorganisms and favor their overgrowth. Refined carbohydrates promote the development of dental caries in many individuals. The significance of caries in the etiology of periodontal disease has already been discussed.

There are several other considerations concerning the diet which are important in the overall dental problem of some patients. The physical nature of the food is important in terms of the degree of stimulation which the periodontal tissues receive while chewing. Rather tough or coarse food massages the gingivae and provides functional stimulation to the attachment apparatus of the tooth. Food of this texture may help to clean plaque off the tooth.

Patients who have habits of eating be-

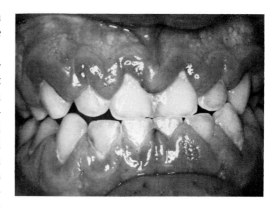

Figure 5–11. Gingival Changes Associated with Leukemia. Enlargement of gingivae due to infiltration of immature leukocytes, hyperplasia, and swelling. Petechial hemorrhage present in gingivae and lips.

tween meals present problems in that they have difficulty in maintaining good oral hygiene. While these patients may brush following regular meals, they are unlikely to do so following snacks. Some children, college students, bachelors, nonmarried women, and elderly individuals are more likely to have poor dietary habits than other patients. The dental health team should be instrumental in encouraging these and other patients to follow a sound dietary regimen.

Blood Diseases

Any pathologic change of the blood or blood-forming tissues may result in alterations of the blood vascular system of the gingiva.

The primary clinical manifestation of acute leukemia, especially the monocytic type, may be presented in the gingivae. The gingivae are ulcerated, necrotic, and hyperplastic (Fig. 5–11). There may be spontaneus bleeding. There is also an increased bleeding tendency of the gingivae in polycythemia, thrombocytopenia, and hemophilia. There may be a necrotizing and ulcerative type of gingivitis in patients with agranulocytosis.

Anemia may result in pallor of the gingivae and oral mucous membranes. In polycythemia the oral mucous membranes have a deep red color.

While some of the oral manifestations of blood diseases reflect changes similar to those occurring in periodontal disease, they do not in themselves cause periodontal disease. Their significance lies in the area of diagnosis of the patient's systemic problem. If any of these conditions is suspected in a patient, the hygienist should confer with the dentist immediately.

Drugs

Many irritating chemical agents such as silver nitrate or phenol may result in ulceration of the gingival tissue if contact is made. Occasionally a patient will place an aspirin tablet next to a painful tooth in the unrewarding hope that it will alleviate the pain. Such practices frequently result in the development of an "aspirin burn" on the gingiva or buccal mucosa.

Ingestion of or exposure to sufficient quantities of certain heavy metals such as bismuth, lead, or mercury results in the formation of a dark line of pigmentation in the marginal gingiva. Implanted fragments of silver amalgam also cause localized gingival pigmentation.

Diphenylhydantoin sodium (Dilantin Sodium) is an anticonvulsant drug used in the treatment of epilepsy. Almost one-half of the patients taking this medication develop gingival hyperplasia. The gingival enlargement is due to a hyperplastic reaction of the connective tissue, apparently to the drug itself. In many of these patients the gingival tissues enlarge to the extent of covering a large portion of the crowns of the teeth. However, good oral hygiene suppresses the extent to which the hyperplasia develops in many patients.

It has been reported that cyclosporine, an immunosuppressive agent, may produce the side effect of gingival hyperplasia and transient perioral hyperaesthesia.

Heredity

Little is known about the influence of heredity on the predisposition of a patient to develop periodontal disease. The prevalence of gingivitis and periodontitis is so high that it is not unusual for several members of the same family to have these problems.

Hereditary gingival fibromatosis, as the name implies, is considered to be hereditary or familial in nature. There is progressive enlargement of the gingival tissues that may become extensive due to hyperplasia of the connective tissue. A positive history must be made and other conditions such as diphenylhydantoin sodium gingival hyperplasia ruled out in order to make a diagnosis.

Unusual Periodontal Diseases

The early periodontal literature described a disease entity referred to as *periodontosis*. This was reported to occur in the young to middle-age groups, more frequently in females. Clinically, few local factors were observed, so it was surmised that the etiology was primarily systemic. Numerous studies have been conducted in attempts to identify the specific etiologic factors. Nothing of a definitive nature was uncovered.

More recently it has been agreed that the condition occurs most frequently in young people, so it has been termed *juvenile periodontitis*. It has been reported to have a genetic background and sometimes is associated with Papillon-Lefèvre syndrome, cyclic and noncyclic neutropenia, acrodynia, mongolism, and scleroderma. Microbiologic investigations have shown a sparse, gram-negative anaerobic flora associated with juvenile periodontitis. The etiology and pathologic nature of this disease or group of diseases are still obscure.

Hypophosphatasia is another rare disease which affects the periodontal tissues. Among other abnormal findings there is decreased formation of the cementum of the primary teeth. Associated with this is premature exfoliation of the involved teeth.

SUMMARY

The etiology of periodontal disease is usually complex in nature for any patient with this problem. The typical patient demonstrates a combination of bacterial plaque, calcareous deposits, inadequate oral physiotherapy, and at least mildly malaligned teeth. Many patients have a history of inadequate or nonphysiologic dental care. Occlusal disharmonies or occlusal habits are secondary factors in the etiology of periodontal disease for many patients. Systemic disease or abnormalities may modify the patient's response to the local irritating factors. Certain specific systemic diseases may necessitate an alteration in the treatment plan for that patient.

The defects which occur in the periodontal tissues as a result of periodontal disease tend to promote the progression of the disease. Inflamed and sensitive gingivae make oral physiotherapy procedures more uncomfortable and more difficult for the patient. Pocket formation allows debris, plaque, and calculus to accumulate at varying depths under the gingiva where they can do the most damage. If gingival recession occurs, the exposed tooth structure may be sensitive and thus interfere with good oral hygiene. The destruction of periodontal ligament and alveolar bone results in mobility and migration of teeth. These lead to food impaction and occlusal trauma.

Periodontal disease is progressive if left untreated. Eventually the teeth are exfoliated or have to be removed because of inadequate support to allow them to perform their normal functions.

BIBLIOGRAPHY

Crandon, J.H., Lund, C.C., and Dill, D.B.: Experimental human scurvy, N. Engl. J. Med., 223:353, 1940.

Daley, T.D., and Wysocki, G.P.: Cyclosporine therapy. J. Periodontol., 55:708, 1984.

Jeffcoat, M.K., and Howey, T.H.: Alveolar bone destruction due to overhanging amalgam in periodontal disease, J. Periodontol., 51:599, 1980.

Reid, J.S., Beeley, J.A., and MacDonald, D.G.: Investigations into black extrinsic tooth stain, J. Dent. Res., 56:895, 1977.

Schour, I., and Massler, M.: Gingival disease in post-war Italy. II. Gingivosis in hospitalized children in Naples, Am. J. Orthodont. Oral Surg., 33:756, 1947.

Tal, H.: Relationship between the interproximal distance of roots and the prevalence of intrabony pockets, J. Periodontol., 55:604, 1984.

Waerhaug, J.: Effect of C-avitaminosis on the supporting structures of the teeth, J. Periodontol., 29:87, 1958.

Wentz, F.M.: Oral manifestation of the blood diseases, J. Am. Dent. Assoc., 44:693, 1952.

CLINICAL DETERMINATIONS

Acquisition of essential baseline information provides the surest method of ensuring that a correct diagnosis is made and appropriate treatment plans are developed. No physician would practice medicine without obtaining such information nor do modern dentists. All subsequent evaluations of health are dependent upon this basic knowledge. Although the dental hygienist is not expected or permitted by law to make diagnoses, nothing prohibits the observation, documentation, and consideration of clinical findings. While these determinants are most commonly made by the dentist, the long-term documentation of the patient's status often is the responsibility of the hygienist. Information that is incomplete or inaccurate or is not recorded is useless and may result in incorrect diagnoses or treatments.

HISTORIES AND RECORDS

A patient's record includes all findings, such as personal data, medical and dental histories, radiographs, diagnoses, and treatment plans. Special forms for recording clinical findings, such as a periodontal chart or dental chart, are integral parts of the patient record. Financial estimates and arrangements and insurance forms are also often included as well. Choice of the form of the patient record depends upon the dentist's own personal preference. Suggestions are offered in this chapter for records that are as complete as possible to guarantee the patient the best health care.

Patient Interview

The initial contact and interview with the patient are usually made by the dentist; however, the hygienist may be charged with this by the dentist. Regardless of the specific procedure employed, the patient should be approached in an unhurried, professional manner in order to allay apprehension and instill confidence. Initial information regarding vital statistics is most commonly obtained by the receptionist. Such information includes the patient's name, address, residence and business telephone numbers, and social security number. Age, including date of birth, sex, race, occupation, and marital status all may be of value to the dentist in the diagnosis and prognosis of the patient's periodontal condition. A sequence of procedures for securing the histories and performing the examination is presented in Table 6–1.

Establishing the availability of a patient

for appointments means conservation of time in setting up future appointments. When active therapy is complete, patient availability must be reestablished for recall maintenance appointments. Patients who are readily available can, for example, be contacted to fill cancelled appointments. This may prevent loss of valuable chair time for the hygienist or dentist.

If a patient is referred, the referring individual's name should be entered into the record indicating whether the referrer is a dentist, physician, friend, relative or another patient. Such referrals should be acknowledged by the dentist. This is an important practice builder since the referring individual appreciates a thank-you note from the dentist, or in the case of a referring professional, a summary of the dentist's findings. In the instance of patient referral from another patient, it is appropriate for the dentist or hygienist to inquire, "May we thank Mrs. Wright for sending you to our office? She is one of our favorite patients."

Time spent on the interview process is time extremely well spent. Communication in the dental office gives a perspective of the patient's desires and expectations. Patients should be encouraged to ask questions and express any fears or misconceptions concerning dental care. During the interview process the hygienist can assess the patient's interests, hobbies, and life style. The value placed on oral health by the patient is extremely important. The interview also provides the health provider an opportunity to express the office philosophy of preventive care. Any unfavorable reaction by the patient toward dental care or to a former dentist is extremely important information for the dentist. Under no circumstances should specific details or names of previous dental care providers with whom the patient is hostile be solicited or recorded. The dentist makes the decisions as to what should be entered in the record regarding this point. If suspicion, mistrust, or hostility seems to pervade the patient's reaction to questions, the dentist should be informed by word of mouth privately, when an appropriate opportunity arises, following termination of the interview. The hygienist may blunt such an approach by saying, "I am sure that Dr. Simpson will want you to tell him about your problem. You will find he is a good listener and very professional."

Fortunately, the interview process seldom is unpleasant, and the hygienist should strive to make it as comfortable and as useful as possible. In the modern dental practice all health professionals are dedicated to the patient's improved health and all should transmit this positive, caring attitude to all patients.

Medical History

The hygienist should be aware of the possible reluctance of some patients to answer questions as personal as those associated with a medical history, however brief they may be. Some patients do not understand that such medical information may be as essential to dental care as it is to medical care. When the patient understands that this information is for her or his own protection and general health, any reluctance or timidity usually subsides.

Many offices provide new patients with a medical questionnaire (Table 6–2; p. 103) to fill out prior to being seen in the dental operatory for interview and examination. The value of this type of history taking is limited since patients may not always understand the questions or the terminology. The hygienist should review the answers on the questionnaire with the patient to be certain the questions were understood. If the patient is unsure about a medical problem, this should be noted and brought to the dentist's attention for further evaluation. Such medical conditions may require contact with the patient's physician for clarification and advice.

The reasons for acquisition of a careful medical history are two-fold. First is, of course, the protection of the patient. The second reason is for the protection of the dental health providers. Certain medical conditions may modify patient management, particularly with regard to periodontal treatment, office asepsis, and use of medications. For example, a patient with a history of rheumatic heart disease must be covered by suitable antibiotic therapy before scaling and root planing in order to be protected from the possibility of bacterial endocarditis that may be initiated by the transient streptococcal bacteremia resulting from these periodontal procedures. Histories of drug allergies, diabetes mellitus, epilepsy, high blood pressure, bleeding disorders, or liver disease are examples of conditions which might modify periodontal therapy.

It has become increasingly important for health providers to protect themselves from medical conditions that patients might bring to the office environment. This may be as innocuous as the common cold or as potentially dangerous to office personnel as hepatitis. Other conditions that should alert the hygienist are tuberculosis, narcotic addiction, venereal diseases, AIDS, or history of mental illness. The dentist will be able to make necessary consultations, suggest protective measures for office personnel and for security, and establish proper asepsis depending upon the nature of the medical condition.

During the acquisition of the medical history and during the interview process, an appraisal is made of the physical status of the patient's posture, gait, facial symmetry, and any lesions or enlargements of the neck, face, or head. Any skin lesion of the face, neck, or scalp may also be observed by the hygienist. Any abnormality should be noted on the patient's record under the medical history section. Such observations, as well as physical limitations of movement, may be of particular value in older patients since this might warrant further follow-up on the part of the dentist.

Blood Pressure

Since hypertension (high blood pressure) is so prevalent and is one of the major causes of stroke, and of kidney and heart disease, arterial blood pressure should be measured and recorded (Fig. 6–1). Hypertension may be insidious, and many patients do not know they are afflicted because symptoms may be absent or unrecognizable by the patient. Patients may visit the dental office more frequently than they visit their physician, and blood pressure determination in the dental office provides a valuable health service.

An inflatable cuff, a manometer for registering pressure in millimeters, and a stethoscope are needed to measure the blood pressure. Auscultation (listening for change in sound or absence of sound) is used to determine blood pressure. After the cuff is placed on the patient's upper arm, the stethoscope is placed on the lower arm near the antecubital fossa. The cuff is inflated until no sound is heard, and then air is slowly released until the first sound is heard (systolic—pumping phase of heart beat). As air is further released from the cuff, a muffled sound just before its disappearance is heard (diastolic—pressure

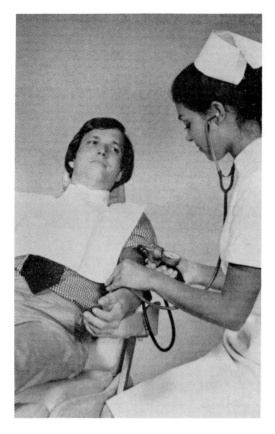

Figure 6–1. Hygienist Taking Patient's Blood Pressure.

when the heart is at rest). Systolic blood pressure is recorded first and diastolic pressure recorded beneath it with a line drawn between: 118/75 would indicate a systolic reading of 118 and a diastolic reading of 75 and would be in the normal range.

A patient with elevated blood pressure, especially elevation of diastolic pressure above 90 on repeated examinations, probably should be referred for medical consultations. In some cases, there may be transient elevations of both systolic and diastolic pressures because of patient anxiety or tension during the first appointment with the dentist and hygienist. Physical exertion, such as climbing stairs to the office, can also result in a transient elevation of blood pressure. The hygienist should simply record blood pressure findings in the

chart. She should not attempt to interpret findings or discuss them with the patient. Elevations should be called to the attention of the dentist.

In patients with a known history of hypertension, even though under control with medication, it is wise to take the blood pressure before starting any dental procedure. During stressful procedures such as surgery, these patients should be monitored periodically, and for a while after termination of surgery until they can be safely dismissed from the office.

A patient's pulse rate is another valuable method of monitoring the regularity of cardiac contraction and should be obtained at the initial visit. The pulse rate can be calculated by finger palpation of contractions of the radial artery just above and on the ventral side of the wrist. The numbers of pulsations per minute can be determined by counting them during the interval of a minute timed by a stop watch, pocket watch, or wrist watch. Seventy to 80 pulse rate per minute is within the normal range. It is slightly higher in women than men. The pulse rate should be entered in the patient's record. The doctor should be alerted to extremely rapid or extremely slow pulse rates.

Body Temperature

Body temperature determined with an oral clinical thermometer may be needed if oral infection of an acute nature is present or suspected or if the patient complains of a fever or sore throat. It is not necessary to routinely take and record the oral temperature. The thermometer should be shaken down until the column of mercury is well below the normal point (98.6°F). It is then placed with the mercury bulb beneath the patient's tongue and the middle of the thermometer sealed by the patient's lips. The patient is cautioned not to bite down because of possible fracture of the glass tube that encases the mercury. After 3 minutes, the thermometer is removed, read, and body temperature recorded in the patient's chart for the dentist's evaluation.

Dental History

The dental history portion of the interview is best performed in the dental operatory with the patient comfortably seated in the dental chair. Initially, the reason prompting the patient to seek dental care should be determined because this chief complaint, if any, should receive the first attention of the dentist. A simple question, "Do you have a specific reason for wanting dental care now?" will provide the opportunity for patient response. If the problem is of an emergency nature, the time of onset, nature, duration, and severity of the chief complaint should be obtained and entered in the patient record and the dentist notified.

Most often the response is that the patient wishes regular dental care, but valuable information can be gained from the answer to this question. Patients may say, "I don't like the way my teeth look," or "my teeth are loose," or "my gums bleed when I brush." Such responses clearly indicate those areas in which the patient is primarily concerned, and may provide cues for further dental examination. Responses should be recorded in the patient record under the chief complaint section.

A short dental history provides assessment of the patient's appreciation of dental health, frequency of dental visits, and oral hygiene habits. Some key questions are listed here.

"1. How often have you gone for recall appointments to your dentist in the past?
2. When were your teeth last scaled and polished?
3. Have you ever had any oral infections or gum abscesses?
4. Have you ever had periodontal surgery?
5. Have you ever had a bad reaction to a local anesthetic?
6. Have you ever had prolonged bleeding after gum treatment?
7. Have you ever had a bad reaction to any medication?
8. When was the last time dental radiographs were taken of your teeth?
9. Are you aware of any oral habit?
10. How often do you brush your teeth?
11. Do you use any particular method in brushing your teeth?
12. Have you ever received instruction in toothbrushing methods?
13. Do you use any dental aids such as dental floss or toothpicks?
14. What do you think your major dental needs are at this time?"

Answers to these questions may be helpful to the dentist in diagnosis, treatment planning, and patient management. The patient, for example, who has gone to the dentist in the past only for emergency treatment may require more dental health education in order to be motivated to accept a total oral health treatment program. Affirmative answers to a history of gum abscesses or periodontal treatment may indicate recurrent periodontal disease. A negative answer to a question on oral habits does not rule out the presence of such habits, but does indicate lack of patient awareness.

The response to questions relating to oral hygiene practices reflect the patient's interest in oral health maintenance but not necessarily the effectiveness of such activity. Such questions do provide a starting point for further discussion and instruction in oral hygiene. Suggestions on increasing interest and motivational methodology are presented in Chapter 8. Summary findings of both medical and dental histories should be entered in the patient record as baseline information for the dentist's evaluation (Fig. 6–2).

Documentation

Emphasis has been placed in this chapter on the recording of findings, and there are valid reasons for this type of documenta-

Patient _John Drake_	Age _52_	Sex _M_	Chart No. _0715_
Dentist _Dr. James Royce_	Address _1108 Fairview Rd._		
Physician _Dr. Ray Martin_	Address _225 E. Broad Street_		

Chief Complaint: _"Gums bleed on brushing"_

Medical History Summary: _Mild diabetes, controlled by diet._
Allergic to penicillin

Dental History / Last Dental Rx: _Extraction #19_

Previously Periodontal Rx: _None. Teeth scaled once a year._

Oral Hygiene: Technic Used: _Bass roll_   No / Day _2_

Auxiliary Aids Used: _Electric toothbrush_

Oral Habits: _Smokes two packs of cigarettes a day_

Extraoral Exam: _Cold sore left corner of mouth_

Intraoral Exam: Soft Tissue

Gingiva: Inflammed		Edematous	✓	Suppuration	
Bleeds On Probing	✓	Abcesses		Hypertrophy	
Recession _facial #20, 21, 28, 29_					
Attached Gingiva: Adequate		Minimal	✓	None	
Frenal Attachments: _high on facial of #24, 25_					
Calculus:	None	Slight		Moderate ✓	Heavy
Plaque:	Slight	Moderate		Heavy ✓	Plaque Score

Figure 6–2. Summary Findings, Medical and Dental.

tion. The patient record represents the permanent history of the individual's experience in the dental office. It should reflect the medical and dental histories, chief complaint, initial oral findings, diagnoses, treatment plan, and record of therapy. In earlier times the dental record might have been less complex, but the expanded concern of the dental providers for the patient's health has dictated a more complete record than previously. Baseline information gained from the new patient establishes the level of health from which all future changes can be measured. As such, it serves as an essential method for monitoring health and prognosticating future health status.

Many dental records are now designed to be problem oriented. This concept, borrowed from medicine, focuses attention on the most significant dental needs. Appropriate sequencing of therapy is dictated by these needs and a priority order of treatment is established. Except in the case of emergencies or caries threatening the dental pulp, periodontal therapy most often should occupy the primary step in the treatment plan.

Another factor that has strongly influenced the use of more complete patient records is the increasing tendency of patients to seek legal redress of real or imagined grievances concerning dental treatment. The patient record is the written documentation of patient treatment and, together with timely obtained radiographs, establishes the dental provider's best defense in any dento-legal matters. Records should contain legible entries neatly written in ink. Notations entered in pencil are not legally acceptable since they can be erased and modified. Should the hygienist make an incorrect entry or misspell an entry, a single line simply is drawn through the incorrect word or phrase. All record entries should be signed by the provider performing the procedure. The importance of accuracy and neatness in writing in the record cannot be overemphasized!

PERIODONTAL EXAMINATION

Lining Mucosa

It should be recognized that while the main objective of this chapter, and the major interest of the hygienist, is a detailed evaluation of the supporting tissues, other areas of the mouth must also be examined. Under the rubric of total patient care, the modern dental care provider must be concerned with all factors that relate to patient health. Hygienists are primarily responsible for oral health and must examine all oral structures.

A strong tendency exists for all of us to overlook obvious lesions while attending the urgent. Thus, a dentist may give insufficient attention to the periodontium while examining the teeth for dental caries. Oral examination need not be excessively time consuming in order to be complete. Systemic appraisal of the lining mucosa will result in no area of the mouth being omitted.

Attention is initially directed toward examination of the patient's lips to note any deviation from normality. Then a survey is made of the entire oral cavity by retracting the lips and inspecting the mucous membrane of the cheek, vestibule, hard and soft palate, and the dorsal surface of the tongue. A gauze sponge is used to grasp and turn the tongue such that the floor of the mouth and ventral surface of the tongue may be examined. Any abnormality such as ulcers, abrasions, growths, or white patches should be noted. White areas should be lightly stroked with a gauze to ascertain that these areas are not just exfoliated epithelial cells or food debris. Growths should be noted in the record for the doctor's attention. Patients should not be unduly alarmed since many patients are cancerphobic. The hygienist should develop a regular routine for examination of lining mucosa always beginning on the right side, then the left side, the palate, tongue, and floor of the mouth.

Charting

Over the years, a wide variety of charts have been developed on which to record clinical findings including those designed for the storing of such information in computers. Many dentists found the comprehensive anatomic chart too detailed and time consuming. Nonanatomic charts with diagrams for noting caries but no provision for periodontal findings became the common standard in many dental practices. Another type of chart simply provided blank spaces in which to write in findings beside the tooth number.

Unfortunately, all of these methods resulted in an underestimation of periodontal disease. It is axiomatic that if findings are not recorded, they are not treated. One study found that of practitioners' charts almost 80% contained records of caries but only 17% contained records of periodontal pockets. The study concluded that "periodontal disease is not being treated because it is not being diagnosed." Another study of hygienists' practice patterns found that less than 50% of them recorded gingival findings on a chart. Although there have been some imaginative efforts to design a simplified method of periodontal examination, there is no substitute for use of an anatomic chart at initial examination. The anatomic chart provides the necessary detail and room to portray accurately and visually the status of the patient's condition at time of entry into the dental practice. A chart such as that illustrated in Figure 6–3 will lead the trained observer to avoid exclusion of any phase of periodontal and dental examination. Unquestionably, the orderly and precise registration of clinical information does require more time, but the value to the patient and the dentist is worth the effort. Few periodontists would treat patients without such a careful registration of oral conditions.

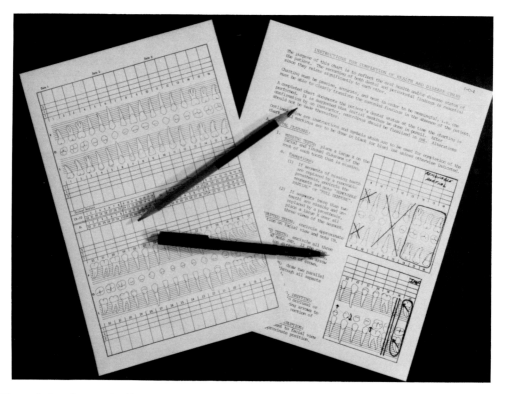

Figure 6–3.   Anatomic Chart with Instruction Sheet.

Missing Teeth

Counting the teeth is an important portion of the oral examination. Recording the missing teeth is an essential first step in the charting. A missing tooth is recorded by drawing an "X" through the tooth figure on the anatomic chart. When a tooth is missing with closure of space by adjacent teeth, this may indicate a possible imbedded tooth, which should be verified on radiographs. Missing teeth, if not replaced, may sometimes cause a disruption of the arch form, extrusion of an antagonistic tooth, and drifting and tipping of adjacent teeth (Fig. 6–4). Such alterations in arch form may result in marginal ridge discrepancies. If a missing tooth has been replaced by a bridge, this finding can be noted by a connecting line drawn between abutment teeth.

Removable dentures can be recorded in writing in the boxes adjacent to the missing

teeth that have been noted by the "X." A full denture is recorded by placing an "X" on all the missing teeth in the arch and writing full *denture* in large letters in the notation box on the appropriate arch.

Gingival Health

Periodontal and dental clinical examination require a dental mirror, a periodontal probe, a dental explorer, a compressed air syringe, saliva ejector, and gauzes. An anatomic chart with provisions for written comments and occlusal analysis should be used. Pens with black ink for recording findings and with red ink for marking areas of bleeding complete the essentials for the examination.

Following the inspection of the lining mucosa, an overall appraisal of the periodontium should be accomplished, noting the amount of attached keratinized gingiva on the facia and lingual aspects of the mandibular arch and facial of the maxilla.

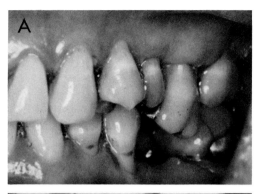

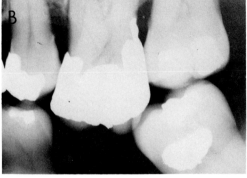

Figure 6–4. Collapse of Dental Arch. Extraction of the mandibular first molar and failure to replace it have resulted in drifting and tilting of the mandibular second molar and extrusion of the maxillary first molar. A, Clinical photograph. B, Corresponding radiograph.

Height of frenal attachments in relation to the masticatory mucosa should be observed by retracting lips and cheeks to provide tension. Sometimes a high frenal attachment exerts a significant pull on the gingival tissues. When this is coupled with a narrow band of attached gingiva, it may result in recession of soft tissue on a tooth or teeth (Fig. 6–5). Recession itself may reduce the amount of attached gingiva to a point where frenal attachments may accelerate the process. Such a condition should be indicated in the appropriate location on the anatomic chart by use of the suggested symbol at the bottom of the chart (Table 6–3).

On the anatomic chart the height and contour of the free gingiva should be drawn with a pen at its location on each tooth. The outline and contour of both the facial and lingual marginal and interproximal gingivae are entered on the chart. Generalized gingival recession may be recorded by drawing a line across the roots of the affected teeth corresponding to the height of the gingival margin. Horizontal lines are printed on the chart over the roots of the tooth figures at 2-mm intervals to aid in accurate gingival level placement. If recession is present on a single tooth, the line would correspond to the gingival contour exactly as seen clinically from either facial or lingual view of the particular tooth. Localized recession can be noted by a "V" shape outlined on the root. Such conditions, coupled with the designation of a frenal attachment, may indicate an area for special attention. If the gingivae are enlarged, the drawn configuration would be located on the crown portions of the teeth to the extent that the enlargement covers the crown.

An assessment of the gingivae includes a complete survey of papillary, marginal, and attached portions. Normal healthy gingiva is light pink except in dark-skinned individuals where melanin is present. Any deviation toward redness or bluish-magenta color should be noted, as these are signs of inflammatory change.

In health, the free or marginal gingiva ends in a thin edge and follows a scalloped appearance around the necks of the anterior teeth facially and lingually. The papillary gingiva ends in a peak and fills the interproximal space between contacts of the anterior teeth. In the posterior region the papillary gingiva fills the interproximal area with a slight depression (col) between facial and lingual peaks (see Chapter 2). With inflammatory change, the architecture of the gingiva is altered, and marginal and papillary gingivae may be rounded or blunted. Sometimes soft-tissue cratering occurs especially if calculus deposits are heavy interproximally or if necrosis of the papillae occurs due to acute inflammation.

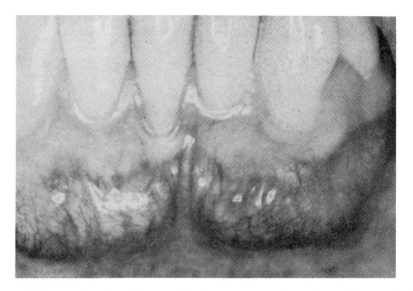

Figure 6–5. High Frenulum Attachment.   Tension on gingival attachment has resulted in recession on lower mandibular central incisor.

Such changes can be noted on the chart using appropriate symbols (Table 6–3).

Healthy gingiva is held snugly to the neck of the teeth and is not displaced by compressed air blown into the gingival crevice. After forceful displacement with a periodontal probe in the crevice, connective tissue resilience brings the gingiva back to its original tight adaptation to the tooth. With inflammation marginal gingival tissues lose this adaptive capacity and displacement of the tissue from the tooth occurs. A compressed air blast into the crevice may cause separation of the marginal gingiva from the tooth, and often reveals the presence of subgingival deposits of calculus. In the presence of severe inflammation even papillary gingiva may also be subject to displacment.

The surface texture of healthy attached gingiva is stippled. Absence of such stippling may persist with fibrosis in more chronic inflammation. Varying degrees of keratinization occur in normal gingiva, and absence of keratinization usually reflects abnormal or pathologic change.

Healthy gingival crevices do not bleed when lightly probed. Bleeding from the gingival crevice represent a parameter that can be relied upon to indicate bacteriologic and histopathologic changes associated with periodontal disease. Since the epithelium of the gingival crevice becomes ulcerated and blood vessels become dilated and engorged during inflammatory changes, one of the earliest clinical signs of a pathologic condition is the tendency of the gingiva to bleed. Bleeding is an earlier indicator of inflammation than redness or swelling of gingival tissues. Bleeding is an extremely objective sign. It is present or it is not. Methods of quantitating the extent of gingival bleeding, recording bleeding scores, and noting bleeding areas on the chart will be presented later in this chapter. Patients often recognize bleeding on brushing as one of the early signs of gingival trouble. Spontaneous bleeding, however, must be distinguished from bleeding brought on by brushing or probing since this sign may indicate a fault in the capillary walls due to systemic conditions or a problem in blood coagulation mechanisms.

Changes in gingivae resulting from inflammation may be recorded on the chart by drawing areas of gingiva enlargement

Table 6–2. Medical Questionnaire

1.	Are you allergic to any medicine? (makes you itch, swell, break out)	Yes	No
2.	Are you taking any medicine or drugs regularly?	Yes	No
3.	Do you have a physician? When did you last see your physician? _____	Yes	No
4.	Have you ever had a reaction to local anesthetic? (fainting, itching, nervous feeling, vomiting)	Yes	No
5.	Have you ever had heart problems? (heart attack, high blood pressure, chest pain, heart murmur)	Yes	No
6.	Have you ever been hospitalized? (operations, pregnancy, emergency)	Yes	No
7.	Do you have any lung problems? (TB, emphysema, pneumonia, shortness of breath)	Yes	No
8.	(Have you ever had liver problems? (hepatitis, jaundice, cirrhosis)	Yes	No
9.	Do you have diabetes? Do any members of your family have diabetes? _____	Yes	No
10.	Have you ever had an excessive bleeding problem? (after a cut, operation, extraction)	Yes	No
11.	Do you have a kidney or urinary problem? (kidney stones, itch, rash, burning)	Yes	No
12.	Have you had a venereal disease? (syphilis, gonorrhea, herpes, AIDS)	Yes	No
13.	Do you have epilepsy? (seizure)	Yes	No
14.	Do you have any emotional problems? (fear of dental care, seen a psychologist or psychiatrist)	Yes	No
15.	Do you have a history of ulcers, diverticulitis, or colitis?	Yes	No
16.	Have you ever had a tumor (cancer, skin swelling)?	Yes	No
17.	Have you ever had radiation treatment?	Yes	No
18.	Have you had rheumatic or scarlet fever?	Yes	No

to delineate the extent and distribution of the swelling. Localized acute inflammatory conditions such as a periodontal abscess and draining fistulas should be recorded by outlining and locating the involved area near the appropriate tooth diagram on the chart. A notation should also be made of such localized areas for the dentist's inspection.

Pocket Recording

Detection of gingival and periodontal pockets involves the use of a periodontal probe. This instrument is calibrated in millimeters and is thin enough to permit its placement beneath the gingiva around all the teeth. The probe placed to the bottom of the pocket is read at the gingival margin

to the nearest millimeter. Such a measurement is termed the pocket depth, which is the distance from the gingival margin to the bottom of the pocket. Until recently such pocket depth measurements were accepted as a reasonable approximation of the extent of attachment loss. Two factors refute this—the variation in gingival margin level and the extent of penetration of the probe into connective tissue.

It has been pointed out that inflammatory changes, systemic conditions, and certain medications may result in swelling of marginal gingiva. Conversely, improper toothbrushing, gingival recession due to anatomic factors or disease, and tissue shrinkage due to healing may cause an apical shift of the gingival margin. Thus the

Table 6–3.   Symbols Used in Periodontal Charting (Refer to Figures 6–8 to 6–13)

The charting must be precise, accurate, and neat in order to be meaningful. It may be noted lightly in pencil prior to confirmation by the dentist, but must then be put in *ink.*

1. *Probing*—to the nearest mm [note the color-coded probe is marked 3, 6, and 8 mm]; blocks are available for measurements; (1) initial [date at top]; (2) presurgical evaluation [date at top]; (3) postsurgical evaluation [date at top].
   The entire dentition should be probed and charted. Note: Mesial and distal depths should be well into the interproximal to get a true representation of the greatest depth, not at the line angles.

2. *Furcation invasion*—indicate an appropriate view—V = Class I; ▽ = Class II; ▼ = Class III (i.e., #3, 14, 18, 19, 30). Class I, incipient; Class II, definitely into furca, but not through and through; Class III, through and through.

3. *Missing teeth*—indicate X (entire three views)—clinically missing (i.e., #1, 4, 13, 16, 31, 32).

4. *Condemned teeth*—indicate two vertical parallel lines through teeth [∥] (entire three views).

5. *Gingival level*—not just a wavy line but an accurate representation of the location and contour of the free gingival margin and papillae. Are the papillae high or blunt? (i.e., #22–27). Also subjective comment in boxes is appropriate.

6. *Mucogingival problem*—wavy horizontal line [~] indicated in areas where it *may* influence the periodontal problem or treatment.

7. *Mobility*—indicate I, II, III. Note on the facial view of tooth if greater than physiologic (i.e., #9–12; 20–27).

8. *Periapical disease or root canal*—circle or depict on facial view of tooth and note in block above.

9. *Diastema*—indicate two parallel lines [∥] between occlusal and incisal view (i.e., #9–19; 11–12).

10. *Weak contact*—indicate wavy vertical line [⟩] between occlusal and incisal view (i.e., #28–29).

11. *Marginal ridge discrepancy*—indicate N between occlusal or incisal view (.e., #14, 15; #29, 30).

12. *Tissue cratering*—indicate : : between appropriate teeth (i.e., #5–6–7; 10–11; 14–15).

13. *Malpositioned teeth*—indicate arrow [↑] to show direction on occlusal view (i.e., #9, 10, 21, 23, 24, 26).

14. *Bridge*—criss-cross lines across facial and lingual views (abutments) and make appropriate comment in block (i.e., #3–6).

15. *Frenal problems*—indicate with prominent V-shaped figure [V] and comment in block.

16. *Overhanging restoration*—indicate with L-shaped drawing [L] (i.e., #14).

17. *Faulty restoration of periodontal significance*—outline restoration.

level of the gingival margin fluctuates, and accurate measurement cannot be made from a variable measuring point. In order to make accurate assessment of the extent of attachment loss, a fixed reference point such as the cementoenamel junction must be used for measurement. Only when the gingival margin coincided with the cementoenamel junction would the probing depth measurement and the attachment loss method be coincidentally the same.

The situation is further complicated by the difficulty often experienced in accurately locating the cementoenamel junction. In young individuals the gingival level may be coronal to the junction. Gingival enlargement due to inflammation also prohibits accurate location of the ce-

mentoenamel junction. When papillae fill the interproximal embrasure, it is difficult to establish the junctional location. Finally, restorations often obscure the cementoenamel junction. For all of these reasons clinical researchers frequently fabricate an acrylic splint, which can be placed on the occlusal surfaces of the teeth, as a permanent fixed reference measuring point.

For years it has been assumed that the tip of the probe identified the level of the more apical cells of the dentogingival epithelium. In healthy tissues with an intact epithelium and collagen fibers are dense, the probe tip probably does terminate in epithelium. When tissues are inflamed the connective tissue barriers are reduced and the probe tip actually ends somewhere in the inflamed connective tissue. Resolution of the inflammation with treatment may result in the construction of new collagen fibers and the probe tip may again terminate in epithelium. Other factors including the thinness of the periodontal probe, the positioning of the probe, and the extent of pressure exerted on the probe are variables which modify the accuracy of measurements. The presence of heavy deposits of calculus beneath the free margin of the gingiva can prohibit the probe reaching the entire depth of the pocket.

The variability of the gingival margin and the inability to accurately determine the location of the probe tip present a vexing problem in clinical measurement. The clinician knows that such measurement as gained from conventional pocket depth measurements are not truly representative of the clinical situation, but some method must be used to assess the status of gingival separation from the tooth. The solution is a compromise in which the clinician recognizes the deviation in accuracy but uses changes in probing measurements as one method of determining change from baseline.

For practical reasons most clinicians still probe periodontal pockets rather than attempting to gauge attachment levels. A systematic placement of the probe is made around each tooth, and an attempt is made to "trace" the attachment level of the tissue to the tooth. A periodontal probe with graduated color-coding is recommended to aid in pocket measurements (Fig. 6–6).

Since bleeding may be involved by passage of the probe tip into the inflamed connective tissue, patients with a medical history of rheumatic fever, rheumatic heart disease, organic valvular defects, organic murmurs, and artificial heart prostheses should not be probed unless covered by appropriate prophylactic antibiotic therapy (refer to Chapter 9). Probing can be accomplished at a second appointment following consultation by the dentist with the patient's physician.

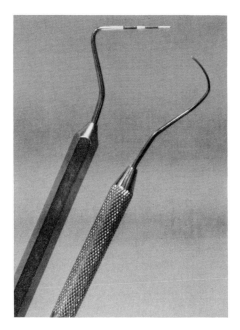

Figure 6–6.   Color-Coded Probe on Left and Nabor's Furcation Probe on Right.

It is a wise plan to have a regular order to the probing sequence. Since the most common tooth numbering system begins with the maxillary right third molar, it is appropriate to start on the facial of the maxillary right quadrant. Probing can then be accomplished on the facial of the maxillary left quadrant, the lingual of the maxillary left, and is completed in the upper arch in the maxillary right. The probing sequence in the mandibular facial proceeds from left to right, while the lingual surfaces are probed from right to left. Such a patterned system of probing is easily recorded.

At least six measurements of pocket depth should be recorded for each tooth: three on the facial and three on the lingual. Should the depth of the gingival crevice be in the 1 to 3-mm range, this is usually not recorded since this represents the normal range of crevicular depth. Any measurement of pocket depth greater than 3 mm should be recorded in the box on the chart corresponding to the facial or lingual representation of the tooth being examined.

An entry should be made for each pocket measurement.

The probe should be inserted to the depth of the pocket with the probe tip against the tooth surface. Firm but gentle pressure should be exerted such that the bottom of the pocket is reached. Timidity at the prospect of causing the patient minor discomfort should not prevent the hygienist from negotiating the pocket. If the patient is informed beforehand regarding the importance of determining the extent of separation of the gingivae from the teeth and are assured that discomfort is slight, no problem is usually encountered.

Patients with acute periodontal conditions should not be probed, but rather examined by the dentist and treated for the emergency situation. Total periodontal charting is deferred to a subsequent appointment. This is also the case where heavy deposits of calculus prohibit subgingival probe placement. Pocket depth recordings may require rechecking by the dentist or hygienist later following preliminary scaling procedures.

Interproximal areas of teeth represent the area where periodontal disease is most likely to develop, and it is the area where pockets are usually the deepest. Unfortunately, the interproximal areas are also most difficult to probe accurately due to the tooth contact areas. To probe these interproximal pockets the probe tip must touch the tooth just apical to the contact area with the probe as near the contact area as possible. The probe must be angled to reach this area. Do not attempt to keep the probe parallel to the long axis of tooth! In order to locate the deepest part of the pocket the probe is "stepped" along the root surface from both facial and lingual to the area beneath the contact. The hygienist is cautioned not to angle the probe too much, which will result in false readings. By keeping the probe near the contact area this error will be minimized. Tooth crown contours must be considered in placement of the probe. This is particularly true in the case of fixed prostheses.

Furcation invasions in which the periodontal pockets reach into the bifurcations and trifurcations of the teeth also present a difficulty in probing. Simple vertical placement of the probe provides only one measurement of such a defect. Use of a Nabor's furcation probe (Fig. 6–6) permits clinical determination of the extent of the furcation defect due to its curved design. A classification for furcation invasion is: Class I, incipient, only slight penetration; Class II, definitely into the furca, but not through and through; and Class III, the probe passes through the furcation to the opposite side of the tooth. Use of the Nabor's probe in a mandibular molar furcation is demonstrated in Figure 6–7.

An example of photographs, radiographs, and charting with appropriate symbols of a patient with periodontitis is presented in Figures 6–8 through 6–13. Please consult Table 6–3 for explanation of symbols.

Plaque Control Record

It has been experimentally proven that bacterial plaque, when allowed to accumulate on the gingival one-third of the tooth crown and in the gingival crevice, results in gingival inflammation. If the plaque is not controlled, gingivitis may lead to more serious periodontal disease. Because the microbial population that comprises plaque plays such a paramount role in the etiology of inflammatory periodontal disease, it is critical that the extent and location of plaque be assessed during the periodontal examination.

Early plaque is invisible to the naked eye and only when there is considerable accumulation can it be visually detected. Therefore, the plaque must be made visible by application of staining agents or dyes. Stained plaque permits identification of location by the hygienist and provides for easy demonstration to the patient. Some of these dyestuffs are currently being inves-

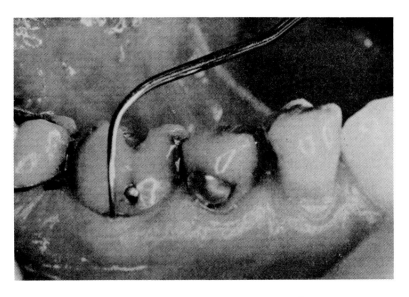

Figure 6–7. Nabor's Furcation Probe in Furca of Mandibular Molar.

tigated because of possible harmful effects, but other products are being developed that will continue to permit hygienists to locate and quantify the extent of plaque. Staining of plaque is a valuable aid in patient education and is discussed in Chapter 8. Materials include a disclosing solution or tablet, an explorer or curette to verify plaque accumulation by scraping, a periodontal probe, and a hand mirror to point out areas of plaque accumulation to the patient (Fig. 6–14).

A useful method of recording plaque was developed by O'Leary, Drake, and Naylor. This plaque control record diagrammatically represents 32 teeth with each tooth divided into four surfaces representing facial, lingual, mesial and distal aspects (Fig. 6–15D). After disclosing solution is applied, the patient is allowed to rinse to get rid of loose material and excess dyestuff. Only the gingival one-third of the crown is considered for periodontal scoring. On the plaque control record missing teeth are indicated by drawing two parallel lines through them. The remaining teeth are counted and this number is multiplied by the four surfaces of each tooth to provide the actual number of surfaces available on which plaque might accumulate. Then a tooth by tooth assessment of plaque is made. It is helpful to establish a consistent order to this plaque survey. It is suggested that the hygienist begin with the maxillary right, then the maxillary left, then the mandibular left, and conclude with the mandibular right. If plaque is found on facial or lingual surfaces of the tooth, a dot is placed on that surface on the record (Fig. 6–15A). If plaque is present on mesial or distal surfaces, from either facial or lingual, only a single marking is made. It may be assumed that any interproximal plaque is probably present through the entire interproximal area. A single mark is thus sufficient to record this (Figs. 6–15B and 6–15C). In Figures 6–15B and 6–15C the clinical representation and record markings are illustrated.

When all surfaces of all teeth have been examined and presence of plaque recorded (Figs. 6–15E and 6–15F), a plaque score for the patient can be computed. This consists of dividing the number of tooth surfaces with plaque by the total number of tooth surfaces available. When this figure is multiplied by 100, the plaque score is presented as a percentage of tooth surfaces with

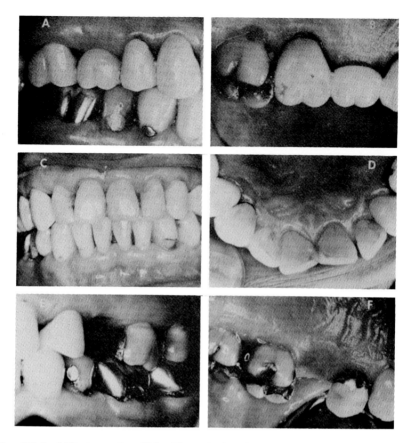

Figure 6–8. Clinical Photographs of Maxillary Arch (facial and lingual) of periodontal patient. (Courtesy of Learning Resources Center, University of North Carolina School of Dentistry, and Dr. Walter Kucaba.)

plaque (Fig. 6–15G). This objective method of assessing plaque accumulation allows for accurate baseline information at the initial appointment (Fig. 6–15H). The patient can be informed of a score in terms that they can understand, "Mr. Johnson, the bacteria in plaque are responsible for gum disease. In your mouth 60% of your teeth have this plaque in the critical area at the gum line."

Plaque scores at subsequent appointments can also be recorded on the plaque control record, and this can be used to monitor patient progress in achieveing effective daily maintenance of oral hygiene (Fig. 6–16). The ideal goal of such patient efforts would be zero, but anything less than 10% would be realistically acceptable.

The plaque control record affords an extremely objective method of quantitating plaque accumulations at each appointment, is a reasonably rapid method of recording such accumulations, is useful in monitoring patient progress, is readily understood by the patient, and provides a goal for the patient to work toward in control of periodontal disease etiology. Other methods of scoring plaque are also available. Both the oral hygiene index (OHI) of Greene and Vermillion and the simplified oral hygiene index (OHIS) have been widely used in epidemiologic studies. Another index frequently used in research studies is the plaque index (PI). None of these methods of quantification have the visual impact of the plaque control record

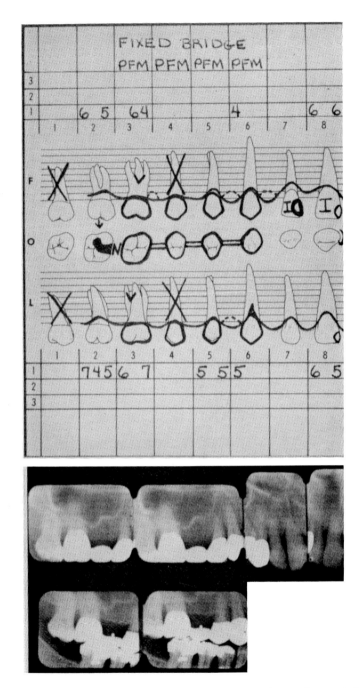

Figure 6–9. Maxillary Right Quadrant (chart and corresponding radiographs). Note furcation invasions on facial and distal of #3 and mobility #7 & 8. (Courtesy of Learning Resources Center, University of North Carolina School of Dentistry, and Dr. Walter Kucaba.)

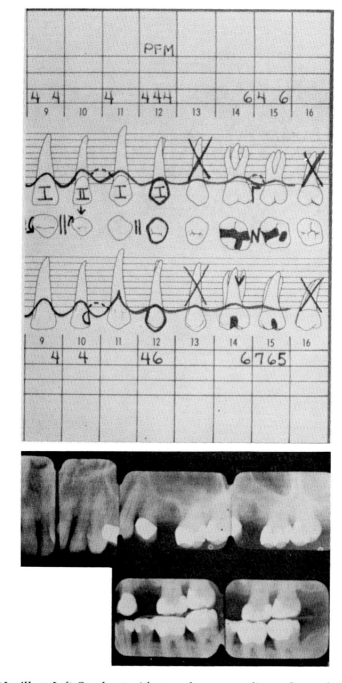

Figure 6–10. Maxillary Left Quadrant (chart and corresponding radiographs). Note overhang restoration distal #14, soft-tissue crater between #14 & 15, and mobility #9, 10, 11, 12. (Courtesy of Learning Resources Center, University of North Carolina School of Dentistry, and Dr. Walter Kucaba.)

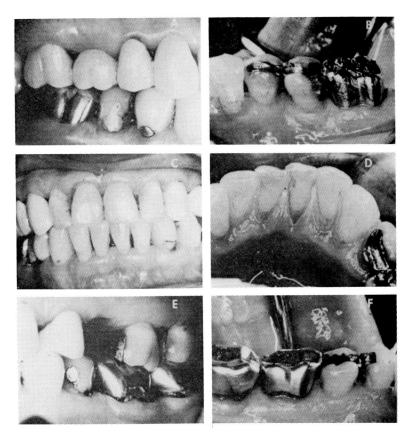

Figure 6–11. Clinical Photographs of Mandibular Arch (facial and lingual) of periodontal patient. (Courtesy of Learning Resources Center, University of North Carolina School of Dentistry, and Dr. Walter Kucaba.)

or use numerical scorings as easily understood by the patient as the plaque control record. Epidemiologic indices are described in Chapter 10.

Calculus

The presence of calculus deposits and their location and extent should be noted during the oral examination. Supragingival calculus is most commonly found on the lingual of lower anterior teeth and facially and interproximally to maxillary molars. In some individuals it may be more generalized. Subgingival calculus is discovered during probing, exploring and on radiographic examination. Written comments on the amount of calculus and its location should be made in the patient's record.

Bleeding Score

Previously the importance of bleeding in periodontal examination was stressed. The bleeding sites can be identified clinically and charted. A variation of the plaque control record can be used to document the areas of bleeding. In actual practice the bleeding scores are obtained at the time of probing and precede the plaque control record. Dyestuffs used to determine extent of plaque obscure the bleeding and thus the bleeding score is recorded before use of the dyes. See Table 6–1 for order of examination.

Exactly the same graphic representation of teeth and tooth surfaces is used for documentation of bleeding as is used in the plaque control record. First, missing teeth

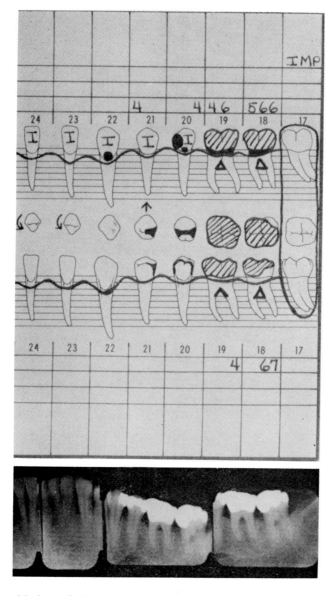

Figure 6–12. Mandibular Left Quadrant (chart and corresponding radiographs). Note furcation invasion facial and lingual of #18 & 19, and mobility #20, 21, 22, 23, 24. (Courtesy of Learning Resources Center, University of North Carolina School of Dentistry, and Dr. Walter Kucaba.)

are noted and crossed out on the bleeding record. Then the periodontal probing is accomplished on either the facial or lingual of a quadrant. Following the probing, the quadrant is examined for areas of bleeding. Any site that demonstrates bleeding is recorded with a dot on the appropriate surface on the record. As with plaque scoring, only a single dot is placed on a proximal surface if bleeding is detected from either facial or lingual aspects. Each quadrant is probed, bleeding noted, and the site recorded until the entire dentition has been examined. By dividing the number of sites

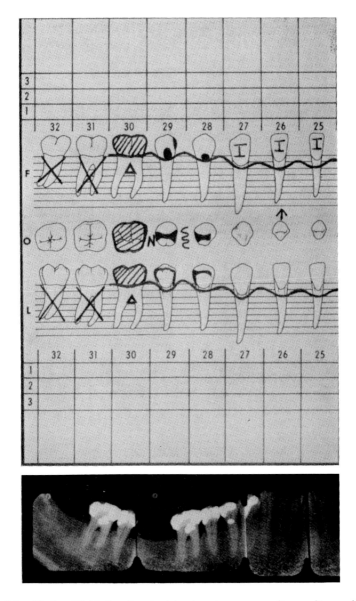

Figure 6–13. Mandibular Right Quadrant (chart and corresponding radiographs). Note furcation invasion mandibular right first molar. (Courtesy of Learning Resources Center, University of North Carolina School of Dentistry, and Dr. Walter Kucaba.)

where bleeding occurs by the total number of available sites and multiplying by 100, the percentage of bleeding sites can be computed.

When both the bleeding sites and the plaque sites are entered on the same record, a graphic comparison of the role of microbial plaque in the inflammatory response of the gingivae is available to demonstrate to the patient. In Figure 6–16 both gingival bleeding and plaque score are presented side by side. This is facilitated by having a record printed with two adjacent diagrams, one for bleeding and one for

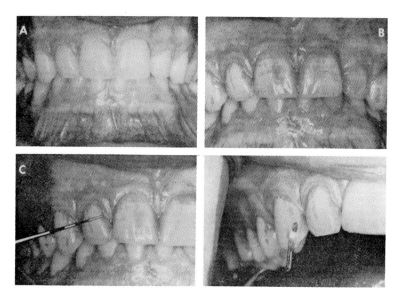

Figure 6–14. Recording Plaque Retention. A, Clinical photograph of patient's teeth to be disclosed for visualization of plaque. B, Visualization of plaque following disclosing solution or tablet. C, Plaque in the gingival third of tooth and sulcus only to be scored. D, Plaque accumulation in gingival third of tooth verified by scraping with a curette. (Courtesy of Walter McFall and Learning Resources Center, The Plaque Control Record Slide-Tape No. 7243. University of North Carolina School of Dentistry.)

plaque. While this is an objective method of identifying the location of bleeding sites, it does not attempt to gauge the amount of bleeding. Written notations in the patient's record, using descriptive adjectives such as profuse, immediate, delayed, or slight, will help to delineate the type of bleeding noted with probing. By observing the charting of pockets, the location of plaque, and the presence of bleeding sites a dramatic picture of the cause and effect relationship of plaque and disease is often revealed. This can be shared with the patient as an extremely effective educational modality. This baseline information establishes the extent of the disease and provides a permanent record of the initial disease state and subsequent improvement with therapy.

Mobility of Teeth

A certain amount of physiologic movement of teeth is necessary such that teeth may "give" with occlusal forces placed upon them. Mobility beyond this physio-logic limit may be the result of excessive forces placed on the teeth, loss of periodontal support, system changes or combinations of these. Thus, it is essential to document the extent of tooth mobiity at the clinical examination.

Mobility of posterior teeth is detected by placing the handle end of the mouth mirror on the facial surface of the tooth and the handle end of the periodontal probe on the lingual surface and then gentle pressure is exerted in a faciolingual direction (Fig. 6–17). For the anterior teeth, the handle of an instrument can be placed on the facial aspect of the tooth, while the side of the index finger or end of an instrument handle is placed on the lingual surface of the tooth. Pressure is applied in a facial and lingual direction. Extent of apical depression should also be ascertained by occlusal pressure with an instrument handle. Care should be taken when assessing mandibular tooth mobility that the mandible is not moving during examination.

Early tooth looseness is generally man-

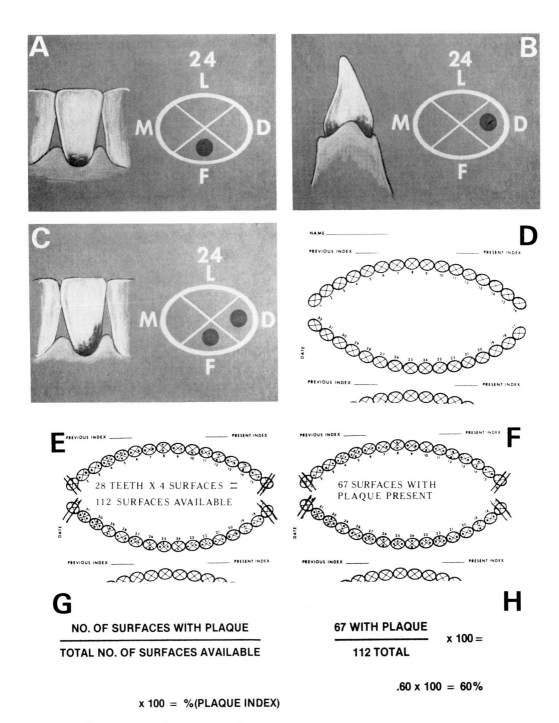

Figure 6–15.   Computation of Plaque Score.

BLEEDING   PLAQUE

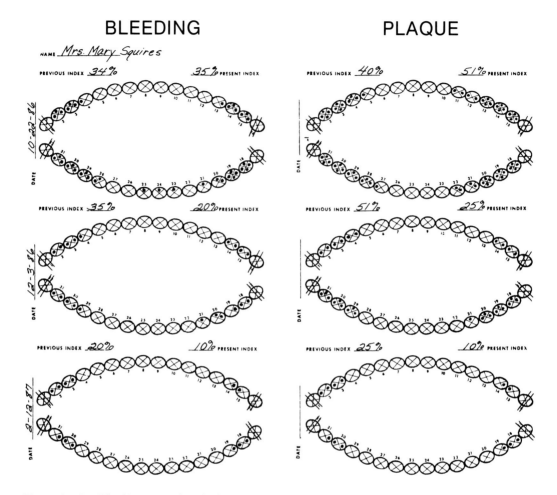

Figure 6–16.   Bleeding Record and Plaque Record.

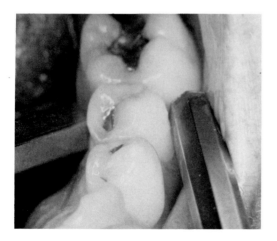

Figure 6–17.   Testing for Tooth Mobility by Use of Instrument Handles.

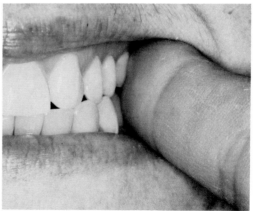

Figure 6–18.   Palpation of Teeth During Jaw Movement.

ifested by faciolingual movement. With progressive loss of support, mobility also occurs mesiodistally, and when teeth can be intruded as well the prognosis of the tooth is usually poor. Different degrees of mobility have been established as Class I, II and III. Class I may be defined as tooth movement greater than physiologic mobility but no greater than 1 mm. Class II is reserved for teeth with greater than 1-mm mobility in a mesiodistal or faciolingual direction. Class III is reserved for teeth with mobility greater than 1 mm in a mesiodistal or faciolingual direction and which can also be rotated or intruded. Charting of mobility can be denoted on the anatomic chart by placing the appropriate Roman numeral on the facial aspect of the affected tooth.

Caries and Faulty Restorations

Fortunately, dental caries is decreasing in prevalence, but it still exists and plays a role in the initiation of periodontal diseases. Carious lesions, whether new or recurrent around old restorations, should be recorded on the anatomic chart. Poorly contoured or poorly contracting restorations should be noted. Weak contacts should be tested by the use of dental floss and indicated on the chart by drawing a wavy line between the affected teeth. Open contacts are indicated by drawing two parallel lines between teeth on the anatomic chart. Faulty restorations, amalgam overhangs, poorly contoured crowns, or broken restorations can be outlined on the chart by drawing these on the tooth diagrams and by written comment in the space adjacent to the spical areas of the diagrams.

Periodontic-Endodontic Considerations

Occasionally, during the acquisition of the dental history or during clinical examination the patient will complain of tooth pain. Bacteria from an infected dental pulp may invade the periapical area of a tooth, which may result in a deep periodontal pocket. Drainage may be through the periodontal ligament resulting in destruction of periodontal ligament to gingival crevice. In other instances the purulent exudate may burrow through bone and soft tissue and present as a draining fistulous tract in lining mucosa or apical areas of masticatory mucosa. Endodontic root canal therapy that removes the infected pulpal tissue often resolves the tract or periodontal pocket without much adjunctive periodontal treatment.

Teeth, particularly multirooted teeth, may contain lateral or accessory canals communicating between the dental pulp and the periodontal ligament. Bacteria in deep periodontal pockets may invade the pulp through these canals. A common anatomic location of these accessory canals is in the furcation area of molar teeth. If bacterial invasion occurs, the pulp may become infected and a combined periodontal-endodontic lesion result.

Complaints of tooth pain, particularly of a lasting nature, require a systematic testing of pulpal vitality of the suspected tooth or teeth. One instrument that can be used by the hygienist is the vitalometer, which sends a mild electric current through the tooth (Fig. 6–19). If the teeth in question have proximal, metallic restorations, rubber dam strips may need to be placed between contacts to prevent the electric current from passing from one tooth to another which might give a false reading. A control on the vitalometer permits the hygienist to slowly increase the current. A severely inflamed pulp will respond to a small amount of current, and the patient will report pain. Teeth, in which most of the pulp is necrotic, will respond only to high current levels or not at all. The vitalometer findings are more reliable on single rooted teeth, since multirooted teeth may respond with contradictory readings. Good periapical radiographs and tooth responses to thermal stimuli are mandatory for the dentist's evaluation and diagnosis. It should be noted that the vitalometer (electric pulp tester) should probably not

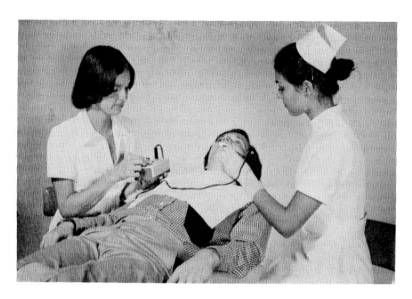

Figure 6–19. Hygienist Testing for Pulpal Vitality with Electric Pulp Tester (vitalometer)

be used on patients with pacemakers for heart trouble (refer to Chapter 9). Another common method of assessing pulpal vitality is the use of thermal stimuli. Both cold stimulus, such as ice or cold water, and hot stimulus, such as hot gutta percha or warmed instruments, may be used.

Teeth with large amalgam restorations, especially molars, are subject to vertical fractures of crown and/or root. Teeth with root canal therapy also are subject to such fracture. An extremely deep pocket on a tooth in a mouth with only mild or moderate pockets may be a clue to such a fracture. The hygienist can have the patient bite down on a rubber polishing wheel on a suspected tooth. If on quick release of biting pressure a sharp pain is experienced by the patient, then a fracture should be suspected. All of the hygienist's findings should be recorded. Final decisions on diagnosis and treatment are made by the dentist.

Sensitive Teeth

Dentin sensitivity may occur with gingival recession and the patient may report discomfort to thermal changes, metallic objects, or sweet or sour foods or liquids.

Usually cold is the stimulus that elicits discomfort. Such sensitivity may be detected clinically by isolating the suspected tooth with cotton rolls and blowing cold compressed air from the air syringe. A quick scratch of the cervical root area with a sharp explorer tine also will induce discomfort if the cause is dentin sensitivity. If no caries is present, then the application of appropriate desensitizing medicaments should be accomplished (refer to Chapters 8 and 10). Written notation of the affected tooth should be made in the patient record.

RADIOGRAPHIC EXAMINATION

Dental radiographs are shadow pictures representing varying degrees of density of structures through which the x-rays pass. Since soft tissue of the mouth lacks density, it appears dark or radiolucent on the radiographs. Gingivae lack density and barely appear on dental radiographs. Radiographs cannot reveal early stages of periodontal disease because these changes are present only in the gingivae. Pathologic alterations in soft tissues may be present for some time before bone changes are detected on radiographs. There is no substitute for accurate clinical examination in the detection of periodontal disease.

Bone tissue and teeth, being more dense, will appear on radiographs as light or white on the film and are termed radiopaque structures. The periodontal ligament is composed of vascularized soft tissue and appears dark. Alveolar bone proper that comprises the wall of the alveolus appears radiopaque and contrasts well with the dark periodontal ligament space. Pulpal tissue, being primarily vascular soft tissue, appears as a dark radiolucent structure.

Three types of radiographs are commonly obtained in dental offices. These are a full periapical series of films, intraoral bitewing radiographs, and panoramic films that permit a view of both jaws and temporomandibular joints. For radiographic examination of the periodontium periapical films are by far the most satisfactory. Bitewing radiographs may be valuable in viewing the crest of the interproximal alveolar bone. All too frequently a horizontal series of bitewings is obtained which does not reveal the bone. Such bitewings are only useful in diagnosis of dental caries. Vertical bitewings can be obtained, which are useful in presenting views of crestal bone. Panoramic films have value as a generalized screening tool, and they may reveal jaw fractures, impacted teeth, bone cysts, or other jaw disorders.

On high quality periapical films the cortical crestal bone appears as a dense white opaque line in the interproximal space, and, in health, the opaque line is intact and unbroken in continuity. Crestal bone rises in height as the apex of a triangle in the anterior maxilla and mandible and becomes flatter progressively from cuspid to premolar and molar areas (Figs. 6–20 and 6–21). Contour of the bone varies with the shape of contacting tooth crowns, the respective heights of adjacent marginal ridges of contacting tooth crowns, and the length of the proximal contacts. The cortical crest height is located 1 to 2 mm below the cementoenamel junction. It has been established that the cementoenamel junction plays a significant role in the shape of the alveolar crest. When the cementoenamel junction of two adjacent teeth are at the same level, then the crest tends to be flat. If a tooth or teeth are tipped, the cementoenamel junctions will not be at the same level and the crestal bone will be ramped accordingly. In case of severe gingival recession, a crestal bone resorption and recession will keep pace resulting in crestal levels some distance apical to the cementoenamel junction, and yet no periodontal pathologic condition in terms of pockets may exist.

Interproximal cancellous supporting bone appears as a spongy network of light interlacing lines with small dark radiolucent areas between. So much variation of the trabecular pattern occurs in cancellous bone that criteria for normality is hard to establish. When heavy forces are placed on posterior teeth, the bone may appear dense and trabeculae are arranged more perpendicularly to the long axis of the tooth. Conversely, when light forces are applied to the teeth then fewer trabeculae are apparent. Periodontal structures seen on periapical films are illustrated in Figure 6–22. For correlation with the normal histology refer to Chapter 2.

Radiographs may provide useful information concerning the length, shape and proximity of tooth roots. Since broad and long roots provide more surface for connective tissue attachment, it is useful to known this in planning therapy. Likewise, widely divergent roots in multirooted teeth enhance prognosis, while fused roots offer less attachment. When roots are in close proximity, there may be little intervening alveolar bone. Periapical radiographs also can reveal how close root apices of maxillary teeth are to the maxillary sinus. Interproximal bone levels as well as bone and periodontal ligament relations can also be obtained from radiographs. These are all advantageous features that can be valuable in diagnosis, therapy and prognosis.

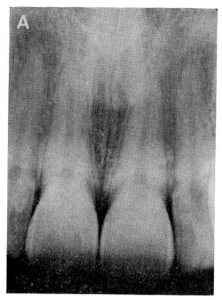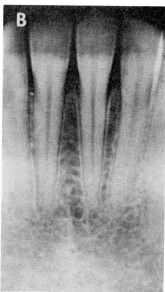

Figure 6–20. Normal Radiographic Bone Height and Contours.   A, Maxillary and B, Mandibular anterior segments. Note crestal cortication and normal distance of crest from cementoenamel junction.

There are, however, some severe limitations to the use of radiographs. Radiographs cannot portray soft tissue-hard tissue relationships since the gingival tissue cannot be visualized. Thus periodontal pockets do not appear on radiographs. It is impossible to view soft tissue recession on radiographs. The structure of the tooth itself effectively blocks study of facial and lingual osseous structures. Some teeth such as premolars have dumbbell-shaped roots that limit even proper viewing of parts of interproximal periodontal ligament, and the palatal root of the maxillary molars prohibit adequate visualization of the trifurcation area. Obviously, no assessment of mobility or inflammation can be gained from radiographs.

Radiographs and Periodontal Disease

Inflammatory processes occur initially in soft tissues, and gingivitis does not result in radiographically identifiable change. With the extension of inflammation alteration of osseous structures can be visualized on radiographs. The earliest change

seen in the radiographs suggestive of the presence of periodontal disease is usually the loss of intactness of the interproximal cortical crest. Coronal portions of the lamina dura also may be disrupted, indistinct or absent. Such early osseous alterations occur with suprabony pockets and should be observed in routine radiographic examination since treatment is more effective in the earlier stages of periodontitis.

In the presence of periodontal pathologic conditions and pocket formation, concomitant bone changes may be seen in the radiographs varying with the severity of the periodontal condition (Fig. 6–23). When assessing the extent of bone loss the cementoenamel junction is used as a reference mark. In the case of generalized periodontitis, the height of the crestal bone is usually reduced rather uniformly, representing what is termed "horizontal bone loss" (Fig. 6–24). When this reduction in crestal bone height is uneven and varies in the extent of reduction from one tooth to the adjacent contracting tooth, the bone loss is characterized as the "vertical type

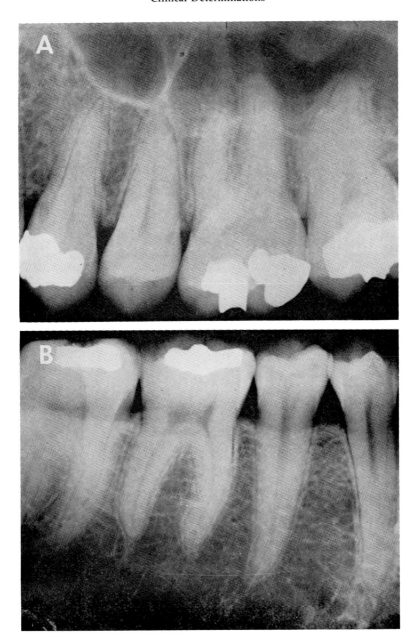

Figure 6–21. Periodontal Supporting Structures. A, Maxillary and B, Mandibular posterior segments. Note crestal cortication and normal distance of crest from the cementoenamel junction.

of bone loss" (Fig. 6–24). This vertical type of bone loss is seen more frequently in severe localized periodontitis on only one or two teeth. Local etiologic factors such as faulty restorative margins, food impaction, or poor tooth contacts may contribute to such lesions. Vertical bone loss, particularly adjacent to molars and incisors in ad-

olescents, may be an indication of juvenile periodontitis. The type of bone defect depends on many factors including the thickness of the bone, the position of the tooth in the bone, and the occurrence of excessive occlusal forces in an area of already damaged periodontal support. Intrabony defects may or may not be discernible on

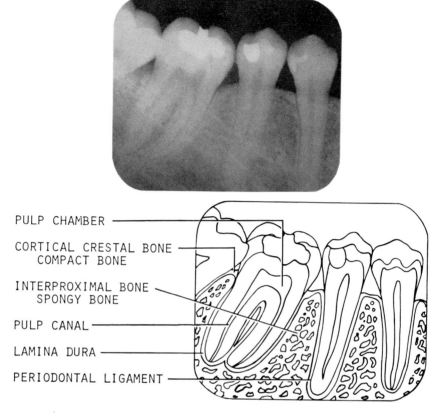

PULP CHAMBER

CORTICAL CRESTAL BONE
    COMPACT BONE

INTERPROXIMAL BONE
    SPONGY BONE

PULP CANAL

LAMINA DURA

PERIODONTAL LIGAMENT

Figure 6–22.   Periodontal Supporting Structures.   This radiograph with its corresponding drawing shows the periodontal ligament, lamina dura, cortical crest bone, and interproximal spongy bone.

radiographs depending on their configuration.

Furcation areas should be carefully observed on radiographs to determine areas of bone loss. Such radiographic changes are more easily viewed in mandibular molars with divergent roots, and are more difficult to ascertain in maxillary molars. Radiographic signs should prompt careful reevaluation of furcation areas clinically.

Relative crown-root lengths should be observed in relationship to bone height on radiographs. Large crowns on short conical-shaped roots are a poor prognostic sign if bone loss has occurred to a significant degree. Conversely, long, broad roots on teeth tend to enhance the prognosis of teeth. Root resorption may occur as result of excessive occlusal force. An irregular or widened periodontal ligament space may reflect the presence of occlusal trauma on a tooth. Clinical examination for tooth mobility and institution of a functional occlusal analysis are warranted with such radiographic evidence.

Bitewing radiographs are especially helpfull in determining true interproximal bone height because this type of picture is made at an angulation to the long axis of the teeth that permits only a minimum of elongation or foreshortening. Calculus deposits, particularly more densely calcified ones, also are well delineated on these films. Poor restorative margins on mesial and distal surfaces are best viewed on bitewings. Interproximal carious lesions are more easily detected in bitewing radiographs.

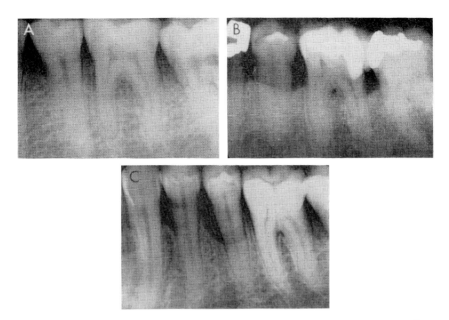

Figure 6–23. Progressive Alveolar Bone Destruction. Radiographic appearance of varying degrees of severity of bone loss in periodontal disease. A, Mild; beginning loss of crestal alveolar bone. B, Moderate; definite loss of interproximal supporting bone. C, Advanced; severe loss of interproximal supporting bone.

All radiographic abnormalities such as radiolucent and radiopaque areas, embedded root tips left in the jaw following extraction of teeth, carious lesions, faulty restorations, and impacted teeth should be recorded in the patient record. Caries and poor restorations can be sketched on an anatomic chart.

Radiographs taken over a period of years do provide a history of the supporting structures for an individual patient. This may provide a picture of healthy stability. In other instances, longitudinal radiographic series provide a record of progressive destruction.

No clinical examination can be consid-

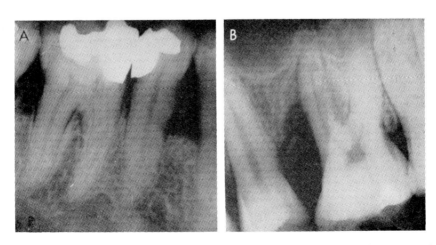

Figure 6–24. Patterns of Bone Loss. A, Horizontal type of bone loss as shown in radiograph. B, Vertical type of bone loss as shown in radiograph.

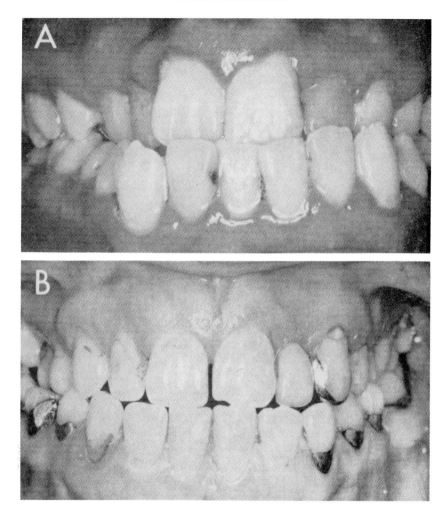

Figure 6–25. Crossbite. These are examples of anterior crossbite (A) and bilateral crossbite relationship in right and left premolar and molar areas in (B).

ered complete without high quality, well-angulated radiographs. Radiographic views often provide information that can be obtained from no other source. Because of the inherent limitations of radiographs, this superb diagnostic tool must be considered secondary to clinical evaluation in diagnosis of periodontal disease. There is a serious danger in too great a dependency on radiographs since periodontal disease may advance without radiographic evidence. The problem with radiographs is that the periodontal lesion may not be re-

vealed until the disease is well established or, more dangerously, it may not be revealed at all.

OCCLUSION

Occlusion represents the dynamic interrelationship of contact between teeth of opposing arches. When jaws are closed together in the habitual position of closure, the teeth interdigitate in maximum intercuspation. The mandibular arch is the contained arch, the maxillary teeth being slightly facial to mandibular teeth. Mandibular buccal cusps and maxillary lingual cusps of the posterior teeth provide the supporting cusps that maintain this contact with opposing fossae, grooves, and marginal ridges.

In a morphologically normal occlusion the mesiobuccal cusp of the upper first molar occludes with the buccal groove of the lower first permanent molar. Deviations from this arrangement represent malocclusions and were classified by Angle as Class I, II or III. Class I is characterized by a normal relationship of maxillary and mandibular first permanent molars. The distal incline of the lower cuspids' incisal edges is related to mesial incline of the upper cuspids' incisal edges. Malocclusion in Class I is due to the presence of rotated, tilted, or overlapped teeth. In Class II the mesiobuccal cusps of the maxillary first molar rests between the buccal cusp of the mandibular second premolar and the mesiobuccal cusp of the mandibular first molar. All lower teeth occlude more distally with their antagonists than in Class I relationship. Sometimes this relationship is associated with a prominent maxilla and a receded lower jaw. In Class III the mesiobuccal cusp of the maxillary first molar rests between the distobuccal cusp of the mandibular first molar and the mesiobuccal cusp of the mandibular second molar. Lower molars and cuspids occlude more mesially than in a Class I relation. Sometimes this tooth malocclusion is associated with a prominent lower jaw. Malocclusion may result from either skeletal malposition or tooth malposition or a combination of both.

Normally the maxillary arch of teeth is larger than the mandibular arch with buccal cusps and incisal edges overlapping mandibular buccal cusps in both a horizontal and vertical dimension. Malrelationships may occur in this arrangement in posterior or anterior teeth. This malrelationship is termed a crossbite. In posterior areas the crossbite occurs when buccal cusps of the maxillary posterior teeth interdigitate in the central fossa of the mandibular teeth. Anterior maxillary teeth may be in linguoversion to mandibular teeth. Crossbite may be unilateral or bilateral (Fig. 6–25). In crossbite situations, smooth mandibular movements may not be possible, excessive forces may be placed on the teeth, or food impaction may occur complicating periodontal therapy.

Other alterations in tooth relationships such as an open bite of the anterior or posterior teeth, malposed, rotated or crowded teeth should be noted on clinical examination. The intactness of the gingivae depends upon the protection of correct tooth morphology and the axial inclination of teeth. Malocclusion alone does not seem to result in inflammatory periodontal disease, but oral hygiene effectiveness is severely limited when teeth are malposed or jumbled. Teeth which erupt and develop too far facially may have insufficient keratinized gingiva. Malalignments of teeth can be indicated on the chart by drawing an arrow on the occlusal view of the affected tooth indicating the direction of displacement. Some abnormal occlusal relationships such as open bite may contribute to tongue thrust habits or an enlarged tongue (Fig. 6–26). Protruding maxillary anterior teeth may be associated with mouth breathing, a habit that causes a drying of the maxillary facial gingivae resulting in irritation and inflammation of the tissue. All of the conditions mentioned are best corrected by orthodontic treatment and concomitant correction of pernicious oral habits, provided that periodontal support is adequate.

Occlusal Positions

Mandibular movements such as opening and closing are controlled by the neuromusculature of the head, face, and neck. The muscles of mastication, medial and lateral pterygoids, masseter, and temporal are principally responsible for the dynamics of mandibular movement. Much of the

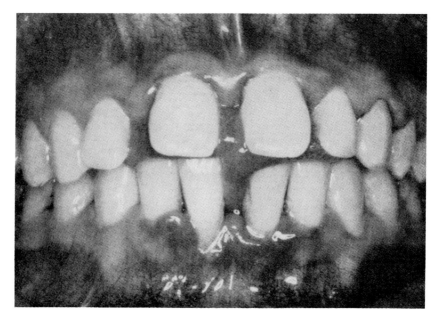

Figure 6–26. Open bite. This is an example of anterior open bite resulting from a tongue thrust habit and loss of periodontal support.

time the mandible assumes a position of physiologic rest in which the teeth are not in contact and the mandibular musculature are in minimal tonic contraction sufficient to maintain the postural position of the mandible against the force of gravity with the head in an upright position. A clearance of freeway space exists between maxillary and mandibular teeth.

Centric relation may be defined as the relation of the mandible to the maxilla (and other cranial structures) at any given vertical dimension when the condyles are in their most superior, concentric, unstrained position in the glenoid fossae. Although centric relation is a jaw to jaw position, when teeth are present it also is a tooth to tooth position. Its importance lies in the fact that it is a stable, reproducible, and returnable point of condyle position and therefore permits reliable functional occlusal analysis and tooth adjustment. When there is harmony in the entire stomatognathic system, the mandible can smoothly arc to and from centric relation.

Centric occlusion refers to the maximum intercuspation or contact of the teeth of opposing arches. It may also be called acquired or habitual centric. If a patient is requested to bite their teeth together, they will habitually close into centric occlusion. Opening and closing movements of the mandible originate from centric occlusion and postural rest position. Centric occlusion and centric relation do not usually coincide, but rather represent different tooth-to-tooth relationships in the centric range, as shown in Figure 6–27. A centric prematurity occurs when a tooth is "high" at centric occlusion.

A centric interference is an occlusal tooth to tooth contact that occurs in centric relation before a stable and balanced jaw to jaw relationship is reached in centric. Such interferences are quite common and do not necessarily indicate any disorder, but if these disharmonies do result in damage to teeth or supporting structures they may need to be eliminated. There is a great amount of adaptability in the stomatognathic system and normal functions of the system such as mastication do not cause

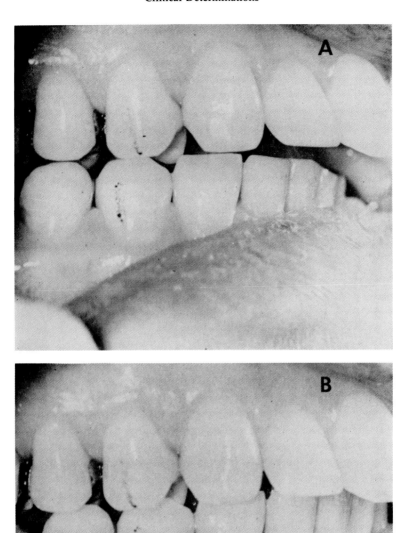

Figure 6–27. Profile Photographs Showing Discrepancy between Centric Relation and Centric Occlusion. A, Centric relation; B, Centric occlusion. Note the shifting of pencil marks on teeth from CR to CO.

injury to the system. Disharmonies in the occlusion may, however, result in damage to any part of the system. Alterations may occur on the teeth, in the supporting apparatus, in the myofascial region, or in the temporomandibular joints. There is considerable variation from patient to patient.

Occlusal Signs and Symptoms

An extensive functional occlusal analysis need not be done for every patient, but it should be recognized that patients with periodontal disease may have lost considerable tooth support. Increased tooth mobility is one of the cardinal signs of occlusal trauma. This may be the result of either loss of attachment apparatus due to destructive inflammatory periodontal disease, or due to excessive occlusal forces on the teeth from noxious habits.

If, during the course of clinical examination, signs of heavy forces on the dentition are detected, an occlusal analysis is indicated. These clinical signs include mobility of the teeth, unusual attritional wear of the teeth, occlusal tables broadened faciolingually, and shiny wear facets (Fig. 6–28). These signs usually indicate clenching, bruxism, or other parafunctional habits.

Fractured teeth or restorations may occur as the result of faulty restorative dentistry or with fatigue of restorative materials (Fig. 6–29). One should, however, be suspicious of noxious grinding habits especially if other signs or symptoms of neurosis are present. Patients may complain of soreness of masticatory muscles. Rigidity or tenderness of the musculature may restrict mandibular movements and may implicate bruxism especially if muscular soreness is reported in the morning. Hypertonicity or spasm of the facial and masticatory muscles can be detected by palpation (Fig. 6–30).

Patients may report tooth mobility, a "wedging" feeling of the teeth, food impacted between teeth, periapical pain or discomfort as symptoms of heavy forces on the teeth. A spouse or roommate may have informed the patient of the sounds of night grinding. Any of these symptoms should be entered in the patient's record and should prompt an occlusal analysis.

In response to heavy and repeated forces on teeth from occlusal habits there may be a building up of bone to compensate. These bony overgrowths are a physiologic process and are seen clinically as exostoses (Fig. 6–31).

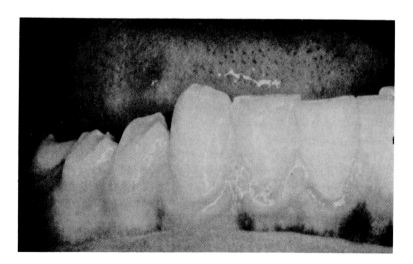

Figure 6–28. Abnormal Wear Facets of Mandibular Premolars and Molars from Clenching and(or) Bruxism.

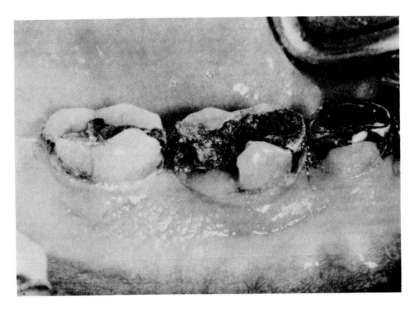

Figure 6–29.   Fractured Distolingual Cusp Mandibular First Molar from Occlusal Forces.

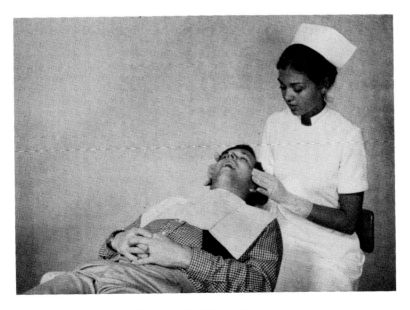

Figure 6–30.   Hygienist Palpating Temporalis Muscle for Spasm.

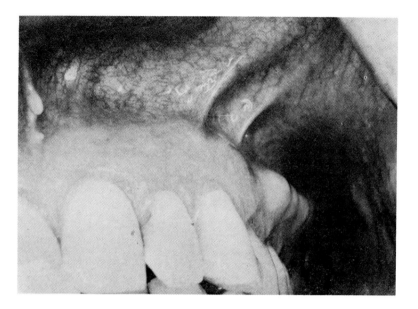

Figure 6–31. Maxillary Exostoses in Premolar and Molar Region from Occlusal Wear.

Clinical signs of excessive force also can be indicators of damage to the attachment apparatus, occlusal trauma. In some instances there is damage to the teeth rather than supporting structures, while in other patients both dental and periodontal attachment lesions may be present. Reported patient symptoms and clinical signs of occlusal stress should be carefully correlated with observations made of periapical radiographs.

Functional Occlusal Analysis

When it is determined that an analysis of occlusal relations is indicated, it is important to establish a reliable starting position of the mandible. Centric relation offers the most stable and reproducible jaw to jaw relation and is the logical starting position in a functional occlusal analysis. This requires manipulation of the mandible in such a manner to ensure the proper position of the condyles in the glenoid fossae. When the condyles are up and back in the fossae, they are braced against bone and ligaments. This represents the terminal position of an arc from which the mandible can open and close without the condyles

leaving their retruded position in the fossae. A hinge movement of the mandible can then be accomplished with the condyles rotating about a central point. Teeth can then be brought together and interferences at centric relation can be determined.

For most patients this maneuver of mandibular manipulation can be accomplished with reasonable ease by the educated hygienist. In other patients manipulation is more difficult, and it should not be attempted on patients with severe muscle hypertonicity, myofascial pain, pain or tenderness in the temporomandibular joint. These clinical findings should be noted by the hygienist, recorded in the chart, and reported to the dentist. Hygienists can perform mandibular manipulation such that accurate tooth contacts can be identified at centric relation. As with most technically precise procedures mandibular manipulation requires experience, patience, and practice. Unless the hygienist is willing to master these techniques of manipulation occlusal analysis should be deferred to the dentist.

It is extremely important that the patient's musculature be relaxed when the analysis is performed. This cannot be achieved if the patient is nervous, tense or fearful because this will result in contraction of the musculature. For this reason, the analysis is best accomplished when no other dental treatment is planned, and many dentists prefer a separate appointment for complete occlusal appraisal. Every attempt should be made to achieve a quiet, relaxing environment for the analysis.

The patient is seated comfortably in the dental chair and the chair adjusted to place the patient in a supine or semisupine position. Patients should be requested to relax their arms and legs and assured, in a quiet voice, that the examination will cause no discomfort. The head rest should be placed beneath the patient's neck such that the chin is tilted up. This permits equilibrium of the head and neck musculature and assists the condyles in assuming a distal position in the fossae. Mandibular positioning is accomplished with the patient's teeth apart and the jaw open in the physiologic rest position.

Detection of Centric Interferences

Operator guidance is required to place the condyles at the terminal hinge posture from the open position. Two methods of operator manipulation have been developed, the anterior guidance method and the bilateral manipulation method. Both methods have been shown to achieve accurate assessment of initial tooth to tooth contact patterns at centric relation.

In the anterior guidance method the operator's thumb is placed against the lower teeth resting lightly on the incisal edges. The operator's fingers are gently placed under the interior border of the mandible and mandibular symphysis so that the mandible can be lifted. The mandible is arced in a closing-opening manner over a short distance of jaw movement to ensured that the condyles are properly placed and only condyle rotation occurs. When the hinge movement is smoothly established,

initial contact is made with the patient's maxillary incisors contacting the operator's thumbnail. The operator slowly moves the thumb down the labial surface of the lower incisors while maintaining the hinge movement. Initial tooth to tooth contact is then permitted and this contact observed.

Usually the patient can detect this area of initial contact and the hygienist can request the patient to point toward the side of the mouth where teeth initially touch. Repeating the procedure can help verify the centric interference. This patient is then requested to "squeeze your teeth together." This will result in a slide from the interference in centric relation to maximum intercuspation at centric occlusion. This slide or deflection skid from centric relation to full occlusal contact may have several components of movement—vertical and anterior or lateral. The direction of movement and length or dimension of the deflection in millimeters can be determined, estimated, and recorded. Articulating paper can then be placed with the hygienist's free hand and the manipulation of the mandible repeated to identify the location of the occlusal incline causing the slide from centric relation to centric occlusion.

With the bilateral manipulation method the hygienist is seated behind the patient. The patient's head is stabilized between the operators side and arm in a way to keep the patient's head from moving. All four fingers of both hands of the hygienist are placed on the lower bony border of the mandible. The hygienist's thumbs are brought together in the midline over the symphysis of the chin. With patient's jaw in an open position, a gentle arcing of the mandible is achieved through thumb pressure. Only a short opening and closing are required to permit condylar rotation and seat the condyles in terminal hinge position. When the hygienist feels this free movement, then upward pressure is applied with the fingers and the patient should be asked if they feel any tenderness in the joint. If they feel any discomfort, the condyles are not braced correctly and the procedure must be repeated until the movement is free and painless. Then the mandible is closed until initial tooth contact occurs.

When the initial contact has been identified several arcs are made to confirm the presence of the interference. Then the patient again may be requested to squeeze the teeth together making the slide into centric occlusion from the interference. Directions and extent of the slide can be determined. Marking the area of interference with articulating paper is more difficult with the bilateral manipulative method since both of the hygienist's hands are required to guide the jaw. A chairside assistant must hold the paper.

Eccentric Determinations

Once centric interferences have been identified, it is possible to determine the lateral and protrusive excursions of the patient's mandible. These excursions are initiated from central occlusion with the teeth in maximal intercuspation or from centric relation. There are three types of functional patterns of tooth-to-tooth contacts. The side to which the mandible moves laterally is the functioning side, while the opposite side is referred to as the nonfunctioning side. In the most common excursive relation the mandibular cuspid and one or more posterior teeth on the functioning side contact their respective antagonists in the maxillary arch. This tooth to tooth lateral functional relation is termed group function since stress is distributed over a group of the teeth. Another common functional tooth contact pattern, particularly in young adults, is the cuspid to cuspid contact. Other anterior teeth also may guide this lateral movement, but no teeth posterior to the cuspids make contact. This pattern is termed cuspid guidance or canine guidance. The third, and least common pattern, is termed balanced occlusion. In this arrangement the majority of posterior teeth contact in lateral excursion. In

the natural dentition this occurs primarily with extensive attribution of the teeth. With the increasing life expectancy of the population, and with bruxism habits, this condition may occur more frequently in older individuals in the future.

As the patient moves from centric occlusion to the lateral excursive cusp tip to cusp tip end-point any mobility of teeth should be noted. Palpation of the teeth during these movements may detect any teeth receiving excessive forces. Articulating paper can be inserted on the functional side and the patient can then move laterally from centric occlusion to mark these areas of heavy contact.

While the patient moves from centric occlusion to lateral excursion on the functioning side, the hygienist should observe the opposite side of mouth for tooth contacts on the nonfunctional side. Ideally, there should be no contacts of teeth on the nonfunctional side because such contacts prohibit smooth, functional jaw movement. Such nonfunctional contacts are rare with cuspid protection but are common with balanced occlusion. Nonfunctional interferences can often be detected visually or by marking them with articulating paper. Such contacts also can be detected by placing dental floss posterior to the terminal molars and having the patient slide toward the functional side. If the floss, when pulled anteriorly, catches on the nonfunctional side then a nonfunctional contact is identified. Thin cellophane strips can also be used to locate nonfunctional contacts.

During protrusive mandibular movements the anterior teeth of both arches should make contact. It is desirable that at the end point of incisal edge tooth contact the forces be distributed over a number of anterior teeth, but this is not always possible. Interferences in the molar or premolar region may cause the jaw to be deflected toward the left or right in protrusive movement. Posterior tooth contact in protrusive movement is not desirable.

Occlusal Analysis

CR-CO	1	2	3	4	5	6	7	8	9	10	11	12	13	14	15	16
	32	31	30	29	28	27	26	25	24	23	22	21	20	19	18	17
RL	1	2	3	4	5	6	7	8	9	10	11	12	13	14	15	16
	32	31	30	29	28	27	26	25	24	23	22	21	20	19	18	17
LL	1	2	3	4	5	6	7	8	9	10	11	12	13	14	15	16
	32	31	30	29	28	27	26	25	24	23	22	21	20	19	18	17
Prot.	1	2	3	4	5	6	7	8	9	10	11	12	13	14	15	16
	32	31	30	29	28	27	26	25	24	23	22	21	20	19	18	17

Figure 6–32. Summary Findings of Occlusal Analysis. Note prematurity #5 and 29 contacting on centric relation (right side). Right lateral excursion shows canine-guided occlusion, #6 and 28 contacting, with no nonfunctional contact (interference) on left side. Left lateral shows group function with #11, 12, 13, 14 contacting #21, 20, 19, 18; a nonfunctional contact (interference) is noted on right side (#2, 31). As mandible moves from centric occlusion to protrusive, teeth #7, 8, 9 are shown contacting #26, 25, 24; occlusal stress is unevenly distributed over all the anterior teeth.

An occlusal chart is necessary to record tooth to tooth contacts in centric, functional, nonfunctional, and protrusive mandibular movements (Fig. 6–32). Interferences in centric relation position are recorded by circling the involved maxillary and mandibular teeth. The direction and extent of centric relation to centric occlusion can be noted on this chart or in the record. Tooth contacts in right or left function and corresponding nonfunction are circled on the appropriate teeth in the excursive portion of the chart. Protrusive tooth relations are circled in the protrusive diagram.

IMPRESSIONS AND STUDY CASTS

Stone study casts are valuable for diagnostic purposes, for patient education, and as a permanent record of the patient's presenting dental condition. The articulation of teeth as well as wear facets, dental attrition, plunger cusps, marginal ridge relations, and the occlusal plane of teeth can often be evaluated and studied more carefully on study casts than during clinical examination.

Increasingly, hygienists are being per-mitted by dental practice acts to secure impressions for the development of study casts. The procedure of impression taking is not difficult, but, as with all clinical procedures, it requires practice and attention to detail to gain accurate impressions that will result in excellent casts.

The patient should be draped with a plastic apron to prevent soiling of the clothing during taking of the impression, and the patient should be seated with the head erect and against the head rest. Chair height should be such that the hygienist will not be strained or stooped during the procedure. A cup of water or mouthwash should be available.

Proper selection of the correct sized metal perforated tray should be made. The largest tray that can be inserted comfortably in the patient's mouth is preferable because it permits a better distribution of impression material and can capture vestibular detail. The upper impression is generally secured first. An examination of the mouth should be made to note the height of the palatal vault and the presence of tori or exostoses. Insertion of the empty tray should be done in order to detect any impingement on teeth or soft tissues.

Mixing and spatulation of impression material is done according to manufacturers' specification. A powder dispenser and water dispenser are usually provided to ensure proper proportions. Use of cold water will cause the impression to set slower. Powder should be rapidly incorporated into the water in a rubber mixing bowl and spatulated until the mixture is cohesive and smooth. The patient may rinse with water or mouthwash just prior to insertion of the tray filled with impression material, or a gauze pad may be used to wipe saliva off the teeth that might result in bubbles in the impression. The preselected tray should be loaded from front to back with more of the material toward the front of the tray. A small amount of the impression material should be rubbed on the occlusal surface of the teeth with the hygienist's finger. Tray insertion is an upward and backward direction due to the labial inclination of the maxillary teeth. Make sure that the rim of the tray is under the patient's lip and impression material is in the vestibule. Care should be taken that the metal of the tray does not touch the teeth. The tray is held by the handle and should be positioned in line with the patient's nose. A saliva ejector can then be placed in the patient's mouth. Continue to hold the tray until the impression material is set.

By testing unused material in the mixing bowl the proper degree of set can be determined for tray removal. Remove the tray with a firm downward motion. A finger of the opposite hand should be placed between the tray and the mandibular teeth to avoid having the tray strike the teeth. As soon as the seal is broken, the tray is removed from the mouth and inspected for accuracy of detail. The tray can then be wrapped in a wet paper towel. Patients may rinse the mouth with mouthwash to remove loose particles of the impression material. Teeth should be examined and remnants of any interproximal material should be removed with an explorer.

Some patients are sensitive to the contact of impression material in the posterior part of the palate. Upper impressions primarily trigger the gag reflex. Admonishing the patient to breathe through the nose may alleviate the gagging symptoms long enough to secure a satisfactory impression. Do not attempt to remove an unset impression. Once gagging starts, the patient's head should be brought forward and lowered and the patient should be encouraged to continue nasal breathing. Another effective diversion is to tell the patient to lift both their legs off the chair and hold them stiff. This places strain on abdominal muscles and decreases gagging. Assure the patient before taking the impression that the material will set during the time one can hold one's breath comfortably. This fact helps eliminate anxiety on the patient's part regarding fear of choking during impression taking.

As with the upper impression, the lower arch should be carefully inspected prior to tray insertion and a tray try-in should be accomplished. Some difficulty is presented by the tendency of the impression material to flow due to gravity. Material should be well mixed, the tray loaded from the lingual aspect, the impression material wiped on the occlusal surface, and then the tray quickly inverted and carried to place. The tray is inserted into the mouth in a sideways manner because of tray width in relation to the average oral aperture of the patient. Once in the mouth, the path of insertion is downward and slightly forward to compensate for the axial inclination of the incisor teeth. As soon as the impression is seated, the patient is asked to stick out their tongue and then relax it thus registering the impression of the floor of the mouth. After the seal is broken and the lower impression is removed, the impression should be inspected for defects before accepting it as satisfactory. Any loose impression material in the mouth, especially interproximal remnants between the teeth, should be removed.

Impressions, placed in wet towels,

should be quickly transferred to the laboratory for pouring in dental stone. The details of carefully pouring of the stone, adequate vibration, and trimming of the hardened stone casts are familiar to all hygienists. The impressions should be poured as soon as possible to prevent distortion.

PHOTOGRAPHS

Clinical color photographs are becoming an integral part of the patient's records in many dental offices. The dentist may use selected oral photographs to plan treatment, document therapy, and for scientific presentations and articles. Many photographs are never taken by the dentist due to the pressures of time, and the hygienist trained in clinical photography can be of tremendous value. Demands on the hygienist for patient care may also prohibit the taking of clinical photographs, but the hygienists who master clinical photography are a valuable asset. Because of the variety of photographic equipment available, no attempt will be made here to describe clinical photographic technics.

Intraoral photography demands excellent photographic equipment, metal retractors, intraoral mirrors of various designs, and a great deal of practice. Extraoral photography, which shows the patient's face, requires patient consent that is best documented in writing by the patient. There is no question that good clinical photographs are an asset in patient and provider education, presentation of treatment plans, and in documentation of therapy. Individual dentists must decide on the value of photography in the office. Films can be filed with the patient record or in an office film library.

SUMMARY

Clinical determinations at initial examination provide an essential baseline from which to judge a patient's progress for years to come. It is a critical step in arriving at a diagnosis and developing a plan of therapy. Dental practices that omit a thorough clinical examination supported by quality radiographs are doomed to provide inadequate therapy based on inadequate information. Today's hygienist is superbly educated to accomplish a complete clinical examination, and this chapter has presented the technics, methodology, and documentation needed for such an examination. If you were to be a patient, in a dental practice would you agree to therapy without such a careful appraisal? The mature hygienist who values herself as a vital member of the dental health team must be willing to perform these demanding and exacting clinical examination procedures.

BIBLIOGRAPHY

Angle, E.H.: Classification of malocclusion, Dental Cosmos, 41:248, 1899.

Carwell, M.L. and McFall, W.T., Jr.: Centric relation determinations: Clinical and radiographic comparisons, J. Periodontol., 52:347, 1981.

Dawson, P.: Occlusal Problems, St. Louis, C.V. Mosby Co., pp. 54–61, 1974.

Geiger, A.: Occlusal studies in 188 consecutive cases of periodontal disease, Am. J. Ortho., 48:330, 1962.

Green, J.C. and Vermillion, J.R.: Oral hygiene index: A method for classifying oral hygiene status, J. Am. Dent. Assoc., 61:172, 1960.

Green, J.C. and Vermillion, J.R.: The simplified oral hygiene index, J. Am. Dent. Assoc., 68:7, 1964.

Greenstein, G.: The roe of bleeding upon probing in the diagnosis of periodontal disease, J. Periodontol., 55:684, 1984.

Hirschfeld, I.: Individual missing tooth: A factor in dental and periodontal diseases, J. Am. Dent. Assoc., 24:67, 1937.

Listgarten, M.A., Mao, R. and Robinson, P.J.: Periodontal probing and the relationship of the probe tip to periodontal tissues, J. Periodontol., 47:511, 1976.

Löe, H., Theilade, E. and Jensen, S.: Experimental gingivitis in man, J. Periodontol., 36:177, 1965.

McFall, W.T., Jr., Hutchens, L.H., Jr., Marshall, T.W. and Holland, J.C.: Periodontal activities and attitudes of dental care providers, J. Dent. Res., 62:228, 1983. Abstract #529.

McFall, W.T., Jr. and Morgan, W.C.: Effectiveness of a dentifrice containing formalin and sodium monofluorophosphate on dental hypersensitivity, J. Periodontol., 56:288, 1985.

Meitner, S.W., Zander, H.A., Iker, H.P. and Polson, A.M.: Identification of inflamed gingival surfaces, J. Clin. Periodontol., 6:93, 1979.

Miller, S.C. *Oral Diagnosis and Treatment Planning*, Philadelphia, P. Blakiston, p. 7, 1936.

Morgulis, J.R., and Oliver, R.C.: Developing a periodontal screening examination, Calif. Dent. Assoc. J., 7:59, 1979.

Norwicki, D., Vogel, R.I., Melcer, S. and Deasy, M.J.: The gingival bleeding time index, J. Periodontol., 52:260, 1981.

O'Leary, T.J., Drake, R.B. and Naylor, J.E.: The plaque control record, J. Periodontol., 43:38, 1972.

Pritchard, J.: *Advanced Periodontal Disease*, 2nd ed., Philadelphia, W.B. Saunders Co., pp. 142–147, 1972.

Ramfjord, S.P. and Ash, M.M.: *Occlusion*, 3rd ed., Philadelphia, W.B. Saunders Co., pp. 301–307, 1983.

Ritchey, B. and Orban, B.: The crests of the interdental alveolar septa, J. Periodontol., 24:75, 1953.

Shefter, G.J. and McFall, W.T., Jr.: Occlusal relations and periodontal status in human adults, J. Periodontol., 55:285, 1984.

Silness, J. and Löe, H.: Periodontal disease in pregnancy. II. Correlation between oral hygiene and periodontal condition, Acta Odont. Scand., 22:112, 1964.

Simpson, D.M., McFall, W.T., Jr., and Jewson, L.G.: Periodontal practice patterns of dental hygienists, J. Dent. Res., 63:307, 1984. Abstract #1228.

7

INSTRUMENTATION

Basic to the treatment of inflammatory periodontal disease is the removal of bacterial plaque and calculus from the surface of the teeth. These are the most frequent irritants and in most situations are the most significant cause of gingivitis or periodontitis. The clinical procedures utilized for the removal of deposits from the teeth are scaling, root planing, and polishing.

Scaling is the procedure designed to remove calculus by mechanically fracturing the deposit from the tooth surface. The removal of gross deposits is relatively simple. The removal of fine deposits, especially those which have formed in deep periodontal pockets, is exceedingly more difficult. The elimination of calculus and the associated plaque reduces greatly the irritation to the gingival tissue and permits the existing inflammatory response to resolve. In the case of edematous gingivitis, the gingivae usually heal completely and no further periodontal treatment is necessary. Where residual periodontal pockets are present, pocket elimination procedures are usually indicated.

Root planing is the procedure designed to eliminate roughness on the root surface and at the cementoenamel junction. Roots may be rough because of fine particles of calculus which remain following scaling, because of necrosis of cementum following the loss of periodontal ligament attachment in the pocket, because of defects in the cementum where Sharpey's fibers were previously inserted, because of areas of cemental resorption, or because of previous improper instrumentation. The cementoenamel junction is usually the roughest area of the tooth because of the imperfect union of enamel and cementum. Any irregularity on the tooth surface facilitates the formation and retention of bacterial plaque and calculus.

Increasing empirical data suggest that bacterial endotoxins either adhering to the cemental surfaces or embedded in the surface contribute significantly to the pathogenesis of periodontal disease. These substances may evoke a chronic inflammatory response in the periodontal tissue or may interfere with healing following debridement, or both. Meticulous root planing can remove the affected cementum and eliminate the associated endotoxins.

Polishing removes soft deposits and stains from the teeth and smooths the root surfaces. This helps prevent the recurrence of plaque and makes it easier for the patient to remove soft deposits by brushing. Prevention of plaque formation is important in controlling the occurrence of both periodontal disease and dental caries.

The clinical procedures of scaling, root planing, and polishing on a routine basis by the hygienist and adequate oral physiotherapy on the part of the patient are the most effective means available to prevent the development of periodontal disease. The greatest services which the hygienist performs are in association with these procedures.

CLINICAL PROCEDURES

Instruments

Hand instruments are divided into a working end or blade; a shank, which is a rigid connector of the blade to the handle; and the handle (Fig. 7–1). Handles are available in a variety of shapes and sizes. Instrument handles should be selected on an individual basis to provide the maximum ease and comfort for the hygienist. Handles approximately the diameter of a pencil with an irregular surface provide maximum control to prevent slipping of the instrument while in use.

The blades of the instruments are designed to perform different aspects of the scaling procedure. On the basis of the blade shape the instruments are divided into curettes, sickle scalers, hoes, files, and chisels.

The curette is a spoon-shaped blade with two sharp edges (Fig. 7–2). The edge of the blade with the greatest curvature is the one usually employed for scaling and root planing. The curettes are paired. One member

of the pair is used on the distal portion of a tooth and the other member is used on the mesial portion of that same tooth. Curettes are available in anterior and posterior sets (Fig. 7–3). The shanks of the posterior instruments are angled to provide access to the surfaces of the posterior teeth.

The curette is the most useful of all hand instruments. Several investigations have shown it to be superior to other instruments for fine scaling and root planing. The larger curettes such as the Younger-Goode instrument are utilized for the removal of gross deposits. Smaller curettes such as the Gracey instruments can be placed subgingivally, to the base of pockets, with minimal discomfort to the patient for the purpose of subgingival scaling and root planing.

The sickle scaler has a triangular-shaped blade with three sharp edges. Because of the relatively large size of the blade it can usually be employed only for supragingival scaling (Fig. 7–4).

The hoe has one working surface which is at a right angle to the shank. The shanks are bent at various angles to give access to different tooth surfaces. The hoe is used primarily for gross scaling, but it will negotiate some large pockets. The edges of the blade of the hoe frequently gouge the root surfaces. Rounding the corners of the edge before use prevents this from happening (Fig. 7–5).

The file has several short fine blades, all at right angles to the shank. The file may be used for root planing, but its most valuable use is for smoothing the cementoenamel junction. One of the main disadvan-

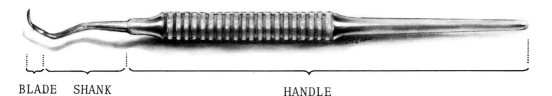

BLADE   SHANK   HANDLE

Figure 7–1.   Basic Parts of Periodontal Hand Instrument.

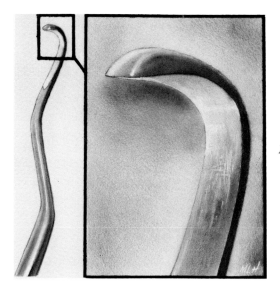

Figure 7–2.   Periodontal Curette.

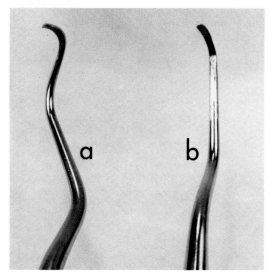

Figure 7–3.   Curettes.   Posterior (a) and anterior (b) curettes. The shank of the posterior instrument is shaped so as to allow access to the posterior teeth.

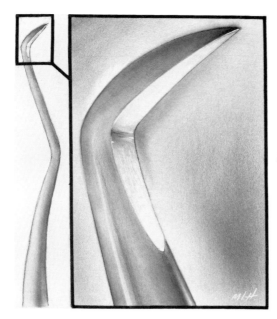

Figure 7–4.   Sickle Scaler.

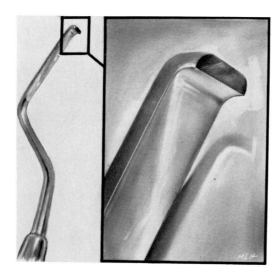

Figure 7–5.   Periodontal Hoe.

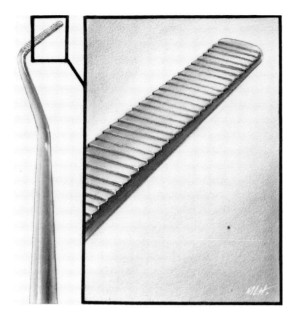

Figure 7–6.   Periodontal File.

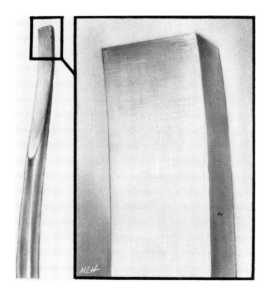

Figure 7–7.   Periodontal Chisel.

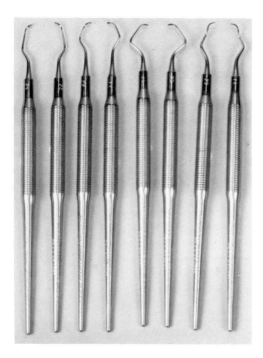

Figure 7–8. Gracey Curettes. This set of four pairs of curettes has been prepared especially for dental hygienists.

tages of the file is that it is extremely difficult to sharpen (Fig. 7–6).

The blade of the chisel is in the same general plane with the shank (Fig. 7–7). It has been used for the removal of gross deposits from the anterior teeth. Because of its limitation in use and potential traumatic capabilities, its use is not recommended.

For all practical purposes the curettes are the instruments of choice for scaling and root planing. They are available in various sizes to meet different clinical demands. They are available in sets so that all aspects of the tooth surface can be reached (Fig. 7–8). They can be easily and accurately resharpened.

Because scaling and root planing are arduous tasks which are quite demanding on the hygienist and the patient, attempts have been made to design *automatic instruments* for these purposes. Several such devices have appeared in the last few years, but the ultrasonic dental instrument (Cav-

itron) has been the most popular and best studied.

The ultrasonic dental instrument is a device for converting electric energy into sound waves. There are a series of metal strips called a stack in the handle of the instrument that are set into vibration because of an electromagnetic field produced by the electric current. The vibration results in the working tip of the instrument moving back and forth (reciprocating action) at the rate of 25 to 42 kilocycles per second. This is above the audible range for humans (greater than 20 kilocycles per second) and thus the term ultrasonics (Fig. 7–9).

Theoretically, the tip is not actually brought into contact with the deposit to be removed. A propagating medium of water or antiseptic solution is employed to transfer the sound waves from the instrument to the deposit. The reciprocating action of the tip creates microscopic bubbles in the propagating medium. This phenomenon is referred to as cavitation. The bubbles explode and the mechanical action produced by the vaporization process fractures the deposit from the tooth surface. In actual practice, the tip must contact the deposit or tooth surface to be effective.

It is extremely important that sufficient coolant be used with the ultrasonic instrument since considerable heat is generated by its action. The heat would result in soft-tissue damage. (A more recent ultrasonic unit has been developed which utilizes a piezoelectric crystal instead of a stack to reduce heat generation.) The propagating medium will serve as the coolant if copious amounts are used. Evacuation of the coolant is necessary. This usually requires a second person to assist the operator. The instrument should be used with light pressure since excessive tooth structure may be removed or gouging of the root structure may occur if pressure is applied directly to the tooth surface. Considerable instruction and practice on extracted teeth is indicated before the instrument is used

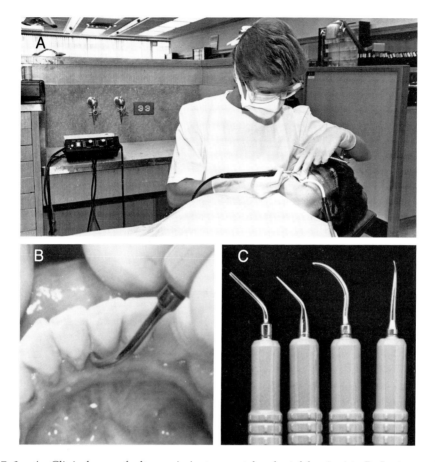

Figure 7–9. A, Clinical use of ultrasonic instrument by dental hygienist. B, Instrument tip in place. C, Assorted instrument tips.

clinically on a routine basis. The hygienist should always wear protective eyeglasses, face mask, and rubber gloves when using the ultrasonic instrument.

Before using the unit, the water line should be flushed of any residual water. The water line should be sterilized. The use of sterile membrane filters has been reported to eliminate microflora from the water for up to 48 hours (Dayoub, Rusilko, and Gross, 1978). Tuning of the instrument should be high enough to produce cavitation but as low as possible to reduce heat production.

The ultrasonic instrument is best used for the removal of gross deposits and stains from the teeth. A variety of tips have been designed in an attempt to provide instruments small enough to scale adequately in pockets. The tip should be directed as parallel to the tooth surface as possible, but at no greater than a 15° angle. This is to prevent roughening the root surface. The tip must be kept in constant contact with the surface and continuously moved with light brush strokes. In most instances, it is impossible to negotiate deep pockets adequately to the extent that fine deposits can be removed or the roots planed. Although the literature is inconsistent on the effectiveness and potential root surface damage of the ultrasonic device, it is our opinion that fine scaling and root planing are best done by hand instrumentation. It has been shown that even when flaps have been raised to gain access to the root surfaces, hand instrumentation was more effective than ultrasonics in removing calculus and smoothing roots (Hunter, 1984). The irrigating effect of the propagating medium is of definite benefit in the treatment of acute necrotizing ulcerative gingivitis. Patient reaction to the ultrasonic unit is favorable in some cases and unfavorable in others.

Several rotary instruments have been proposed as scaling devices. These are essentially modified burs used in a rotary type handpiece for the mechanical removal of deposits from the teeth. These instruments have not been studied sufficiently that their use clinically could be recommended. Preliminary studies indicate that they may remove too much tooth structure to be of practical application.

While the ultrasonic and rotary instruments have not proved themselves to be the answer to the clinical problems associated with scaling and root planing, they have opened avenues that may be more fruitful in the future.

HAND SCALING AND ROOT PLANING TECHNIQUES

General Considerations

The hygienist should approach each patient with a definite plan of what is to be accomplished on that particular appointment. Patients' needs vary with their clinical problem. Patients seen on recall appointments will probably receive a complete mouth scaling and oral care review in one appointment. A patient with advanced periodontitis will need several appointments of scaling and root planing prior to the other aspects of therapy.

There are several general considerations, however, that should be adhered to regardless of whether the treatment will be accomplished in one visit or in a series of appointments. First of all, it must be ascertained that there are no contraindications for performing the scaling procedure. Scaling results in the development of a

transient bacteremia in the majority of patients with gingival inflammation. Special precautions must be made for patients with certain medical problems to protect them from bacteremia (see Chapter 10).

The patient should be seated in a comfortable reclined position in the dental chair. The height of the chair is dependent on whether the hygienist prefers to operate in a standing or sitting position. The hygienist will find that she is less tired at the end of the day if she performs the major part of her treatment while sitting. Standing at intervals, however, is relaxing. Whether standing or sitting, the hygienist should maintain a good posture with her back straight. While standing, the body weight should be equally distributed on both legs.

The operating light should be adjusted to provide maximum intraoral illumination. If the hygienist is seated, most areas of the mouth can be viewed directly. This is desirable since scaling and planing can usually be accomplished faster and more efficiently if performed directly, rather than by operating while looking in a mouth mirror.

Eyeglasses and removable dental appliances should be removed from the patient prior to starting the scaling procedure. The hygienist should assume a position so that the working arm is below the level of her heart. This prevents the hand and arm from getting excessively tired.

The mouth should be divided into segments and each area scaled and planed in an orderly fashion. This procedure can be followed if all the teeth are to be scaled in one appointment or if it is going to take several appointments. Skipping from one area to another results in wasted time and does not insure complete removal of all deposits. A logical division of the arches is anterior and right and left posterior segments since most instruments are designed to be used either in the anterior or posterior area. Greater efficiency is gained if an instrument is used in all places indicated by its design before changing to another instrument.

Locating Deposits of Calculus

Drying the teeth with a jet of warm air helps expose supragingival calculus. Directing the jet into the sulcus aids in the visualization of subgingival deposits. The operating light should be sharply focused in the area under treatment. Areas where clinical signs of inflammation are evident should be carefully examined for subgingival calculus. Deposits in periodontal pockets usually cannot be seen, and the operator must rely on her tactile acuity to locate deposits on the root. The insertion with a light touch of explorers or sharp fine curettes into the pockets will disclose the roughness of deposits on the root surface. Grooves leading into furcation areas and concavities on the root surfaces are the most difficult areas for the location and removal of deposits. This is especially true in deep pockets.

Scaling and Root Planing

The application of topical anesthetics to the gingivae makes subgingival scaling and root planing more comfortable for the patient. The use of topical antiseptics, such as iodine lotion, may help reduce the frequency of bacteremias.

After the calculus is located, the instrument is carried to place to remove it. In general, instruments should be held with a modified pen grasp. This allows a firm grip to insure control of the instrument. It also provides fingertip acuity to assure adequate removal of the calculus.

Either the third or fourth fingertip, or both, should be used for the finger rests. These fingers should rest on teeth as close as possible to the one being scaled. This provides maximum control while the deposits are being removed. The teeth used for the rest should be kept dry to prevent slippage during the scaling stroke. Loss of control may result in laceration of the soft tissues. A gauze sponge may be placed over the teeth if keeping them dry otherwise is problematic.

Calculus should be removed by a short forceful stroke. The blade of the instrument is placed at the apical aspect of the deposit. The blade should form a 75 to 85 degree angle with the tooth (Fig. 7–10). A more acute angle will result in the blade slipping over the deposit. A more obtuse angle may result in gouging of the root. After the instrument is in position, the wrist is rotated so that the hand and the instrument blade are rotated coronally. Scaling by mere finger action is difficult and fatiguing. Deposits on the interproximal surfaces are usually removed by vertically directed stroke. Lingual or facial deposits may be removed by vertical or horizontal strokes (Fig. 11).

Patients present with various amounts of calculus deposition. Gross supragingival calculus, if present, should be removed first. These deposits are easy to locate and relatively easy to remove unless they have been present a long time. The larger curettes, sickle scalers, hoes, or the ultrasonic unit should be employed for the removal of gross deposits. Fine curettes may fracture if used to remove large, tenacious deposits. After sufficient experience it usually does not take long to gross scale the complete mouth.

After gross scaling, the mouth is divided into segments for subgingival scaling and root planing. Fine sharp finishing curettes are used for this purpose. It is not possible to insert large blades into the narrow confines of periodontal pockets to smooth the root surface adequately. The blade of the curette is inserted into the orifice of the sulcus or pocket and a light push stroke is used to carry it to the base. At the base of the pocket the blade is opened to form the 75 to 85 degree angle with the tooth. With a firm but gentle stroke, the instrument is held against the tooth and pulled to the cementoenamel junction. This is repeated until the root is smooth, indicating that it has been planed free of deposits and

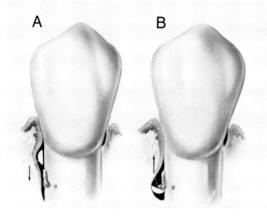

Figure 7–10. Removal of Subgingival Deposits. A, The instrument is carried with the blade closed to the apical aspect of the deposit. B, When in place the blade is opened to form a 75 to 85 degree angulation with the root surface and is then pulled coronally.

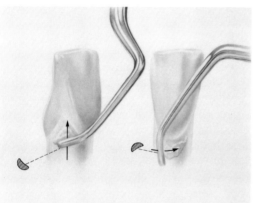

Figure 7–11. Basic Scaling Strokes. A, Vertical stroke—usually employed on proximal surface. B, Horizontal stroke—usually employed on facial and lingual surfaces.

roughness. The root planing strokes likewise are produced by the rotation of the wrist. The removal of subgingival calculus in the anterior area is shown in Figure 7–12 and in the posterior area in Figure 7–13.

Having the appropriate instruments arranged in an organized manner on the instrument table or stand will aid in performing an efficient scaling procedure. For example, if the anterior teeth are to be planed first, it is advisable to have the anterior curettes readily available in the order to be used. The instrument is placed on the aspect of the canine for which it is designed to be used and the planing is accomplished. It is then used on the lateral incisor and eventually on the canine on the other

side of the arch. It is used from both the lingual and facial aspects. Then the opposing anterior teeth are scaled and planed in a similar fashion. The other member of the pair of curettes is used to scale and plane the other aspect of the anterior teeth. Several different pairs of curettes may have to be used before the teeth are satisfactorily planed.

In some instances it is necessary to smooth the cementoenamel junction with files. The blade of the file is placed on the roughness and several short rapid strokes in a vertical or horizontal direction are applied to smooth it. This is followed by curetting to remove the scratches made by the file.

After the anterior teeth have been satisfactorily scaled, and planed, the proceduring is repeated on the posterior teeth using the curettes designed for that purpose. The placement of instruments on the teeth in various areas is demonstrated in Figure 7–14A through K.

Curettes which have been reduced in size because of several previous sharpenings should be available for use where teeth are crowded or malaligned to the extent that regular sized instruments are too large to gain access to the interproximal surfaces. In certain situations malaligned anterior teeth may be best planed by using posterior curettes. Likewise, the lingual surfaces of lingually inclined anterior teeth may be more easily planed with the contra-

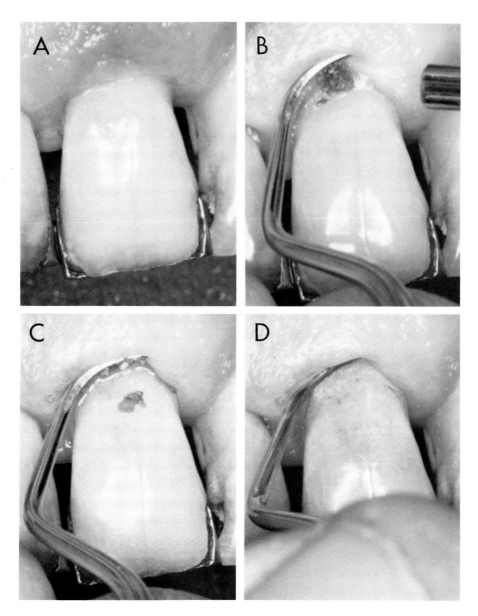

Figure 7–12. Removal of Subgingival Calculus in Anterior Area.   A, Calculus hidden on facial of tooth by gingiva. B, Exposure of deposit with curette in place to remove it. C, Large deposit is fractured from tooth. D, Fine scaling and root planing to remove all of deposit.

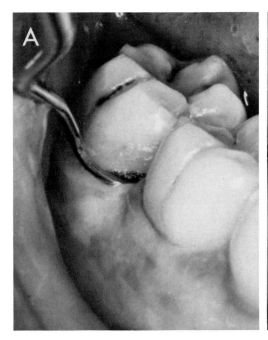 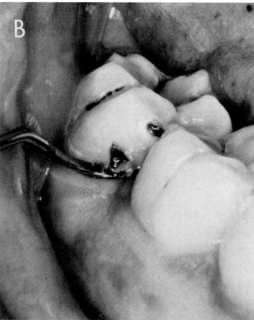

Figure 7–13.   Removal of Subgingival Calculus in Posterior Area.   A, Curette in place exposing deposit on mesial of second molar. B, Deposit of calculus and plaque is removed from tooth.

angled posterior instruments. In any situation where access is difficult to obtain with a straight shanked instrument, an instrument with an angled shank should be tried.

Frequently patients with periodontal disease will require several appointments to complete the scaling and root planing. One segment of the arch is treated in one appointment and the other segments in subsequent appointments. The areas previously treated should be reevaluated at the next appointment. Shrinkage of the gingival tissue which usually follows scaling may disclose deposits still present on the teeth. These deposits should be removed at the time. The areas previously scaled should be examined carefully under good light and in a dry field. Small fragments of calculus left behind are irritants and serve as centers for further calculus formation.

RESULTS OF STUDIES OF TISSUE RESPONSE FOLLOWING SCALING

Studies have indicated that teeth can be adequately scaled and root planed if a proper technique is employed. Sharp curettes have been shown to produce the smoothest root surfaces.

The inflammation in the connective tissue of the gingivae resolves within a few days following scaling. Chronic inflammatory cells will still be present at the base of periodontal pockets. Fragments of calculus and tooth tissue as well as debris and clumps of bacteria may be implanted into the gingival tissue.

Varying amounts of crevicular epithelium are removed by the scaling procedure. Reepithelialization occurs within 1 to 2 weeks following scaling.

Clinical studies have clearly shown that periodontal health is restored following scaling and root planing procedures if instituted adequately and before pockets have reached depths which make it impossible to gain access to the entire root structure. It has been shown also that long term beneficial results can be obtained (Ramjford, 1981; Badersten, 1981, 1984). With thorough root planing in pockets 5 to

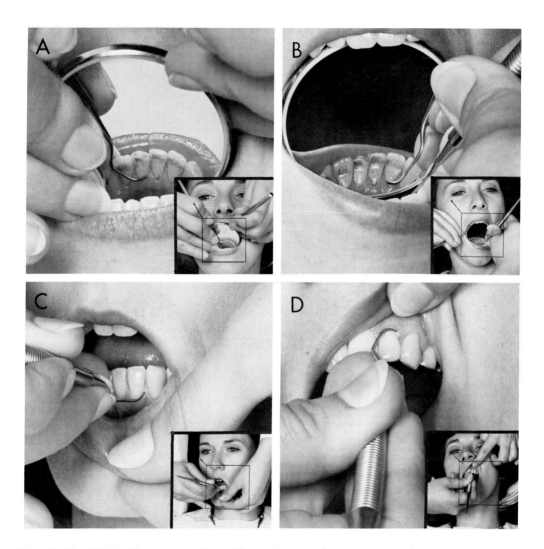

Figure 7–14. Clinical Instrumentation. These photographs demonstrate the instrument grasps, finger rests, patient's head positions, and lip and cheek retraction for scaling and planing in various areas of the mouth. The instruments are in the starting positions and would be moved by wrist and finger action to remove deposits from the appropriate aspects of the teeth. The positions of the instruments, finger rests, etc., would be the same for subgingival instrumentation.

A, Mandibular anterior lingual area. Direct approach. (The oversized mirror is used for demonstration purposes. Normally a conventional mirror is used to reflect light and displace the tongue.) B, Mandibular anterior lingual area. Indirect approach. Hygienist is in right front position looking into mirror. C, Mandibular anterior facial area. D, Maxillary anterior facial area. Facial aspect of left anterior teeth.

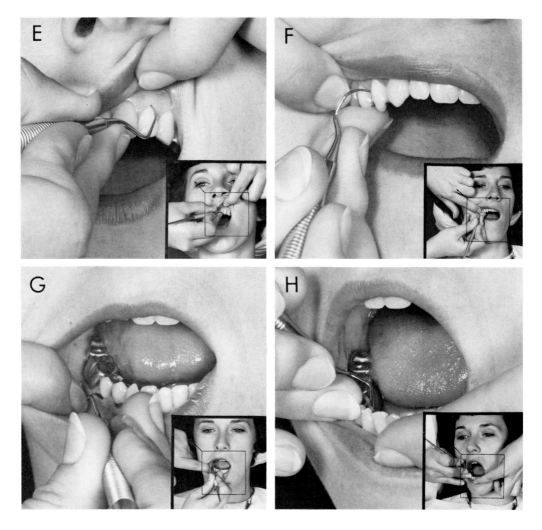

Figure 7–14. (Cont'd.). E, Maxillary anterior facial area. Mesiofacial aspect of left anterior teeth. F, Maxillary right posterior area. Facial and mesial aspects. G, Mandibular right posterior area. Facial and mesiofacial aspects. H, Mandibular right posterior area. Lingual aspect.

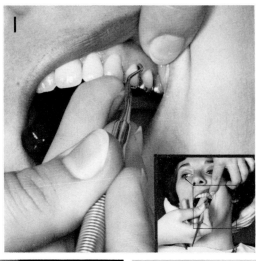

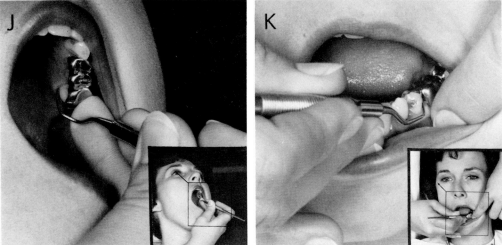

Figure 7–14 (Cont'd.). I, Maxillary left position area. Distal aspect. J. Maxillary left posterior area. Palatal aspect. K, Mandibular left posterior area. Distal aspect.

12 mm in depth, it was shown that gradual and marked improvement of the periodontal condition occurred over the 9-month period when plaque control was maintained (Badersten, 1984). In a study of 17 subjects more shallow pockets were produced when root planing was accomplished utilizing Widman or reversed bevel flaps, but that root planing alone produced slightly more gain of attachment (Isidor, 1984).

In time bacterial plaque will reestablish on the coronal and root surface. In a controlled study it was demonstrated that large numbers of spirochetes and motile rod organisms reestablished as early as 4 to 8 weeks. It was stated that these organisms were probably not completely eliminated by the original scaling and root planing (Magnusson, 1984).

PATIENT CONSIDERATION

The hygienist must constantly remember that she is performing a procedure on a human being. Extreme care must be given to prevent provoking the patient by a too rigorous approach to the clinical task. Extreme care must be given so that the tooth or the soft tissue around the tooth will not be injured. Several microscopic studies following scaling have shown that particles of calculus may be implanted into the gingival tissues. Care in scaling and frequent irrigation of the pockets while scaling will help prevent this from occurring.

A thorough scaling and root planing can be accomplished only if sharp instruments are used. The use of dull instruments results not only in an inadequate procedure, but in a waste of time and effort. Instruments should be checked at daily intervals and sharpened if needed. It may be necessary to sharpen instruments with a sterile stone during the course of the scaling procedure or to discard an instrument for a sharp one.

During the scaling procedure, the instruments will need to be wiped clean of fragments of calculus, plaque, and debris from time to time. A gauze sponge held in the nonoperating hand provides a convenient means of accomplishing this. Patients find it disagreeable to have instruments wiped on the towel draped around their necks. Frequent rinsing with warm water helps keep the area under treatment free of hemorrhage and debris and thus aids in making the tooth surfaces more visible. A dental assistant should assist the hygienist with patients who pose special problems in oral evacuation.

Adequate cheek and lip retraction with the mouth mirror will aid in gaining access to the different areas of the mouth. However, too vigorous retraction is uncomfortable to the patient. This will usually result in the patient contracting the facial muscles, making it extremely difficult to gain access to the teeth. If the patient does become tense, the hygienist should reassure the patient and ask him to relax. A very light retracting force will usually result in the patient relaxing the musculature.

Some patients experience sensitivity of the gingivae or teeth following scaling. Frequent rinsing with hot water for a day or two will allay gingival sensitivity. The management of dental sensitivity is discussed in Chapter 10.

POLISHING

The purpose of polishing is to remove stains and plaque from the teeth. Since this is usually done following scaling and root planing, it is a relatively simple procedure. Gross and tenacious stains should be removed with the ultrasonic unit or hand instruments. Sharp amalgam carvers or large curettes serve this purpose well (Fig. 7–15).

Most polishing agents consist of flour of pumice, glycerin, and coloring and flavoring agents. Flour of pumice alone mixed with water to a putty consistency may be used. Zirconium silicate has also been employed as a polishing agent.

The polishing agent applied to the teeth

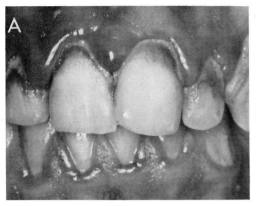

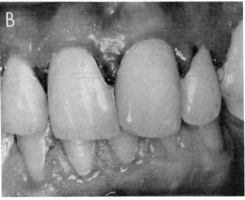

Figure 7–15. Polishing. A, Clinical situation of young patient with green stain and gross plaque on teeth. B, Three days following oral prophylaxis.

in a rubber cup or on a bristle brush in a prophylactic handpiece provides the most efficient way to polish the teeth. A slow speed and light pressure should be employed to reduce the amount of heat generated. Care must be taken not to let the rotating device damage the soft tissue. A systematic routine should be followed to assure that all areas will be polished. The rotation of the cup or brush often slings polish out of the patient's mouth. For this reason, the patient should be adequately draped to protect clothing.

In many instances the interproximal areas cannot be reached with the cups or brushes. These areas can be polished by placing the polishing agent in the facial and lingual embrasures and carrying it into the interproximal area with linen strips or dental tape. Portepolishers may also be used for this purpose. The wooden tips can be carved so that they fit the individual embrasures. These same methods of polishing may be used to polish around pontics or under solder joints of fixed restorations.

A customized handpiece, the Prophy-Jet, has been introduced as a more effective way to remove plaque and stains from the tooth surface. The handpiece emits an air jet which propels sodium bicarbonate particles in a 100°F water stream. It is recommended that the stream be applied about 1 cm from the tooth surface in 3 blasts of 5 seconds each. It has been reported that this device removes plaque and stains as effectively as conventional means but in less time (Weaks et al., 1984). In an in-vitro study of the use of the Prophy-Jet on root surfaces, it was reported that root structure was removed, leaving a smooth surface free of debris and connective tissue fibers (Atkinson, 1984).

It must be remembered that one of the primary purposes of polishing is to produce a smooth tooth surface to prevent plaque and calculus formation. It is important that all dental surfaces be polished.

Removable dental appliances should be examined to see if they need cleaning. Gross calculus deposits should be removed by careful scaling. The ultrasonic cleaning devices designed especially for the cleaning of removable appliances are excellent for further cleaning. The appliance may be repolished on a lathe or with a handpiece utilizing a watery mix of flour of pumice as the polishing agent. Extreme care must be taken to prevent distortion of the metal framework or clasps.

FINISHING OF DENTAL RESTORATIONS

It has previously been mentioned that restorations with nonphysiologic contours are frequent causes of local irritation to the gingival tissues. In some instances the only

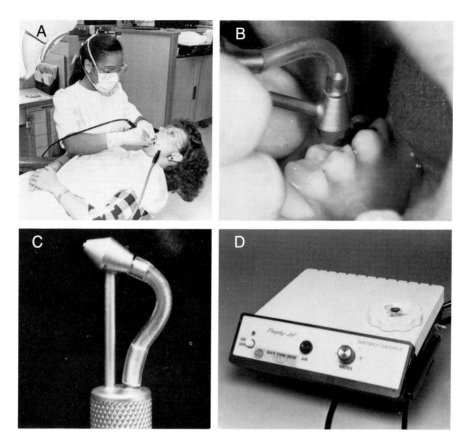

Figure 7–16. A, Clinical use of Prophy-Jet by dental hygienist. B, Placement of instrument in association with tooth surface. C, Instrument head. D, Control unit.

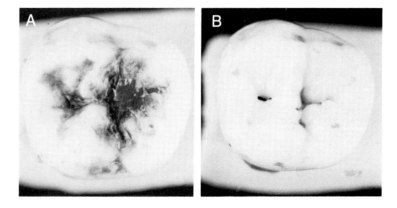

Figure 7–17. *Demonstration of stain removal from molar by Prophy-Jet.* A, Before. B, After.

solution is replacement of the restoration. In many instances, however, the discrepancy in the restoration can be corrected.

Gingival overhangs of amalgam restorations are the most frequently encountered defects which can be corrected. The presence of the overhang can be determined by careful study of the radiographs or by running the tine of an explorer over the margin. A sharp amalgam knife or sickle scaler is used to remove the overhang. The blade of the instrument is placed apically to the defect. A short, coronally directed stroke will shave off part of the overhang. This is repeated until the restoration is carved into harmony with the tooth surface. The margin is then finished with sandpaper strips and linen strips. The margin should be carefully examined with a sharp explorer to ascertain that the overhang has been completely removed and that the cavity preparation has not been exposed.

Most of the occlusal and proximal margins of restorations can be finished with large round burs or stones. The rotary instrument should be run at moderate speeds and a light pressure used. Only the excess marginal restorative material should be removed. The occlusal anatomy of the restoration is redefined using small round burs and finishing burs. This consists primarily of creating the central fossal groove and mesial and distal grooves. These grooves aid in the excursion of food from the occlusal surface of the tooth. Marginal ridges should be formed and trimmed to be at the same level of the marginal ridges of the adjacent teeth. Occlusal embrasures, if not already present, should be created. These features help to prevent food impaction from occurring interdentally.

After the anatomic considerations are fulfilled, the restoration should be polished. The surface is smoothed using a watery mix of flour of pumice applied in a rotating rubber cup. Tin oxide or zirconium silicate is likewise applied to produce a glossy polish to the amalgam restoration (Fig. 7–18).

Restorations tarnish and require repolishing from time to time. Whenever restorations are finished or polished, care must be taken that the occlusal relationship with the opposing teeth not be altered.

INSTRUMENT SHARPENING

Proficient instrumentation depends primarily on two basic factors: the skill of the operator and the quality of the instruments used. The most important quality of an instrument is its degree of sharpness. The time required to sharpen instruments is greatly compensated for by the time saved while scaling and root planing. The clinical procedures are made considerably easier for the operator and the patient.

The sharpness of a scaling instrument is dependent upon the acuteness of the angle formed by the two sides of the blade which meet to form the cutting edge. An instrument becomes dull when this edge is rounded over by use and the acute angle is lost.

The sharpness is regained by removing enough metal from the blade to recreate the edge. This may be accomplished on a hand stone, by use of a rotary sharpening stone or a combination of both. Several types of hand stones are available in various shapes. Arkansas, diamond grit hones, and aluminum oxide ceramic are most popular. Cylinders of different sizes and shapes as well as flat, contoured, and grooved stones have been designed to facilitate the sharpening of different instruments. All will sharpen instruments if used correctly. Most manufacturers provide excellent instructions with the sharpening device. It has been demonstrated that if the original shape of the instrument is maintained, a 20% reduction can be made without significantly weakening the instrument (Murray, 1984).

It is recommended that a neophyte practice initially on instruments to be dis-

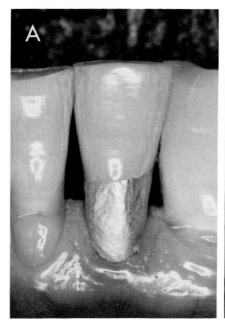
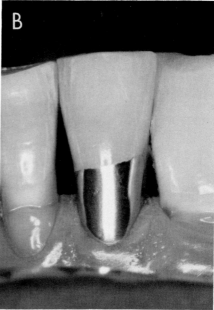

Figure 7–18. Finishing Amalgam Restoration. Class V restoration of mandibular incisor. A, Before polishing. B, After polishing. (Courtesy Dr. W.D. Strickland, *The Art and Science of Operative Dentistry.* The Blakiston Division, McGraw-Hill Book Co., 1968.)

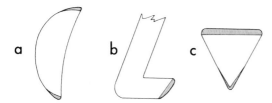

Figure 7–19. Sharpening Periodontal Scalers. The cutting edges have become rounded by use and are dull. The shaded areas indicate the metal which must be removed to create a new sharp edge. a, Curette, b, Hoe, c, Sickle scaler.

carded. The sharpening tool and instrument should be firmly grasped. A good light source should be utilized. Uniform reduction of the blade and retention of the original design prevent weakening of the instrument. The shaded areas in Figure 7–19 show how the various scaling instruments should be sharpened. A 70° to 80° cutting edge should be obtained for scalers. This provides optimal scaling efficiency. Care must be taken not to oversharpen. This results in creating a point at the end of the blade. It is most important not to grind the face of the curette since this weakens the instrument.

The most efficient way of determining if an instrument is sharp is by visual examination. Dull instruments present a blunt, rolled cutting edge. The cutting edge is not readily visible on a sharp instrument because of the acuteness of the angle. The ease with which a plastic test stick or an extracted tooth can be planed is another test for sharpness.

Instruments should be sharpened frequently. If this suggestion is adhered to, only a few strokes are necessary each time to keep instruments in good operating condition. A sterile sharpening stone should always be available to sharpen instruments in use at the dental chair. The backlog of dull instruments may be sharpened between patients or when there is a cancellation.

SUMMARY

The removal of deposits from the surfaces of the teeth is essential in the prevention and treatment of periodontal diseases. The degree to which the inflammatory process will resolve is dependent upon the thoroughness with which the deposits are removed. To be effective the scaling and planing procedures must be done with meticulous methodology and with small, sharp instruments.

BIBLIOGRAPHY

Atkinson, D.R., Cobb, C.M., and Killoy, W.J.: The effect of an air-powder abrasive system on in-vitro root surfaces, J. Periodontol., 55:13, 1984.

Badersten, A., Nilveus, R., and Egelberg, J.: Effect of nonsurgical periodontal therapy. 1. Moderately advanced periodontitis, J. Clin. Periodontol., 8:57, 1981.

Badersten, A., Nilveus, R., and Egelberg, J.: Effect of nonsurgical periodontal therapy, J. Clin. Periodontol., 11:63, 1984.

Clark, S.M.: The ultrasonic dental unit. A guide for clinical application of ultrasonics in dentistry and dental hygiene, J. Periodontol., 40:621, 1969.

Dayoub, M.B., Rusilko, D.J., and Gross, A.: A method of decontamination of ultrasonic scalers and high speed handpieces, J. Periodontol., 49:261, 1978.

DeNucci, D.J. and Mader, C.L.: Scanning electron microscopic evaluation of several resharpening techniques, J. Periodontol., 54:618, 1983.

Green, E., and Seyer, P.C.: Sharpening Curets and Sickle Scalers, 2nd Ed., Berkeley, Ca., Praxis Publishing Co., 1972.

Hinrichs, J.E., et al.: Effects of scaling and root planing on subgingival microbial proportions standardized in terms of their naturally occurring distribution, J. Periodontol., 56:187, 1985.

Hunter, R.K., O'Leary, T.J., and Kafrawy, A.H.: The effectiveness of hand versus ultrasonic instrumentation in open flap root planing, J. Periodontol., 55:697, 1984.

Isidor, F., Karring, T., and Attstrom, R.: The effect of root planing as compared to that of surgical treatment, J. Clin. Periodontol., 11:669, 1984.

Magnusson, I., et al.: Recolonization of a subgingival microbiota following scaling in deep pockets, J. Clin. Periodontol., 11:193, 1984.

Moskow, B.S.: The response of the gingival sulcus to instrumentation: a histological investigation. 1. The scaling procedure, J. Periodontol., 33:282, 1962.

Murray, G.H., et al.: The effects of two sharpening methods on the strength of a periodontal scaling instrument, J. Periodontol., 55:410, 1984.

Pameijer, C.H., Stallard, R.E., and Hiep, N.: Surface characteristics of teeth following periodontal instrumentation: A scanning electron microscope study, J. Periodontol., 43:628, 1972.

Rabbani, G.M., Ash, M.M., and Caffesse, R.G.: Effectiveness of subgingival scaling and root planing in calculus removal, J. Periodontol., 52:119, 1981.

Ramfjord, S.P.: Longitudinal evaluation of periodontal therapy, Quintescence International, 12(V):43, 1981.

Rogosa, M., et al.: Blood sampling and cultural studies in the detection of postoperative bacteremias, J. Am. Dent. Assoc., 60:171, 1960.

Suppopat, N.: Ultrasonics in periodontics, J. Clin. Periodontol., 1:206, 1974.

Van Volkinburg, J.W., Green, E., and Armitage, G.C.: The nature of root surfaces after curette, cavitron, and alpha-sonic instrumentation, J. Periodont. Res., 11:374, 1976.

Weaks, L.M., et al.: Clinical evaluation of the Prophy-Jet® as an instrument for routine removal of tooth stain and plaque, J. Periodontol., 55:486, 1984.

Willmann, D.E., Norling, B.K., and Johnson, W.N.: A new prophylaxis instrument: Effect on enamel alterations, J. Am. Dent Assoc., 101:923, 1980.

Chapter

8

ORAL PHYSIOTHERAPY

Microbial plaque plays a dominant role in the causation of both dental caries and periodontal disease. Most preventive measures are directed toward the elimination of plaque or the minimization of its effects. One of these methods is oral physiotherapy.

Oral physiotherapy refers to those procedures practiced on a regular basis by the individual to maintain mouth health. Effective oral care activity on the part of the patient is critical for the maintenance of health of the teeth and periodontium. The dental hygienist has a strategic role in teaching and promoting patient self-care.

Physiologic Cleansing Factors

Certain natural cleansing mechanisms are provided in the design of the tissues and fluids of the oral cavity. Prominent among these is muscular activity of cheeks, lips and tongue which in combination with salivary flow throughout the mouth provides a flushing mechanism that aids in the removal of food debris. In addition to the mechanical flushing action, saliva also possesses bacteriostatic properties that help control the harmful effects of bacteria. Normal occlusal embrasures in contact areas serve to direct food lingually or facially during mastication facilitating oral clearance and preventing food impaction.

Some foodstuffs such as apples and carrots have been cited as having natural cleansing properties. It has been demonstrated that such detersive foods do not remove plaque or promote gingival health in the absence of adequate oral hygiene measures. The inclusion of fibrous foods in the diet is beneficial to substitute for softer plaque-promoting foods especially those containing sucrose. Detersive foods also provide greater stimulation of the periodontal tissues and enhance salivary flow and in this way promote a healthier environment. The nutrient value of fresh fruits and vegetables in promoting periodontal health is also a consideration.

Athough natural factors may help in maintaining mouth hygiene, these physiologic mechanisms are not sufficient in themselves to protect oral tissues from local irritants (Fig. 8–1).

Objectives of Oral Physiotherapy

Diligent oral care techniques accomplish both a cleansing action and gingival stimulation, which are required in order to achieve the highest level of health.

As indicated in Chapter 3, bacterial

158

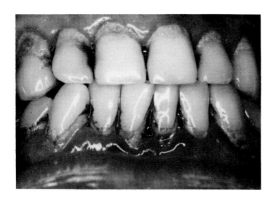

Figure 8–1. Poor Oral Hygiene. This patient has neglected his mouth for some time and has severe periodontal disease.

plaque is primary in the etiology of periodontal inflammation as well as of dental caries. Oral physiotherapeutic efforts should be directed toward removal or prevention of plaque accumulation. With the advent of the use of antimicrobial substances directed against specific oral pathogens, an additional objective could be the reduction of plaque pathogenicity.

Rate of plaque formation, the microbial quality of plaque and susceptibility to its harmful effects all vary considerably on an individual basis. The design of an oral hygiene regimen for a given patient should be based on careful consideration of these factors on an individual basis:

Definite psychologic and social benefits accrue from an active oral physiotherapy program. These include improved appearance, refreshed breath and taste, and a sense of personal cleanliness.

Gingival stimulation is a secondary benefit from effective oral physiotherapy measures. Massage of gingival tissues either with soft tissue bristles or adjunctive aids increases blood circulation and promotes a healthier gingival tone, texture and topography.

TOOTHBRUSHES AND TOOTHBRUSHING

The fundamental tool for oral physiotherapy is the toothbrush. The type of toothbrush recommended depends on method employed, intraoral limitations to access and manipulative ability of the patient. For general use, a toothbrush with a straight handle about 5 to 6 inches long with soft polished nylon bristles of equal length and approximately ½ inch in height is preferred. The size of the brush head may vary somewhat, but, in general, it should be small enough to reach crowded areas of the arch yet large enough to include several teeth in the brushing stroke. Variations in size and design are appropriate to accommodate individual needs and preferences as long as effective use without tissue damage can be taught and demonstrated.

Most toothbrush bristles are made of nylon filaments ranging in texture from soft to firm. Bristle types may be polished or unpolished. Bristles may exhibit 2 or 3 rows of spaced tufts or may be multitufted with 4 or 5 rows of closely spaced tufts (Fig. 8–2). Hard natural swine bristles also may be available and many patients may prefer this type of brush. It has been demonstrated, however, that when used improperly, the hard bristle brush can cause extensive gingival recession and abrasion of exposed root surfaces. Patients should be discouraged from using the hard bristle brush since nylon bristles have been shown to have equal or greater cleaning ability. Careful instructions in proper use of a hard brush should be provided for patients who continue to be resistant to such a recommended change.

Frequency of Toothbrushing

Recommendations for frequency of tooth cleansing have ranged from several times per day to once every 2 days in order to control harmful effects of bacterial plaque. The state of oral health, susceptibility to oral disease, diet and presence of contributory factors such as reduced salivary flow are considerations in determining an optimal frequency of toothbrushing for an individual patient. One study conducted for

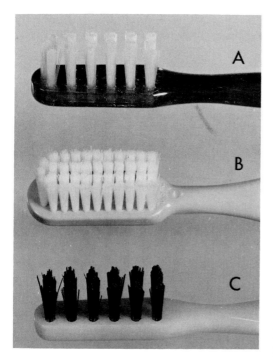

Figure 8–2. Toothbrushes. A comparison can be made between A, a soft nylon brush; B, a medium multitufted nylon brush; and C, a hard natural bristle brush.

6 weeks using dental students as subjects determined that plaque removal every other day was adequate to maintain gingival health in this population. Gingival index scores routinely increased with less frequent oral hygiene. Even once per day may not, however, be effective in preventing dental caries in a susceptible patient nor in maintaining periodontal health in a different patient group.

Optimally, plaque removal after any intake of food or carbohydrate-containing beverage should occur. This approach should be strongly encouraged for any patient who has a demonstrated risk for dental disease. For patients who are at low risk for oral disease, emphasis should be placed on thorough plaque removal twice per day.

Toothbrushing Patterns

Although some minimal amount of time is required for adequate toothbrushing, there is not necessarily an increase in effectiveness with an increase in time. It is more important that a systemic sequence of brushing be established by the patient and that this is followed using multiple and overlapping strokes on all surfaces to ensure cleaning. In a study conducted by MacGregor and Gunn, 115 subjects in two age groups (11 to 13 years and 18 to 22 years) were observed brushing their teeth unaware that this activity was being recorded on videotape. Patterns of brushing in both groups were similar. Most subjects initiated brushing on anterior facial surfaces and used more brushing strokes on these surfaces. Of particular note was that lingual surfaces were rarely brushed in either group.

A suggested pattern can be given to the patient. One such method is to instruct the patient to start with the lower right posterior area on the lingual surface. As indicated in the above study, this is an area often ignored by many individuals. The lingual surfaces of the mandibular anterior and left posterior areas are then brushed. The same pattern is then followed on the facial surfaces. Brushing the occlusal surfaces of the lower teeth completes the mandibular brushing cycle. A similar technique is followed in the maxillary arch.

Several methods of toothbrushing have been suggested in order to fulfill the objectives stated previously. Selection of brushing techniques is dependent upon the clinical situation and the ability and motivation of the patient.

Bass Method

The Bass method of toothbrushing is designed to minimize accumulation of plaque and to cleanse the gingival crevice. An extremely soft nylon bristled brush is used in order not to injure delicate soft tissues. Bristles are inserted into the crevice at approximately a 45 degree angle to the long axis of the tooth and a jiggling or stimulatory motion is exerted. Each placement of the brush covers an area of about two teeth. Several short strokes should be made for each placement. The brush is moved around both dental arches until all teeth are reached.

The Bass toothbrushing method, also referred to as sulcular or intrasulcular brushing, effectively removes and prevents subgingival plaque in accessible crevices (less than 2.5 mm). Use of this method has been shown to increase the level of keratinization of crevicular epithelium although the significance of this to establishing a stronger barrier to toxic bacterial products is questionable. When compared to a roll method of toothbrushing, no overall difference in plaque removal was noted; however, the Bass method was more effective in the cervical thirds of teeth.

Regular removal of supragingival plaque has been demonstrated to prevent gingivitis and the extent to which additional subgingival brushing is indicated is not clear. If subgingival plaque accumulates as an extension of supragingival plaque as has been proposed, then the greater emphasis should be placed on supragingival techniques, especially for patients exhibiting healthy gingiva with shallow crevices.

The potential for damaging the gingival tissue using intrasulcular brushing techniques has been documented. Histologic evaluation of gingiva after periods of intrasulcular brushing revealed a mild to moderate inflammatory infiltrate in the absence of plaque and some detachment of junctional epithelium. Neither of these alterations were associated with loss of attachment. Mastery of the Bass toothbrushing technique is difficult for most patients to achieve. In studies just described, it was noted by the investigators that intensive instruction and reinforcement were needed before dental student subjects could adequately practice this technique. A further observation was that lighting conditions in the home environment compromised the ability of the individual to brush efficiently at home using the Bass method although proficiency could be demonstrated in the office setting.

A modification of the Bass method of toothbrushing often referred to as Modified Bass has gained widespread popularity in recent years. This alteration employs a supplemental rolling stroke after the application of the intrasulcular short vibratory strokes described by Bass.

The utilization of the Bass method or its modification should be recommended to patients only after careful consideration of the patient's ability and motivation. A commitment should be made to reevaluate the patient's use of this technique as well as assess for tissue damage and effectiveness in plaque removal on a regular basis.

Other Brushing Methods

Press-roll methods of toothbrushing are well-suited for healthy mouths in which the interproximal tissues fill the embrasure areas. These techniques, for example the modified Stillman or McCall method, employ pressure on the gingiva followed by a roll of the brush head to cleanse the teeth. A medium textured nylon brush is used with these techniques.

Spaces may occur interproximally as the result of disease, gingival recession, or periodontal surgery. Such areas represent a more apical gingival position and the open areas may trap food. Charter's method is a desirable technique in this type of mouth and in cases of cervical erosion or crater formation subsequent to necrotizing ulcerative gingivitis.

In this technique, the brush is positioned so that the bristles are pointed occlusally at a 45 degree angle. The sides of the bristles, rather than the points, should be placed against the soft tissues. Vibratory movement extends the bristles into the interproximal spaces. Four to six applications of the brush for each embrasure with this same vibratory motion are sufficient for massage and cleansing. Progressive repositioning of the brush is required. Occlusal surfaces are cleansed with rotary motion.

This method is most suited for the facial surfaces of the teeth and is a difficult one for the patient to master. It should not be used when papillae fill the embrasure and gingiva is at normal levels.

Various other toothbrushing methods have been suggested in order to accomplish better oral cleanliness. In the Fones method the teeth are held together and facial surfaces are scrubbed with the brush moving circularly and the bristles directed perpendicularly to the long axis of the teeth. In a technique termed the "Physiologic Method," a soft brush rotated from occlusal edges toward the gingiva simulating food passage is utilized.

More permissive brushing methods have recently been developed which depend upon use of disclosing agents. With these systems the patient is urged to remove the plaque which has been dyed to allow its visualization. These methods stress more self-control on the part of the individual. Usually a soft nylon bristled brush is employed, and any stroke which accomplishes plaque removal is acceptable.

For the maintenance of periodontal health, the objectives of toothbrushing are to prevent plaque accumulation at the gingival margin without causing traumatic damage to oral tissues. Although the Bass method appears to be slightly superior in removing plaque at the gingival margin, other methods also may be adequate to fulfill these objectives. Selection and recommendations for toothbrushing should in all cases be based on individual needs, ability and motivation. Reinforcement and reevaluation are key features in the implementation of an effective oral hygiene program on the part of the patient.

No toothbrushing method has been demonstrated to adequately clean proximal surfaces. Supplementation with interproximal cleaning aids is necessary for achievement of total plaque removal.

Habitual brushing of the masticatory mucosa of the hard palate and specialized mucosa of the tongue has been shown to improve overall mouth hygiene. Bacteria are retained on these surfaces which contribute to increased numbers of microorganisms in the mouth. Generally brushing of these surfaces also limits plaque deposits on the teeth.

Brushing of the palate and tongue should be accomplished with the brushing stroke from the back of the mouth toward the front. This minimizes the tendency for gagging. Individuals with heavy smoking habits may particularly benefit from this brushing technique. Mucosal brushing reduces halitosis, decreases stain on the tongue, and improves periodontal health.

Automatic Toothbrushes

Automatic toothbrushes have been developed in number and have caught the fancy of the general public. Although expensive when compared with conventional brushes, these automatic devices have gained wide acceptance and many brands are now available.

Automatic toothbrushes may employ arcuate (up and down), horizontal (back and forth), or elliptic (oval) types of stroke action. The arcuate motion simulates the action of the Modified Stillman-McCall method of brushing, while the horizontal mechanism somewhat resembles the Modified Charter's brushing method. The elliptic type of motion represents a combination of brushing actions.

Power is gained for brush movement by either battery source or electric current. Many of the automatic brushes employ the principle of rechargeable energy source such that the brushing device is not connected directly to the current. Battery-operated toothbrushes offer safety, but have the disadvantage of requiring the periodic replacement of batteries.

Most automatic brushes have a relatively small brush head. While this limits the number of teeth covered by the bristles in any one area, it does offer the advantage of access in constricted areas. This feature may be of particular value on the lingual surface of mandibular teeth where calculus is prone to form.

Patients should be instructed to follow a definite sequence of brush placement with the automatic toothbrushes. Many more strokes are accomplished in a shorter span of time with the automatic brushes. There is a tendency to move the automatic brushes too rapidly thus skipping areas. It is suggested that the patient bring the brush to the office and demonstrate the brushing method employed.

With the power generated by the automatic brush the potential for damage to either tooth or gingiva may be increased. This chance of damage is greater if hard bristles are used. Firm bristles are available, but most of the bristles are of the medium or soft nylon type.

While there have been reports of the superiority of automatic brushes when compared with ordinary brushes, most of the long-term studies have not shown the automatic brushes to be any more effective. Evaluation of histologic changes does not demonstrate any appreciable difference in tissue response when manually operated and automatically powered brushes are compared.

In certain individuals the automatic brushes do appear to offer some special advantages. These brushes may be of value in encouraging children or hygienically lazy adults to brush their teeth. Also automatic brushes are helpful in handicapped or debilitated individuals.

A newer type of automatic toothbrush which utilizes small rotating brush heads designed to reach specific areas of the teeth is now available. One reported study comparing this and a conventional brush using a Bass brushing technique found no significant difference in plaque removal. Additional investigations are ongoing.

AUXILIARY AIDS

In addition to the toothbrush, many products have been developed to assist either in cleansing or in gingival stimulation. These ancillary aids are intended to supplement the action of the toothbrush, *not to supplant it.*

Disclosing Stains and Tablets

In order to help visualize the bacterial mass a variety of stains have been developed to color the teeth where the plaque exists. Originally this was intended for chairside instruction of the patient, and solutions containing dyes were applied with cotton swabs. These solutions included basic fuchsin, iodine, and Bismark brown.

Development of disclosing tablets using a dyestuff, erythrosin, ushered in a new method of patient education and motivation. With the use of the tablets the individual is able to judge his own brushing efficiency at home.

By chewing, the tablets are broken down and dissolved in the saliva. The mixture of dyestuff and saliva is swished around the mouth. Wherever bacterial plaque is present, a bright red stain appears. The color fades within an hour because the dye is water soluble (Fig. 8–3).

With the utilization of these tablets the patient's toothbrushing method may be modified to simply scrubbing off all of the red material. The frequency of tablet use is dependent upon the effectiveness of the individual in brushing. Those who practice good oral care habits may need to check themselves only once a week. Less proficient brushers may need to use the tablets more frequently.

In order to avoid gingival laceration or tooth abrasion with this "free" brushing style, a modified medium or soft nylon brush is employed. This multitufted brush has bristles of uniform length which have rounded ends. Such a brush causes a minimal amount of damage yet provides suitable brushing efficiency. A comparison of bristles can be made by looking at them under a magnifying glass or dissecting microscope.

Erythrosin stain is now also available in

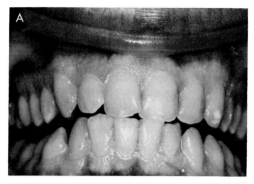

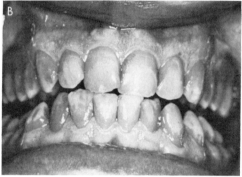

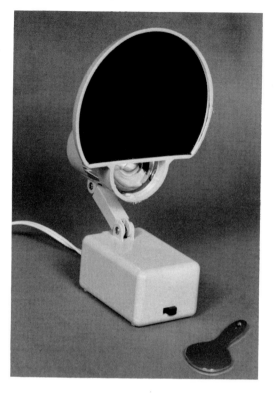

Figure 8–3. Value of Disclosing Stain. A, Appearance of the patient prior to the use of disclosing stains. B, Presence of heavy bacterial plaque.

Figure 8–4. Tools for Patient Self-Examination. With the use of a light source with a mirror attachment and an intraoral mirror, the patient can closely evaluate his oral physiotherapy.

an easily used liquid form. Other dyestuffs may stain plaque blue or purple to provide contrast with gingival color. One dyestuff, fluorescein, is only visible when a special filtered light is used.

Effectiveness in oral physiotherapy is increased when an individual is able to view the stained material on the teeth. Inexpensive mirrors can be supplied the patients to facilitate personal intraoral examination. Light sources equipped with mirrors can also be successfully used by the patient (Fig. 8–4).

Interproximal Plaque Removal

A number of devices have been developed to aid in the removal of interdental plaque. Even diligent use of the toothbrush may not be sufficient to adequately eliminate plaque occurring between the teeth. When papillae fill the gingival embrasures,

plaque may accumulate in the col areas and contribute to the start of disease processes. Often due to positional relations, there may be spaces, diastemas, or open contacts between the teeth. Gingival levels may be located in a more apical position on the teeth as the result of periodontal disease or surgery.

Dental floss and tape are the most useful interproximal cleansing aids. Other aids include interproximal brushes, soft balsa wood wedges, and modified toothpick holders. All can have specific application dependent upon the individual's particular needs (Fig. 8–5).

DENTAL FLOSS AND TAPE. For most patients the use of dental floss or tape to supplement toothbrushing is adequate to achieve complete plaque removal. A num-

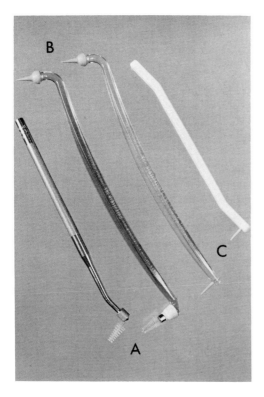

Figure 8–5. Interproximal Dental Aids. A, Small interproximal brushes. B, Interdental stimulator tips. C, Holders for wooden tips. All may be useful in interproximal care.

ber of studies have compared the plaque removal ability and effects on gingival health of waxed and unwaxed floss and have essentially found no differences in their effectiveness. Recommendations should be based on tightness of contacts, restorative quality, patient preference, and reevaluation of effectiveness.

In providing instructions in the use of dental floss, patients should be cautioned against "snapping" the floss through the contact areas and potentially injuring gingival tissues. The floss or tape should be "wrapped" to adapt to the contour of the proximal surface and used in an up and down motion to clean the surface extending into the gingival crevice (Fig. 8–6). Special floss-holding devices are available for individuals who have difficulty mastering this technique (Fig. 8–7).

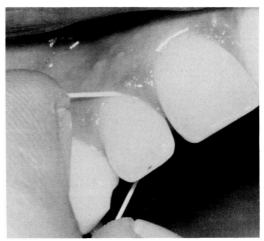

Figure 8–6. Use of Dental Floss. The correct use of dental floss for interproximal cleaning is illustrated.

The use of variable diameter dental floss (Super Floss) appears to be comparable in effectiveness to that of unwaxed floss and can be recommended to patients who prefer it or to those with open gingival embrasures.

OTHER INTERDENTAL DEVICES. Supplemental or alternative aids may be indicated for some patients to accommodate special needs. Although the use of unmounted

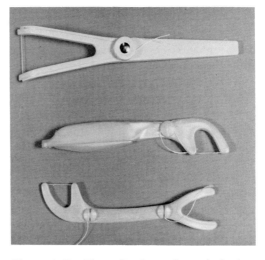

Figure 8–7. Floss Carriers. Several devices have been developed to aid individuals in the utilization of dental floss.

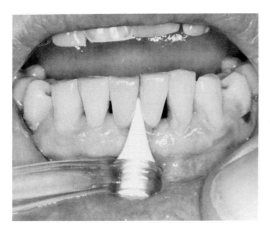

Figure 8–8. Interdental Stimulation. The stimulator tip is properly positioned for interproximal massage.

toothpicks has been shown to be reasonably effective in plaque removal from proximal surfaces, they are difficult to apply lingually. For this reason and because of the potential for tissue trauma, their use is generally contraindicated.

The use of Stimudents or other rubber or plastic tip stimulators (Fig. 8–8) may be useful in providing additional stimulation of interdental tissues. This type of massage is particularly effective in molding desirable papillary form post-surgically.

Mounted toothpick tips (Fig. 8–5) are useful in adapting to irregular root surface contours in areas of recession on all tooth surfaces. The wooden tip should be softened and splayed slightly to improve cleaning ability and reduce the potential for tissue trauma. These aids are especially useful in areas of bifurcation or trifurcation exposures.

Interproximal brushes (Fig. 8–5) are indicated only in areas where interdental papillae have been lost. Use of these devices has been shown to be equal and perhaps superior to dental floss in cleaning exposed proximal surfaces.

Irrigation Devices

A number of devices utilizing water irrigation have been developed. These instruments are designed to flush out debris from between the teeth by water pressure. It is possible for bacteria, necrotic cells, and food particles to lodge between the teeth in the interdental col or in the crevice and not be reached by the toothbrush. Hydrotherapy may provide a useful adjunct to the brush in ridding the mouth of these undesirable accumulations.

The simplest irrigation devices are the glass or rubber-bulbed syringes. Commercial instruments which utilize faucet water or a pulsating stream of fluid produce a stronger spray and greater cleansing efficiency. Some gingival stimulation also may be accomplished through hydrotherapy. Family oral hygiene centers combining water irrigation devices and automatic toothbrushes are available.

The development of intrasulcular irrigation techniques that can be used to deliver chemical antiplaque agents to the depth of the crevice is being investigated and may well become part of routine adjunctive therapy in the future.

Dentifrices

The selection of an appropriate dentifrice is becoming increasingly challenging because of the rapid development of products that provide or claim to provide therapeutic benefits.

Ingredients of toothpastes which are considered inactive (no antimicrobial or other therapeutic effect) are those that determine their consistency, taste, foaming ability, stability, abrasiveness, and general acceptance or appeal. Although dentifrice abrasivity does not appear to be as significant in dental or gingival wear as toothbrush type and technique, some consideration should be given to this factor in the presence of recession.

Active ingredients are those that are therapeutic. Dentifrices that claim a therapeutic value are eligible for and subject to review by the American Dental Association Council on Dental Therapeutics. Such products are not automatically reviewed by this council, but those that do gain approval may display the A.D.A. seal of approval for that product. For dental health professionals, this mechanism for evaluation of commercially available products provides a good guideline to assist in making recommendations to patients.

The benefits of fluoride-containing dentifrices in the reduction of dental caries have been well documented. Guidelines for gaining Council approval of fluoride dentifrices have been modified so that toothpastes with the same basic formulation as one already approved may present substantial animal and other laboratory data to gain approval without extensive clinical studies. Some dentifrices marketed for the treatment of dentinal sensitivity have been shown effective in this regard and now have Council approval. The role of these in the managment of hypersensitive teeth will be discussed in Chapter 10. More recently, a dentifrice that retards calculus formation has received Council approval.

The incorporation of antimicrobial agents into dentifrices has been investigated. These agents will be discussed in the next section on chemical plaque control. Although mechanical plaque removal is still the primary focus of toothbrushing, the established and potential therapeutic benefits of dentifrices behooves the dental profession to carefully consider their patients' specific needs and make informed recommendations in this regard.

CHEMICAL PLAQUE CONTROL

Use of chemical agents for control of plaque and gingivitis is an attractive supplement to mechanical plaque removal which often is inadequate. Extensive research has been devoted to the identification of a safe and effective agent and products which claim this therapeutic value are being widely marketed.

Criteria for Acceptance

The A.D.A. Council on Dental Therapeutics has developed criteria by which such agents may be reviewed and potentially approved. Of concern relative to periodontal health is that a plaque control agent not only controls gingivitis, but also has a significant impact in inhibiting the development and progression of periodontitis. Since the microorganisms involved in dental caries and periodontal disease are different, demonstrated efficacy against periodontal pathogens and subgingival plaque accumulation is necessary if this objective is to be met. Potentially, superficial control of plaque and gingivitis could mask underlying destructive processes and delay adequate therapy.

Methods of Application

Antiplaque agents once developed may be applied in a variety of fashions. They may be incorporated into dentifrices or mouthwashes or be available as gels or solutions. Topical application may occur in the dental office similarly to fluoride application. Agents applied in this manner are likely to be of higher concentrations and exert an effect that would last for weeks or months. Use of intrasulcular irrigation techniques using a blunted hypodermic syringe would probably require professional application. Self-application of antiplaque agents could be used to replace or supplement professional application. Weaker solutions and more frequent use of the agent would generally be recommended for self-application. It is likely that several different products or agents may prove to be beneficial and that there will be some available over-the-counter while others will require a prescription and monitored use.

Specific Agents

Mouthwashes containing sanguinarine and antimicrobial essential oils are currently being marketed as plaque control agents. Other commercially available mouthwashes contain agents such as cetylpyridinium chloride, fluoride and/or alcohol that also have proven antibacterial capabilities. Statistically significant reductions of plaque and gingivitis have been reported when these and other agents have been tested in clinical studies. Some caution, however, is indicated in assessing clinical significance particularly with respect to long-term periodontal health.

CHLORHEXIDINE. The most extensively studied antiplaque agent is chlorhexidine gluconate. Chlorhexidine applied topically or used as a mouthrinse inhibits plaque formation and gingivitis even in the absence of other oral hygiene measures. It has also been shown to eliminate existing plaque and resolve gingival inflammation. The use of chlorhexidine for plaque control post-surgically has been suggested. Daily subgingival irrigation with 0.2% chlorhexidine reduces the numbers of spirochetes and motile rods and changes in this regard are still apparent 2 months after suspension of irrigation. Application of 0.05% chlorhexidine with a jet irrigator appears to be slightly more effective than mouthrinsing using a 0.1% solution. The optimal lowest concentration applied with a jet irrigator was found to be 0.02%. For topical application a 2.0% concentration is usually used while mouthrinses are ordinarily 0.2%.

The effectiveness of chlorhexidine is accounted for in part by its ability to adsorb to tooth surfaces. It is gradually cleared from the mouth. This characteristic is also responsible for the uptake of stain, one of the primary undesirable side effects with the use of chlorhexidine. The addition of oxidizing peroxymonosulfate to the chlorhexidine solution reduces the staining without affecting plaque preventive capacity. Also, use of chlorhexidine rinsing at night has been shown to produce less staining than morning rinses. This relates to periods of food or beverage intake responsible for staining.

Other than the tendency to increase staining and the inducement of slight taste changes, other important side effects have not been identified. Chlorhexidine has been in clinical use in European countries for a number of years and is used in the United States on a limited basis. Although marketed as the active ingredient of a skin germicide, chlorhexidine has not yet been approved by the Food and Drug Administration for use in oral care. It is anticipated that this will occur in the near future and that the selective use in this regard will become an important responsibility of the dental profession.

STANNOUS FLUORIDE. In addition to enhancing tooth resistance to decay, fluoride compounds, especially stannous fluoride, have also been shown to exert antimicrobial effects against plaque bacteria. The use of stannous fluoride in a mouthrinse or a dentifrice has been shown effective in plaque reduction, and to have variable influence on gingival health. These effects were not, however, maintained long term. Submarginal irrigation with stannous fluoride reduces the numbers of spirochetes and motile rods. Although this reduction was not apparent after 2 days, subgingival irrigation with stannous fluoride may be appropriate as part of initial pocket therapy.

SALT AND BAKING SODA. The use of baking soda with and without salt has frequently been recommended for use as a dentifrice. In some preventive programs, the addition of hydrogen peroxide is recommended for routine home care. Although these ingredients potentially inhibit bacteria or their toxic products, additional scientific data need to be accumulated before these or other ingredients may be considered effective in controlling periodontal disease.

SPECIAL PROBLEMS IN ORAL PHYSIOTHERAPY

Some clinical situations require particular oral care management. Where extensive

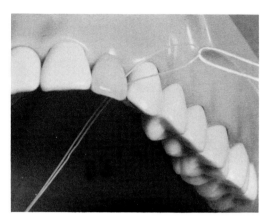

Figure 8–9. Cleaning Under Bridge. With the aid of a plastic floss aid dental floss may be passed beneath a fixed bridge to aid in oral physiotherapy.

restorative dentistry in the form of fixed bridgework is present, toothbrushing alone will not suffice. Dental floss must be passed beneath the bridge to insure that the gingival area of the pontics is cleansed. Plastic loops are available to help facilitate passage of the floss (Fig. 8–9). The irrigating devices are also helpful in cleaning around restorations.

Orthodontic bands may serve as irritants to the gingival tissue and also cause the retention of food and bacteria. Patients undergoing orthodontic therapy, therefore, must practice an energetic oral physiotherapy program. Interdental stimulators may be used to inhibit hyperplasia of the tissues, while waterspray instruments may rinse out debris. These same tools are of value when teeth are temporarily splinted together with wires or bands in periodontal therapy.

Where teeth are crowded or overlapped, conscientious use of dental floss, small-headed toothbrushes, and irrigation is indicated (Fig. 8–10). The automatic brushes, because of the small size of the brush head, are particularly valuable in areas where the dental arch is constricted. Isolated teeth are also difficult to brush, and dental tape, gauze wipes, and even washcloths can be

utilized to keep these teeth clean (Fig. 8–11).

In areas of gingival recession, supplementation with the use of mounted toothpicks may be indicated (Fig. 8–5), particularly when abrasion or erosion is present. The patient should be cautioned against the use of abrasive tools, techniques or agents on these surfaces. A fluoride dentifrice and/or mouthrinse should also be recommended to help protect against root surface caries.

Patients with Periodontal Disease

Individuals with periodontal diseases present problems with oral physiotherapy before and following treatment. Oral physiotherapy instruction usually must be delayed until gross irritants have been eliminated and acute inflammation resolved. Patients with periodontal conditions may be unaware of the presence of disease or that their own lack of oral care has contributed to its presence. Once causative factors are explained these patients may be strongly motivated in performing measures which preserve the teeth (Fig. 8–12, A–C).

Prior to surgical therapy, an initial phase is devoted to removal of etiologic factors. The patient's ability and motivation for self-care should be established during this phase before surgical procedures are undertaken. Frequently this is so successful that a surgical procedure is not indicated when the patient's needs are reevaluated.

During surgical phases of periodontal treatment patients are extremely prone to relapse in their oral care. The mouth may be sore, surgical areas should not be brushed during initial healing, and soft foods substituted for comfort contribute to local irritation. The cumulative effect may be an atrocious drop in oral care by the patient. At this point the hygienist can provide understanding and reassurance as well as reinforcing the cause and effect relation of local irritants. Judicious scaling and polishing may be beneficial. Nutri-

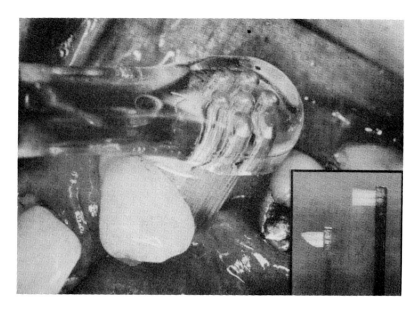

Figure 8–10. End-Tufted Brushes. Small-headed end-tufted brushes may be used for areas difficult to reach with a conventional brush. Brush to clean distal aspect of a tooth beside an edentulous space. Inset, Types of end-tufted brushes.

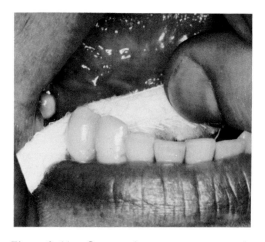

Figure 8–11. Gauze. A gauze sponge can be effectively utilized to clean where there is spacing or around an isolated tooth.

tional counseling, use of soft brushes, warm saline solution rinses, and auxiliary aids all may assist the patient during this active phase of therapy. The potential for use of chlorhexidine for plaque control during this period has been suggested.

Following the surgical period of perio-dontal treatment the hygienist assumes a strategic role. In Chapter 11 the wide range of periodontal surgical procedures is presented. Each operation presents a situation requiring specialized oral physiotherapeutic efforts. A blending of several procedures may be accomplished on a single patient. Careful consultation with the dentist is required in order for the hygienist to stylize oral care methods for each individual.

After surgical intervention the soft tissue level is more apical on the teeth and open spaces may exist between the teeth. With induced recession, cemental exposure occurs and root sensitivity may result. The patient might avoid brushing the sensitive areas and a vicious cycle is established which invites increased bacterial accumulation and, in turn, causes further sensitivity and periodontal damage. Agents and techniques for management of root sensitivity are discussed in Chapter 10. The creation of open gingival embrasures through surgical therapy may necessitate the use of special interproximal aids discussed earlier in this chapter. It is imperative that the

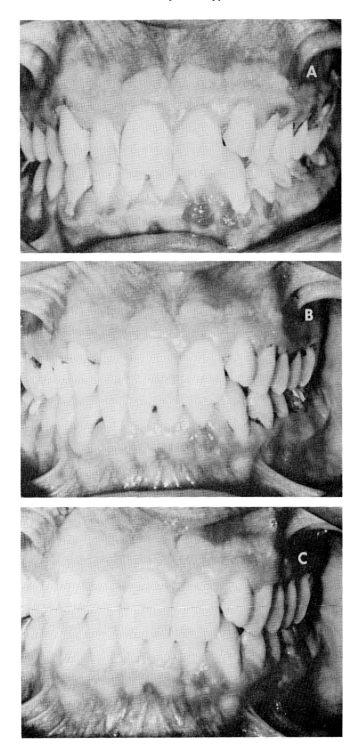

Figure 8–12. Results of Oral Physiotherapy. A, Edematous gingival condition at initial appointment. B, Two weeks of cleansing have exposed calculus. C, One month after continued brushing the teeth were scaled and polished. Note the dramatic change from A. (Courtesy of Dr. Dan H. Barefoot.)

treated periodontal patient apply diligent oral care methods. All of the tools mentioned previously may be required in order to reach a high level of oral cleanliness.

TEACHING ORAL HYGIENE

Motivation

The extent to which patients can be motivated to assume responsibility for their oral health may be dependent to some degree upon the locus of control facet of their personalities. The individual with an "external" locus of control generally feels that luck, chance or fate will determine what happens to him, whereas one with an "internal" locus of control believes that their ability and effort are important determinants of outcomes. Although it is impractical to administer locus of control questionnaires to each patient, an understanding of this concept may help guide the dental hygienist in designing personalized preventive programs. The education of patients in developing proper oral hygiene habits and in appreciating their own role in maintenance of their teeth and supporting structures is the most important and perhaps the most challenging function the dental hygienist has.

Most human behavior is learned and based on need. In order for an individual to perform an action a need must first be perceived by that individual. It is the hygienist's task, in her role as a health educator, to demonstrate and explain to the patient the need for personal oral physiotherapy.

Oral hygiene measures represent an extension of knowledge in control of the oral environment and in maintenance of health. This knowledge can be taught by the hygienist and learned by the patient. Oral physiotherapy instructions are best communicated when the hygienist possesses a high level of enthusiasm and personal conviction.

The result of the educational effort extended by the hygienist is reflected in the response by the patient. When the patient understands the need for oral physiotherapy and incorporates these procedures into his or her own behavior, the transfer of this knowledge is successful.

Wide variation exists in patient attitudes concerning oral health. Some individuals are easily encouraged to take care of their teeth. These people place a high value on the maintenance of their teeth and take pride in their personal hygiene and appearance. Such patients generally respond well when preventive measures are presented. Other patients have lazy oral care habits. This indifferent type of patient requires more stimulation of interest than those more highly motivated. Occasionally there is a patient who will be actually antagonistic to advice on oral physiotherapy. These individuals require patience on the part of the dentist or hygienist. Unfortunately, individuals of this type are prone to relapse and repeated instruction is required.

Research has shown that providing information about the periodontal disease process and preventive procedures is important in patient motivation but for many patients additional factors affect their compliance with recommendations. Periodic assessment and reinforcement of oral hygiene practices are necessary for most people to establish and maintain effective levels of self-care.

An attempt should be made to determine what factors will stimulate the patient to practice daily oral physiotherapy. In some individuals an appeal can be made on the basis of esthetics. Other people may be encouraged by explaining the role of mouth health as related to bodily health. Social acceptance, body cleanliness, and business success are other approaches which may be utilized to get the patient to keep his mouth clean. The patient must find some reward in oral physiotherapy, for ultimately the responsibility for health maintenance rests with the individual.

Introducing Plaque Control

Plaque control education is an ongoing process which should occur throughout treatment. For most patients, the application of the principle of small step learning is likely to produce the most successful results. Based on feedback cues from the patient, the dental hygienist should introduce new information or techniques so that the patient is not overwhelmed and discouraged early in treatment. Acceptance and mastery of basics, such as a new toothbrushing technique, are important to accomplish before introduction of instruction in the use of adjunctive aids such as special interdental cleaners.

Initial introduction of oral physiotherapy is often best accomplished prior to any therapy. At the first appointment with a patient in generally satisfactory mouth health, the hygienist can explain the causes or oral disease. With the patient holding a mirror, local irritants in the patient's mouth are demonstrated. Visualization of plaque is achieved with disclosing stains and tablets. The patient is reminded that the dyestuff actually stains bacteria and that any area thus stained represents a multitude of bacteria. Particular emphasis should be placed on plaque that accumulates in the critical area at the gingival margin where inflammatory periodontal disease originates. A phase contrast microscope through which the patient may view microorganisms obtained from his own plaque has proven to be an effective motivational device.

The patient can than be provided with an appropriate toothbrush and encouraged to attempt removal of the stained plaque. Many dental offices are now equipped with special sinks and lighting to assist the patient in oral physiotherapy procedures, but any convenient sink and mirror may be used (Fig. 8–13A). The toothbrushing effort is then mutually evaluated by the hygienist and the patient. While the patient views in a mirror, the hygienist points out those areas insufficiently cleansed (Fig. 8–13B). Some areas frequently skipped are the terminal teeth in both arches, the canine teeth, and the facial of lower anterior. If the general performance is good, the patient should be praised for accomplishing this goal. Praise is extremely powerful as a motivating factor and provides encouragement to continue good oral physiotherapy.

Selection of the brushing method to be taught the patient is based on factors discussed earlier. Whichever method is selected the objectives should be carefully explained to the patient. The hygienist should demonstrate the method with brush placement and movement in the patient's mouth (Fig. 8–13C). Manipulation of the brush is then accomplished by the patient, while the hygienist observes and offers suggestions (Fig. 8–13D).

Scaling and polishing procedures may then be completed at this appointment. Prior to being dismissed the patient should be provided with toothbrushes, disclosing tablets, and appropriate literature for home study. The patient should be informed that an evaluation of his performance will be made at subsequent appointments (Fig. 8–13E).

Introduction of auxiliary physiotherapy aids is often best delayed until a subsequent appointment. There is usually insufficient time at a single appointment to explain fully the value of these aids and a toothbrushing method. The patient might be confused by being provided with too many devices. An exception to this occurs when the patient has already demonstrated a high level of proficiency with the toothbrush.

Children require special education with accompanying illustrations, teaching aids, and prizes. Appeal to the child through posters of familiar cartoons, comic books, or television characters. The child's parents should be invited to hear and see proper brushing techniques and, in young children, the parent should supervise the oral

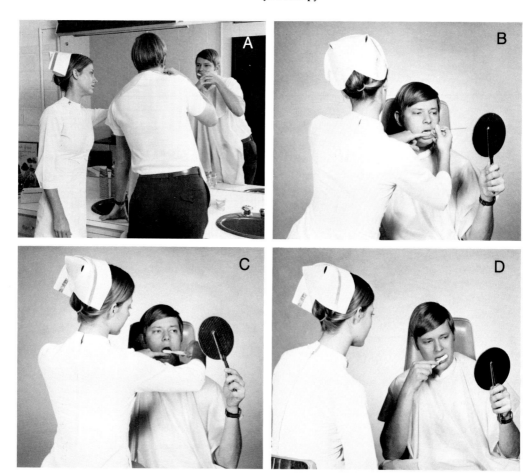

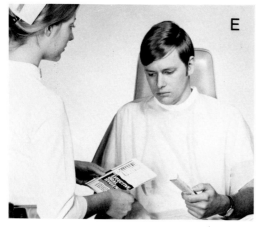

Figure 8–13. Introducing Plaque Control. A, Patient demonstrates usual toothbrushing method in plaque control area. B, The hygienist points out areas poorly cleaned. C, A toothbrushing method is demonstrated. D, The patient learns a brushing method under supervision. E, Helpful literature and brushes are supplied the patient.

care. In both children and adults the disclosing wafer provides a useful form of self regulation.

Adaptation of techniques to accommodate patients with special needs related to health and/or manual dexterity will be discussed in Chapter 9.

SUMMARY

Oral physiotherapy provides the most important method of control of periodontal disease that the patient can practice. While many systems and instruments have been introduced to aid in oral physiotherapy, in the final analysis it is the patients' motivation that ultimately determines their level of effective oral care.

BIBLIOGRAPHY

Abby, M. et al.: The effect of single morning and evening rinses of chlorhexidine on the development of tooth staining and plaque accumulation. A blind cross-over trial, J. Clin Periodontol., 9:134, 1982.

Abelson, D.C. et al.: Evaluation of interproximal cleaning by two types of dental floss, Clin. Prevent. Dent., 3:19, 1981.

Ashley, F.P. et al.: Effect of a 0.1% cetylpridinium chloride mouthrinse on the accumulation and biochemical composition of dental plaque in young adults, Caries Res., 18:465, 1984.

Bay, I. and Rolla, G.: Plaque inhibition and improved gingival condition by use of stannous fluoride toothpaste, Scand. J. Dent. Res., 88:313, 1980.

Bergenholz, A. and Olsson, A.: Efficacy of plaque-removal using interdental brushes and waxed dental floss, Scand. J. Dent. Res., 92:108, 1984.

Bergenholz, A. et al.: Role of brushing technique and toothbrush design in plaque removal, Scand. J. Dent. Res., 92:344, 1984.

Council on Dental Therapeutics, Guidelines for the acceptance of fluoride-containing dentifrices, J. Am. Dent. Assoc., 110:545, 1985.

DeRenzis, F.A.: Endotoxin-inactivating potency of hydrogen peroxide: Effect on cell growth, J. Dent. Res., 60:933, 1981.

Eriksen, H.H., Solheim, H. and Nordb, H.: Chemical plaque control and prevention of extrinsic tooth discoloration in vivo, Acta Odontol. Scand., 41:87, 1983.

French, C.I. and Friedman, L.A.: The plaque removal ability of waxed and unwaxed dental floss, Dent. Hyg., 49:449, 1975.

Fry, H.R. and App, G.R.: Histologic evaluation of the effects of intrasulcular toothbrushing on human sulcular epithelium, J. Periodontol., 49:163, 1978.

Gibson, J.A. and Wade, A.B.: Plaque removal by the Bass and roll brushing techniques, J. Periodontol., 48:456, 1977.

Hardy, J.H., Newman, H.N. and Strahan, J.D.: Direct irrigation and subgingival plaque, J. Clin. Periodontol., 9:57, 1982.

Katz, S.: The use of fluoride and chlorhexidine for the prevention of radiation caries, J. Am. Dent. Assoc., 104:164, 1982.

Kent, G.G., Matthews, R.M. and White, F.H.: Locus of control and oral health, J. Am. Dent. Assoc., 109:67, 1984.

Khoo, J.G.L. and Newman, H.N.: Subgingival plaque control by a simplified oral hygiene regimen plus local chlorhexidine or metranidazole, J. Periodont. Res., 18:607, 1983.

Lamberts, D.M., Wunderlich, R.C. and Caffesse, R.G.: The effect of waxed and unwaxed dental floss on gingival health. Part I. Plaque removal and gingival response, J. Periodontol., 53:393, 1982.

Lang, N.P., Cumming, B.R. and Löe, H.: Toothbrushing frequency as it relates to plaque development and gingival health, J. Periodontol., 44:396, 1973.

Lang, N.P. and Raber, K.: Use of oral irrigators as vehicle for the application of antimicrobial agents in chemical plaque control, J. Clin. Periodontol., 8:177, 1981.

Lang, N.P. and Ramseier-Grossmann, K.: Optimal dosage of chlorhexidine digluconate in chemical plaque control when applied by the oral irrigator, J. Clin. Periodontol., 8:189, 1981.

Leverett, D.H., McHugh, W.D. and Jensen, E.: Effect of daily rinsing with stannous fluoride on plaque and gingivitis: A final report, J. Dent. Res., 63:1083, 1984.

Lindhe, J., et al.: Influence of topical application of chlorhexidine on chronic gingivitis and gingival wound healing in the dog, Scand. J. Dent. Res., 78:471, 1970.

Lobene, R.R. et al.: The effect of cetylpridinium chloride on human dental plaque and gingivitis, Pharmacol. Ther. Dent., 4:33, 1979.

Löe, H. and Rindom Schiott, C.: The effect of mouthrinses and topical application of chlorhexidine on the development of dental plaque and gingivitis in man, J. Periodont. Res., 5:79, 1970.

Löe, H. and Rindom Schiott, C.: The effect of suppression of the oral microflora upon the development of plaque and gingivitis. In: McHugh, W.D. (ed.): Dental Plaque. Edinburgh, E. and S. Livingstone, 1970, pp. 247–255.

MacGregor, I.D.M. and Rugg-Gunn, A.J.: A survey of toothbrushing sequence in children and young adults, J. Periodont. Res., 14:225, 1979.

Mazza, J.E. et al.: Clinical and antimicrobial effect of stannous fluoride on periodontitis, J. Clin. Periodontol., 8:203, 1981.

Menaker, L. et al.: The effects of Listerine® antiseptic on dental plaque, Ala. J. Med. Sci., 16:71, 1979.

Neimi, M., Sandholm, L. and Ainama, J.: Frequency of gingival lesions after standardized brushing as related to stiffness of toothbrush and abrasiveness of dentifrice, J. Clin. Periodontol., *11*:254, 1984.

Odman, P.A., Lange, A.L. and Bakdash, M.B.: Utilization of locus of control in the prediction of patient's oral hygiene performance, J. Clin. Periodontol., *11*:367, 1984.

Rayant, G.A. and Sheiham, A.: An analysis of factors affecting compliance with tooth-cleaning recommendations, J. Clin. Periodontol., *7*:289, 1980.

Southard, G.L. et al.: Sanguinarine, a new antiplaque agent: Retention and plaque specificity, J. Am. Dent. Assoc., *108*:338, 1984.

Stevens, A.W., Jr.: A comparison of the effectiveness of variable diameter vs. unwaxed floss, J. Periodontol., *51*:666, 1980.

Tinanoff, N. et al.: Microbiologic effects of SnF$_2$ and NaF mouthrinses in subjects with high caries activity: Results after one year, J. Dent. Res., *62*:907, 1983.

Vogel, R.I., Alfano, M.J., and Manhold, J.H.: The effect of intrasulcular brushing on sulcular epithelial permeability, J. Peridontol., *52*:244, 1981.

Waerhaug, J.: Effect of toothbrushing on subgingival plaque formation, J. Periodontol., *52*:30, 1981.

Walsh, T.F. and Glenwright, H.D.: Relative effectiveness of a rotary and conventional toothbrush in plaque removal, Community Dent. Oral Epidemiol., *12*:160, 1984.

Westfelt, E., et al.: Use of chlorhexidine as a plaque control measure following surgical treatment of periodontal disease, J. Clin. Periodontol., *10*:22, 1983.

Wolffe, G.N.: An evaluation of proximal surface cleansing agents, J. Clin. Periodontol., *3*:148, 1976.

Chapter

$$\boxed{9}$$

MANAGEMENT OF SPECIAL PROBLEMS

Each patient needing dental care is unique. In order to provide successful therapeutic and preventive services, it is important that attention be given to individual needs, abilities and attitudes and that personalized treatment be planned accordingly. Patients with complicating medical histories, the handicapped, the chronically ill, the elderly or other patients with unusual problems require special consideration. Modifications to treatment may involve anticipation and prevention or management of emergency situations, accommodation of physical disabilities or limitations, protection against disease transmission, special prevention measures, and alterations in appointment scheduling and therapeutic approaches. An additional consideration which could influence patient acceptance of dental therapy is the emotional impact of an illness or disability of the patient.

All of these complicating situations require an understanding of basic principles involved, often, consultations with attending physicians or dentist and sometimes ingenious approaches to successfully meet dental needs.

MEDICAL EMERGENCIES

Preparation for emergencies involves two aspects. Complete information regarding health status should be obtained from each patient. This will permit taking precautions to prevent an emergency and will facilitate the management of an emergency should it occur with a given patient. The second aspect is obtaining the necessary skills and establishing a protocol to deal with emergencies even when no forewarning exists.

Preventive Measures

Often patients are not aware of the impact that a particular health problem may have on their dental health or dental treatment and may not provide important relevant information unless it is solicited. Patients having positive histories of medical problems should be questioned as to the severity of the condition. Frequently, consultation with the patient's physician is indicated prior to initiating treatment. Some type of alert system should be used to clearly indicate on a patient's record the presence of a medical condition requiring special consideration.

MEDICAL HISTORIES. Although formats of medical history records vary considerably, some general information that should be obtained is as follows:

1. Name of physician and date of last physical examination.

Table 9–1. Major Illnesses or Conditions to be Included in Health History*

1. Sensitivities or allergies
2. Reactions to anesthesia
3. Abnormal bleeding
4. Blood disorders
5. High or low blood pressure
6. Rheumatic fever
7. Heart disease/prosthesis
8. Diabetes (patient or family)
9. Epilepsy
10. Tumor/cancer
11. Radiation treatments
12. Hepatitis
13. Under care of physician
14. Medications
15. Other significant illness or condition

*This list is not comprehensive but reflects conditions most commonly encountered that are pertinent to dental treatment. It should be reviewed and updated at regular intervals.

2. Whether the patient is under the care of the physician for a particular problem.
3. Serious illnesses or hospitalization.
4. Prescribed drugs or medications being taken for any condition.
5. Over-the-counter medications, e.g. aspirin, being taken on a regular basis.
6. Previous problems subsequent to dental treatment.

Positive responses to any of these questions should be thoroughly discussed with the patient.

A suggested medical history form is illustrated and discussed in Chapter 6.

Specific conditions that the patient should be questioned about are listed in Table 9–1. More extensive questions regarding symptoms of disorders may assist in identifying undiagnosed health problems and referral of patients for health care if indicated.

COMPLIANCE WITH MEDICATIONS. If medications have been prescribed for the patient, it is important to ascertain the level of patient compliance in taking the medications as prescribed, especially in relation to the dental appointment. For hypertensive drugs or insulin, the regularity of medication and time of previous dose should

be noted. A prescribed amyl nitrate medication should be checked for expiration date and placed for easy access during a dental appointment. If premedication such as antibiotics has been prescribed for a patient prior to a dental appointment, confirmation that the drug has been taken according to the recommended regimen should be noted on the patient's treatment record.

EMERGENCIES. Preparation for management of a dental office emergency begins with establishing a protocol with which all office personnel are familiar. A supply of emergency drugs should be available, well-marked and monitored frequently for currency. An oxygen supply should be available, checked regularly and replaced as needed. Individual responsibilities for maintenance of emergency supplies and in the management of emergencies should be well-delineated. Ideally, rehearsal with mock emergency situations involving all office personnel should occur routinely. The posting of emergency telephone numbers and basic instructions is recommended to enhance the expediency with which an emergency can be handled.

Some states now require certification in cardiopulmonary resuscitation (CPR) for maintenance of licensure in dental hygiene and dentistry. Courses are readily available in most communities through the Red Cross, American Heart Association or other organizations. It is a professional responsibility of the health care provider to maintain current CPR certification.

MEDICAL CONDITIONS OF SIGNIFICANCE

There are a number of health conditions that can significantly impact upon periodontal health or treatment. Some major disease entities and their potential implications for dental management are summarized in Table 9–2.

Table 9–2. Some Diseases and Medical Problems of Significance in Dental Management

Disease or Condition	Possible Complications	Special Management
Diabetes mellitus	Lowered resistance to infection; poor healing	May require antibiotic coverage if uncontrolled or if patient is a brittle diabetic.
Rheumatic heart disease (with valvular damage or history of rheumatic fever); defects or prostheses	Bacterial endocarditis	Antibiotic coverage mandatory during treatment (consult Regimens of American Heart Association).
Coronary thrombosis (sodium warfarin or other anticoagulant therapy)	Bleeding problems	No curettage or surgical procedures unless prothrombin time is at a safe level. Delay treatment until six months after thrombosis.
Epilepsy	None, if patient is well controlled, but refer to text under "Epilepsy"	May require short appointments and special care in emergency situation.
Hepatitis	Transmission to operator or other patients	Special handling of all instruments by effective sterilization. Surgical rubber gloves to be worn during scaling procedures.
Hemophilia	Bleeding problems	Hospitalization and whole plasma transfusion to raise antihemophiliac factor in blood. Special care in scaling not to lacerate tissue and promote bleeding.
Leukemia	Bleeding; lowered resistance to infection	No treatment can be given except on advice of physician (palliative or emergency); antibiotic coverage.
Drug idiosyncrasy	Dermatitis to anaphylaxis	Offending drug or material cannot be used on patient. Alternate drug must be chosen.
Kidney transplants	Impaired disposal of metabolic waste products and drugs.	Antibiotic coverage to level prescribed by physician.
Cortisone therapy (long term) and (or) cessation of therapy	Possible infection and (or) lack of adequate adrenal support under stress	Consult physician as to need of antibiotic coverage and (or) support by cortisone before therapy or anesthetics.
Cirrhosis of liver	Bleeding and inadequate detoxification of drugs.	Only maintenance with scaling and root planning. Short appointments.
Long-term aspirin (salicylate use in arthritic patients)	Possible bleeding problems, especially in surgical procedures.	Bleeding time should be checked. Patient's physician should be consulted regarding management.

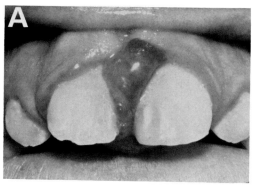

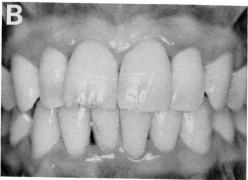

Figure 9–1. Gingival Changes Associated with Juvenile Diabetes. A, Uncontrolled diabetes. Note the gingival abscess between central incisors and generalized redness and edema of marginal gingiva. B, Controlled diabetes. Inflammatory response of marginal gingiva to plaque irritants is more comparable to that expected for a non-diabetic individual.

Diabetes Mellitus

In this disease healing may be delayed and susceptibility to infection increased. The extent to which these features exist are dependent upon the level of control of the diabetic condition (Fig. 9–1). Periodontal disease is generally more prevalent and more severe in a diabetic population than in a healthy group due primarily to a compromised defense capacity against periodontopathogens. Consequently, meticulous oral hygiene is extremely important to maintaining periodontal health in the diabetic.

A prominent feature especially in juvenile diabetes is polymorphonuclear leukocyte (PMN; neutrophil) dysfunction (see Chapter 3) which relates significantly to the occurrence and severity of periodontal disease. Similar dysfunctions have been observed in destructive periodontitis such as juvenile periodontitis and frequently these individuals, though not diabetic, report a family history of diabetes.

The severity of periodontal disease in the diabetic is significantly dependent upon the age of onset of the diabetic condition. Juvenile diabetes is generally more severe than adult-onset diabetes and is more difficult to control. Gingivitis in this group is common prior to the onset of puberty and the progression into periodontitis is likely to occur once the post pubertal years have been reached. The long-term periodontal prognosis is poor unless intensive oral hygiene regimens are followed.

Vascular changes and abnormal collagen metabolism also occur in diabetes and can affect the general resistance and healing capacity of the periodontium.

An altered oral microflora favoring potentially more pathogenic bacteria has been reported to occur frequently in diabetic patients. This alteration is related to reduced defense capacity particularly to PMN deficiencies.

Treatment considerations, in addition to an intensive preventive program, may include antibiotic coverage for treatment or delaying treatment, especially surgical procedures, until better diabetic control has been attained. Consultation with the patient's physician is indicated.

Other considerations in treating a diabetic patient involve determining the form of control, diet or insulin, and questioning the patient relative to the most recent food intake and medication. Should an emergency arise during treatment, this information can assist in providing adequate emergency care.

Hepatitis and Cirrhosis

A patient with a history of either hepatitis or cirrhosis may have liver damage which interferes with his ability for drug detoxification. Administration of drugs such as antibiotics or anesthetic agents should occur only after consultation with the patient's physician. Liver damage resulting from hepatitis is variable and this information should be determined prior to treatment. Excessive bleeding may be a problem associated with cirrhosis. Treatment should be limited to conservative therapy such as scaling and root planing procedures.

A primary concern in the treatment of a patient with a history of hepatitis is the possibility of transmission especially from infective carriers of the virus. It is good practice to refer any patient reporting a history of hepatitis for testing to determine if he or she is a carrier. If so, extra care should be taken to protect against transmission of the virus to office personnel or to subsequent patients (see Table 9–3). Treatment of a patient with active infection or in the initial recovery period should be deferred if possible.

Several findings have resulted from surveillance studies of the distribution of hepatitis B that have profound implications for dental practices. Numerous cases are relatively asymptomatic and not diagnosed. Carrier rates are likely to be somewhat higher in this particular population. Frequently the diagnosis of Hepatitis A is based on clinical symptoms and many such patients are later found to be positive for Hepatitis B virus particles. Transmission of Hepatitis B can occur during the incubation period before the disease is diagnosed. The greater threat may therefore be from treatment of patients not reporting a positive history of Hepatitis B than of those that do.

Hepatitis B viruses are transmitted through body secretions including saliva. The exposure, infection, and carrier rates are several times higher in dental personnel, especially in oral surgeons, than in the average population. Repeated exposure particularly involving contact with blood increases the chances of contracting hepatitis. Dental hygienists are therefore at a special risk.

Optimal aseptic procedures should be practiced on a routine basis for reasonable protection of patients and practitioners. A Hepatitis B vaccine is now available and should be seriously considered by all dental health professionals.

Hypertension (High Blood Pressure)

Many patients do not know they have high blood pressure and have never consulted a physician. Routine measurement of blood pressure of dental patients may detect previously undiagnosed hypertensive conditions. Such patients should be referred immediately for control by a physician of their choice. Hypertensive patients should not be stressed by pain or anxiety during scaling and root planing. A local anesthetic should be administered in case of anticipated pain or anxiety from this procedure.

Epinephrine in the local anesthetic is usually safe, provided that the patient is premedicated to lower the rate of endogenous production by the adrenal glands and that epinephrine is used sparingly and injected slowly, avoiding direct venous penetration. Epinephrine should not be used in patients being treated with adrenergic-blocking agents nor in patients on tricyclic antidepressants and monoamine oxidase inhibitors. The patient's physician should be consulted in the overall management of each patient with high blood pressure.

Hypertension may occur in children, especially if there is a family history of this medical problem. A small cuff is required for registering the blood pressure. Since blood pressure may vary with the age and sex of the child, a critical evaluation is required by the child's physician in case of suspected transient hypertension.

Cardiac Disease (Heart Disease)

Dental treatment should be delayed at least 6 months after an episode of coronary

Table 9–3. Maximum Precautions for Treating an Infected Hepatitis Patient or Hepatitis Carrier*
(Courtesy of Dr. James Crawford, Department of Endodontics, University of North Carolina School of Dentistry.)

1. Wear a cloth gown that can be sterilized thereafter or a disposable paper gown.
2. Wear glasses with side shields that can be disinfected.
3. Wear surgical gloves and wear a surgical tie-on mask (as recommended by public health authorities). Double gloving may be preferred.
4. Avoid procedures that have a high risk of injury to clinicians' hands, if possible. If injuries occur, wash well with soap and water and hydrogen peroxide. Consult a physician.
5. Schedule the patient as the last one to be treated in that operatory for the day to permit adequate cleanup time thereafter.
6. Place a large plastic drape over the bracket table and over the supports for the hand piece, water syringe, and suction hose.
7. Operate hand controls through the covers.
8. Drape the lamp handles and other handles with aluminum foil or plastic wrap.
9. Wrap the air-water syringe handle with plastic wrap.
10. Cover other surfaces used for instruments with plastic film, including the X-ray head and controls. Use paper or plastic covers on counter tops.
11. Use a plastic or paper drape over the chair buttons held in place with plastic tape.
12. Carry out the treatment without touching undraped surfaces such as hoses. Ideally, hoses should have smooth plastic surfaces so they can be cleaned and disinfected.
13. Exposed x-ray plastic film packets can be submerged in iodophor detergent. Scrub 1:1 in alcholol (0.5% iodine) for 30 min. Rinse the iodine solution off with clean hands and dry the packet before taking it to the darkroom. Alternatively, wrap packets with plastic wrap prior to use.
14. Prosthodontic devices, appliances, splints, and rubber-base impressions can be rinsed and immersed in iodine 0.5 to 1% or hypochlorite solution for 30 minutes before rinsing and taking them to the laboratory with clean hands. Handle alginate impressions with gloves; pour up the stone model and sterilize the model with ethylene oxide gas or heat.
15. Prior to cleaning instruments after treatment, place all instruments and water syringe tip loosely in a pan of detergent solution and heat to boiling; or autoclave; or soak in tuberculocidal disinfectant for 30 minutes. Then wash and scrub instruments and sterilize by normal procedure. Wear heavy gloves to handle sharp and soiled instruments.
16. The handpiece should be heat-sterilized (see manufacturer's instructions) or sterilized in ethylene oxide prior to reuse. Note that all handpieces should be equipped with a device, e.g. one-way valve, to prevent aspiration of saliva into handpiece.
17. Any other items that will be reused must be sterilized by one of the above methods prior to reuse.
18. All disposable covers are heat sterilized or are placed with other disposables into a plastic bag containing about 10 ml of formalin solution, tied and discarded.
19. Disinfect any surfaces touched that were not draped, using an EPA registered tuberculocidal germicide to scrub the surface. Then, rewet the surface and leave it unused for the time indicated by the manufacturer of the disinfectant.
20. Disinfect eyeglasses in plain iodine, scrub, and wash face and hands with plain iodine detergent. Scrub, lathering and rinsing 3 times.

*Many of these procedures may be implemented routinely to protect the clinician, especially if not vaccinated, family members, patients, and other office or laboratory personnel since most infective patients cannot be identified.

thrombosis (heart attack). Only emergency treatment should be rendered after consultation and careful planning with the patient's physician. Some patients with a history of thrombosis are on constant anticoagulant therapy, which may produce a bleeding problem during scaling procedures. The patient's physician should be consulted as to the need of reducing the dosage of sodium warfarin to bring the prothrombin time to safe levels. Patients with varicosities and predisposition to embolism sometimes cannot have the anticoagulant reduced with safety, and under these conditions, periodontal treatment may have to be severely compromised. Antibiotics are not usually needed for patients who have recovered from a coronary thrombosis.

Patients with angina usually tire easily and are poor surgical risks. Short appointments are best and a nitroglycerin tablet placed sublingually should precede the injection of the local anesthetic and subsequent dental procedure.

Patients with a history of rheumatic fever, rheumatic heart disease, cardiac birth defects, or artificial heart valves require careful preparation and management. The patient's physician should be contacted regarding protection during dental procedures. Adequate antibiotic coverage prior to, during, and following scaling procedures is mandatory in order to prevent bacterial endocarditis. The 1984 American Heart Association's Recommendations for the prevention of bacterial endocarditis should be followed (Table 9–4). For patients on continuous oral penicillin for secondary prevention of rheumatic fever, either erythromycin or one of the parenteral regimens should be used. The danger of bacterial endocarditis in patients with artificial heart valves or prosthesis is so great that multiple antibiotic coverage is required for protection. A combination of ampicillin and gentamicin given parenterally is recommended.

Cardiac conditions for which antibiotic prophylaxis is recommended or not recommended are listed in Table 9–5. For patients with indwelling transvenous cardiac pacemakers, there apparently is not a high risk for endocarditis, but dentists may choose to provide antibiotic coverage for dental procedures.

Patients with sensitivities to all recommended antibiotics for the prevention of bacterial endocarditis should have an alternate regimen of antibiotic protection prescribed by their physician.

Epilepsy

Sedation may be required if the epileptic patient is anxious or tense in order to forestall a seizure in the dental chair. The hygienist should first inquire as to all medications being taken by epileptic patients on a routine basis, since they are usually taking sedatives such as barbiturates as well as diphenylhydantoin sodium (phenytoin, Dilantin).

If, however, a grand mal seizure does occur in the dental chair during treatment, the dentist and allied health professionals should be prepared to deal with it. The chair should be lowered and tilted back and all objects that might be injurious to the patient should be moved out of the way. A piece of cloth towel can usually be placed between the teeth to prevent self-injury from tongue biting. The patient may need to be restrained during the seizure. Further dental therapy should be postponed.

Many patients on diphenylhydantoin therapy experience gingival overgrowth that increases the problem of removing plaque effectively. This tissue enlargement was previously called dilantin hyperplasia but is more accurately termed phenytoin-induced gingival overgrowth since it is not a true hyperplasia. Preventive measures in oral hygiene have been shown to help minimize overgrowth. As soon as a diagnosis of epilepsy is made, a planned preventive program in flossing and brushing, treatment of caries and replacement of faulty restorations should be commenced, and maintenance recall instigated on a routine basis. Planned fluoride therapy for control of caries also should be established. Pit and fissure sealant therapy is indicated in caries-susceptible patients.

In patients with long-standing enlargement of the gingiva, surgical correction may be required to establish architecture that can be cleansed by flossing and brushing. Instruction in the skills of oral physiotherapy is needed prior to surgical intervention in order to minimize recurrence of the overgrowth. If the patient is unable to floss and brush effectively, the family can be instructed in helping in daily oral hygiene. Pressure appliances have also been

Table 9–4. American Heart Association's 1984 Revised Recommended Regimens for the Prevention of Bacterial Endocarditis in Patients with Valvular Lesions, Defects, and Prosthesis. (Copyright by the American Dental Association. Reprinted by permission of the American Heart Association, Inc.*)

Standard Regimen	
For dental procedures that cause gingival bleeding, and oral/respiratory tract surgery	Penicillin V 2.0 g orally 1 hour before, then 1.0 g 6 hours later. For patients unable to take oral medications, 2 million units of aqueous penicillin G IV or IM 30–60 minutes before a procedure and 1 million units 6 hours later may be substituted
Special Regimens	
Parenteral regimen for use when maximal protection desired; e.g., for patients with prosthetic valves	Ampicillin 1.0–2.0 g IM or IV *plus* gentamicin 1.5 mg/kg IM or IV, one-half hour before procedure, followed by 1.0 g oral penicillin V 6 hours later. Alternatively, the parenteral regimen may be repeated once 8 hours later
Oral regimen for penicillin-allergic patients	Erythromycin 1.0 g orally 1 hour before, then 500 mg six hours later
Parenteral regimen for penicillin-allergic patients	Vancomycin 1.0 g IV *slowly* over 1 hour, starting 1 hour before. No repeat dose is necessary

Footnotes to Regimens:

**Pediatric doses:* Ampicillin 50 mg/kg per dose; erythromycin 20 mg/kg for first dose, then 10 mg/kg; gentamicin 2.0 mg/kg per dose; penicillin V full adult dose if greater than 60 lb (27 kg), one-half adult dose if less than 60 lb (27 kg); aqueous penicillin G 50,000 units/kg (25,000 units/kg for follow-up); vancomycin 20 mg/kg per dose. The intervals between doses are the same as for adults. Total doses should not exceed adult doses.

†In unusual circumstances or in the case of delayed healing, it may be necessary to provide additional doses of antibiotics even though bacteremia rarely persists longer than 15 minutes after the procedure. Penicillin V is the preferred form of oral penicillin because it is relatively resistant to gastric acid.

‡For those patients taking an oral penicillin for secondary prevention of rheumatic fever or for other purposes, viridans streptococci relatively resistant to penicillin may be present in the oral cavity. In such cases, the physician or dentist should select erythromycin or one of the parenteral regimens.

*J. Am. Dent. Assoc. *110*:98–100, 1985. Prevention of bacterial endocarditis: A committee report of the American Heart Association, Council on Dental Therapeutics.

devised to discourage gingival overgrowth. These have met with some success when coupled with a good regimen of daily oral hygiene. The patient must wear the appliance several hours a day and at night.

Some of the newer anticonvulsive drugs such as valproic acid may have side effects in some patients such as interference with the coagulation mechanisms of the body. These patients taking valproic acid should have a bleeding time and platelet function test before undergoing periodontal procedures.

More research is needed to discover a drug equivalent to diphenylhydantoin for control of seizures that does not cause the unfortunate gingival and other systemic side effects.

Venereal Diseases

Serious infection may be contracted after contact with oral lesions that are components of venereal diseases. Careful assessment of health history, evaluation of suspicious lesions, and routine use of rubber gloves and optimal aseptic procedures provide the best protection against this type of cross infection either to dental personnel or to other patients.

Herpes Infections

Herpetic gingivostomatitis is described in Chapter 4. These lesions, whether caused by Type I or Type II *Herpes simplex* virus are highly infectious. Though not a frequent occurrence, an infection of fingers

Table 9–5. Recommendations for Endocarditis Prophylaxis Relative to Specific Cardiac Conditions*
(Copyright by the American Dental Association. Reprinted by permission. Reprinted by permission of the American Heart Association, Inc.‡)

Endocarditis Prophylaxis Recommended:
    Prosthetic cardiac valves (including biosynthetic valves)
    Most congenital cardiac malformations
    Surgically constructed systemic-pulmonary shunts
    Rheumatic and other acquired valvular dysfunction
    Idiopathic hypertrophic subaortic stenosis (IHSS)
    Previous history of bacterial endocarditis
    Mitral valve prolapse with insufficiency

Endocarditis Prophylaxis Not Recommended:
    Isolated secundum atrial septal defect
    Secundum atrial septal defect repaired without a patch six or more months earlier
    Patent ductus arteriosus ligated and divided six or more months earlier
    Postoperative coronary artery bypass graft (CABG) surgery

---

*This table lists common conditions but is not meant to be all-inclusive.
†Definitive data to provide guidance in management of patients with mitral valve prolapse are particularly limited. It is clear that in general such patients are at low risk of development of endocarditis, but the risk-benefit ratio of prophylaxis in mitral valve prolapse is uncertain.
‡J. Am. Dent. Assoc. *110*:98–100, 1985. Prevention of bacterial endocarditis: A committee report of the American Heart Association. Council on Dental Therapeutics.

termed Herpetic Whitlow may result from contact with active lesions. This condition is very painful and can affect one's ability to practice dentistry or dental hygiene for varying lengths of time. Additionally, infections can be transmitted to subsequent patients. One report described an outbreak of herpetic gingivostomatitis in 20 of 46 patients that were treated by a dental hygienist over a 4-day period. Although the hygienist had noted some dermatitis which most likely facilitated the subsequent herpes infection, Herpetic Whitlow was not diagnosed until after the patients had been infected.

Acquired Immune Deficiency Syndrome (AIDS)

This disorder which is presumably viral in origin is characterized by debilitation of certain components of the immune system. Subsequent susceptibility to often fatal opportunistic infection accounts for the high mortaity rate (70 to 100%) associated with this syndrome. It predominantly (75 to 85%) occurs in homosexual males but other identified high-risk groups are intravenous drug abusers, hemophiliacs, and female prostitutes. The potential for transmission by blood-borne agents or from salivary secretions is of great concern to dental personnel especially when treating an undiagnosed patient. Routine optimal aseptic procedures with rigorous adherence when treating patients in the high-risk groups is recommended. Opportunistic oral infections such as herpetic lesions or candidiasis are common in the AIDS patient. This observation, especially in combination with a fever of unknown origin and perhaps other factors, should alert the dentist or dental hygienist to the possibility of AIDS, and appropriate referral should be made.

Blood Dyscrasias

Leukemia may bring the patient to the dental office with gingival complaints before seeking medical attention. The oral manifestations of acute leukemias are gingival hyperplasia, bleeding, and ulceration. Sometimes this condition is confused with necrotizing ulcerative gingivitis and thus careful case history and blood counts are necessary to rule out leukemia. Usually the patient with acute leukemia will give a history of malaise, loss of appetite, and other systemic symptoms such as fever and chills and spontaneous bleeding from the gingivae. No periodontal treatment should be done for these patients until a careful medical examination has been made by a physician.

Hemophilia and hemophilioid diseases also present a problem in management. If the patient has ever required hospitalization and transfusions because of a tooth extraction or cut, intensive investigation by the patient's physician before dental treatment is required to determine the exact nature of the coagulation defect.

Drug Idiosyncrasies

Harmful side effects of drugs are becoming more frequent with the extensive use of antibiotics and other medications now available for use in dental practice. It is important to note such allergic type reactions and the offending drug on the patient's record so that it can be avoided and alternate drugs used for the required therapeutic purpose. An example is a patient who has had a skin or oral rash from penicillin therapy in the past. Another antibiotic should be chosen for control of a dental infection in this instance. Some patients may be allergic to common dental remedies such as iodine preparations and aspirin. All patients should be questioned regarding sensitivity to any specific drug or medicament.

Aspirin (acetylsalicylic acid) has been shown not to be the completely innocuous drug it was once thought to be. It is now known to interfere with the coagulation mechanism through interference with vitamin K-dependent clotting factors (sodium warfarin-like effect). It may also interfere with platelet function. There is a large variation in the severity of the reaction (prolongation of bleeding time) from individual to individual. In patients receiving therapeutic doses, such as patients with rheumatoid arthritis, a bleeding time should be determined. If prolonged, an alternate analgesic such as acetaminophen should be prescribed by the patient's physician in anticipation of periodontal treatment.

Kidney Disease, Transplants, or on Dialysis

These patients have a problem of mineral imbalance and inefficiency of elimination of waste products. Antibiotics are usually needed before scaling and root planing. The dosage of the antibiotic must be carefully regulated according to the efficiency of kidney output. Consultation with the patient's physician is mandatory before any treatment is rendered. Blood pressure should always be taken prior to treatment. Timing of appointments and length of appointment should be determined by consultation with the patient's physician.

Cortisone Therapy

Patients on long-term cortisone therapy require appropriate antibiotic coverage because of lowered resistance to infection. Any patient who has had systemic cortisone therapy within the past 2 years or cortisone withdrawal for a period of less than 2 years should be regarded as dependent on the drug. Cortisone support is needed to enable the patient to adjust to stress during dental procedures. The patient's physician should be consulted on a specific regimen of management.

Tuberculosis

This disease is still a major problem although better treatment and control measures are now available to its victims. Health personnel, including dental hygienists, coming in daily contact with patients can protect themselves with BCG vaccine if they wish. If not, they should have a tuberculin test annually with appropriate follow-up examination if the test is positive. The danger of contracting tuberculosis is not as great from a known tubercular patient as from an undiagnosed patient. Precautions should be taken in treating the known tubercular patient. The use of a surgical type face mask is helpful.

PATIENT MANAGEMENT

Difficult Patients

Some patients may be uncooperative during dental treatment because of previous dental experience or because of attitudes or personality traits. Often it is the dental hygienist who spends the most time with a patient on a regular basis and thus is in a position to discern the presence of such problems and how they may be best managed. A sensitivity to the underlying reasons for uncooperative behavior is essential to reaching a satisfactory resolution or compromise. Patients who are emotional, frightened, angry, or complaining may have had past experiences which were unpleasant or may be having a difficult time in other aspects of their lives. Extra time may be required to develop a rapport with the patient and to reduce the anxiety of the patient. Delaying treatment or compromising a therapeutic approach may be indicated. Anxiety reduction usually can be best accomplished through patience and understanding. For some patients premedication with sedatives or use of nitrous oxide/oxygen analgesia may be necessary at least during initial treatment. Often a team effort is required to deal with the most difficult management problems.

Though more frequent in some geographic areas than in others, it is likely that foreign speaking patients will be encountered in practice. If there is no one who can act as an interpreter, then other means of communication must be used. This usually involves using body signals or illustrations to convey messages. If possible, learning or having available appropriate phrases in the foreign language could facilitate communication and make the patient more comfortable.

Children and Adolescents

The attitudes of child patients may be influenced by previous experiences, fear of the unknown or concepts transmitted by contact with adults or other children. Very important in the management of a non-receptive child patient is that the initial appointments be positive experiences in which some treatment is rendered in a non-threatening manner. More time and extra appointments are often needed to develop trust and establish good rapport. Explaining procedures in a straightforward and honest manner will help develop trust even if the procedure is unpleasant or painful. While bargaining or promising rewards may bring short-term cooperation, the potential for renegotiation at subsequent appointments is established and the cooperative spirit may be lost.

Although periodontal diseases are of relatively minor concern in a pediatric population, many habits, both good and bad, are established which could have an impact on future periodontal health. While prevention of periodontitis is much too abstract as a motivator for good oral hygiene habits, the removal of bacterial plaque can be a tangible goal for children to achieve and can be visualized with the use of disclosing agents and phase microscopy. Care should be taken not to create an unreasonable fear of plaque germs but to establish a rational respect for the possible consequences of failure to remove plaque.

Adolescence brings with it an almost overwhelming set of physiologic, psychologic and social changes in an individual's life. Establishing motivation for good oral hygiene habits during this growth stage can be extremely frustrating. Accepting the teenage patient as an individual and making personalized recommendations that will fit into his or her lifestyle is important in establishing good plaque control habits. Often appeal to friends especially of the opposite sex can be a strong motivator for the adolescent.

PERIODONTAL DISEASE IN CHILDREN. It is most unusual to observe periodontitis in child patients. Gingivitis frequently occurs, but is less apparent in prepubertal years than thereafter. Some serious blood disorders such as leukemia or cyclic neutropenia are accompanied by inflammatory or degenerative processes in the periodontium. These oral manifestations may be some of the earliest signs of the disease and detection in the dental office of any un-

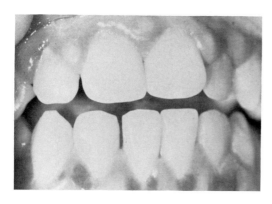

Figure 9–2. Pubertal Gingivitis. Exaggerated inflammatory changes in response to plaque and calculus in a 14-year-old boy.

usual periodontal changes indicate the need for referral to a physician.

Juvenile periodontitis has already been described in Chapters 3 and 4. It affects primarily permanent first molars and incisors and occurs circumpubertally. Routine probing especially of the commonly affected teeth may permit early detection of this disease. Gingival inflammation is often not apparent and cannot be relied upon as an indicator.

Pubertal gingivitis is also associated with the circumpubertal years and reflects the influence of hormones in enhancing the inflammatory response to plaque irritants (Fig. 9–2).

The observation of periodontal inflammation in children or adolescents may be an indicator of susceptibility to periodontal disease. In these cases increased efforts to promote preventive oral care should be made.

MANAGEMENT OF SPECIAL CHILDREN. Handicapped children present a particular problem in management of their oral health. Children with Down's syndrome, cerebral palsy, cystic fibrosis, as well as those who are emotionally disturbed, autistic, and mentally retarded all require both preventive and restorative dental therapies. In many instances these children can be managed in the dental office.

Some patients can be transferred from their wheelchair to the dental chair by the use of a sliding board with the aid of parents or carried bodily by parents. If not, the wheelchair can sometimes be positioned behind the dental chair utilizing adjustable head supports attached to the handles or reversing the headrests of the regular operating chair.

For patients who can be transferred but with whom intraoral radiographs are difficult to obtain, panoramic radiography can be helpful. Many handicapped children, after confidence in the operator has been established, can be treated as regular patients. Severely mentally retarded or emotionally disturbed patients may require restraining materials to arms and legs and, in addition, drug sedation. Two health professionals may be needed in order to prevent quick body or head movement that might result in injury to the patient or operator. Parents and patient, if possible, should understand the rationale for use of restraints and bite blocks, and these should never be utilized in a manner to connote punishment or discipline. Many severely retarded or emotionally ill children are in institutions and require expert professional teamwork to manage each particular problem. The treatment planning should be tailored to the special needs and requirements of the patient. Sometimes a toothbrush prophylaxis for the patient in bed or wheelchair is the best that can be accomplished.

It is a source of great satisfaction that general and oral health care of the less severely handicapped children and adults has been shifted more and more to community health centers, regional institutions, hospitals, and the home. Portable items such as automated polishing devices, electric toothbrushes, floss holders, and irrigating devices can be carried to both hospital and home. Disclosing solutions can be used to identify plaque and its effective removal. Floss holders are valuable adjuncts to patients who are unwilling or unable to learn flossing techniques.

Good visibility and adequate light and space are necessary for both patient and parent to evaluate the effectiveness of plaque removal, whether done by patient or parent. The parent can stand behind the wheelchair patient, bracing chair and head with one hand and brushing or using floss holder with the other. Another position could be with parent in chair and patient seated on floor, tipping head into parent's lap.

Some preventive measures such as scaling, topical fluoridation, and sealants for pits and fissures are best accomplished in a dental office and should be scheduled as regular preventive recall appointments at intervals determined by the oral health needs of the patient.

If the patient is willing and is enthusiastic about playng a game such as brushing off plaque, he or she should be rewarded by praise and(or) a small gift (not candy). Most handicapped children and adults are dependent and can best develop self-esteem by accepting some responsibility for their own oral health care.

The hygienist has an unparalleled opportunity in learning to relate to handicapped patients and helping them with preventive oral health measures. Preventive measures carried out by patients, parents, attendants, hygienists, or nurses can be rewarding, since extensive reparative treatment under general anesthesia in a hospital may be emotionally costly to the patient and both emotionally and financially costly to the parents.

Geriatric Patients

The numbers of people in the geriatric population is steadily increasing and this age group now constitutes a major population segment. Furthermore the proportion of people in this group who are dentulous is increasing. In epidemiologic studies the association between periodontal disease and age has consistently shown a strong positive correlation. Consequently the dental profession is confronted with increasing need for periodontal treatment in a growing population group. Definitive research in periodontal disease activity patterns in the elderly has not been extensive and criteria for determining therapeutic approaches are still somewhat subjective.

The consistent association between age and periodontal disease suggested that there might be a decrease in resistance as part of the aging process. Although some physiologic changes do occur in aging, it is now generally recognized that these changes do not contribute significantly to disease processes in the periodontium. The susceptibility of an individual appears to be determined early in life and does not increase in a normal aging process.

Much of the periodontal destruction seen in an elderly person has developed at a slow rate over a longer period of time and reflects an accumulation of disease. If compared to a younger person exhibiting a similar amount of tissue destruction, it could be concluded that the overall rate of disease activity is slower and the periodontal prognosis better in the older person. The significance of this comparison is important in planning therapeutic approaches. While somewhat aggressive therapy may be indicated for the younger individual, the older one has demonstrated a degree of resistance to periodontal disease and may in fact be at a stage where the disease is inactive. Treatment needed may only consist of conservative preventive therapy and maintenance recall.

Some health-related changes are more likely to occur in a geriatric population and these could adversely affect periodontal health. Such changes should be thoroughly assessed in order to plan and render effective dental treatment. Health problems and associated medications are more prevalent in an older population. These factors can affect general attitudes and ability for self-care. A number of medications cause reduced salivary flow.

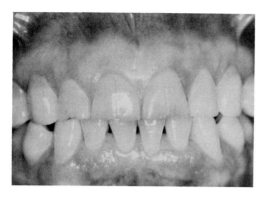

Figure 9–3. Healthy Gingiva in a 70-Year-Old Patient. Gingiva is pink with slight generalized atrophy of marginal gingiva. Recession extending apical to the cementoenamel junction is seen on facial of right premolars and is probably related to traumatic brushing habits.

Changes in social interactions, manual dexterity, vision and hearing, diet, mental alertness and psychologic outlook are all factors that could influence the older patient's interest and ability to maintain good plaque control. As in any age group, influencing factors should be assessed and considered in determining a personalized therapeutic and preventive plan.

Gingival recession is a frequent observation in older patients due to cumulative factors that have contributed to tissue wear or disease over a long period of time. It is not thought to be part of the normal aging process (Fig. 9–3). Exposure of cementum

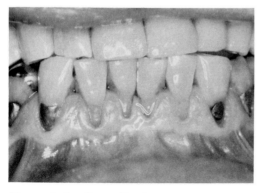

Figure 9–4. Generalized Recession and Restored Root Surface Caries in a 65-Year-Old Patient.

predisposes to the occurrence of root surface caries (Fig. 9–4). For patients exhibiting root surface exposure, the use of daily fluoride mouthrinses or gels should be recommended to protect against root surface decay.

Pregnancy (Normal)

If the patient has had good preventive dental care and is well motivated in daily flossing and brushing, the chances of avoiding caries and pregnancy gingivitis are considerably enhanced. Routine preventive care will probably suffice during this period. If not, caries control measures and definitive scaling may be required to reverse disease trends.

The safest period for any necessary dental treatment in the normal pregnant patient is the second trimester of pregnancy. Radiographs should be restricted to emergency dental problems and even then to a minimum number. The patient's physician should be consulted before prescribing any medication such as antibiotics, analgesics, and anodynes. Tetracyclines should be avoided because of the danger of staining the developing teeth of the fetus.

The third trimester of pregnancy carries with it the danger of premature delivery. Although necessary dental treatment may be rendered, all elective procedures should be deferred until after delivery. Appointments should be short. Nutritional counseling, if needed, can be done in cooperation with the patient's physician.

A new dimension in the medical case history in recent years is the widespread use of oral contraceptives that induce hormonal changes similar to those in pregnancy. While short-term use of these medications has not been proven harmful, their long-term use is suspect as regards alterations in gingival tissue resistance to bacterial plaque and consequent gingivitis.

Periodontal Emergencies

There are a few emergencies of a periodontal nature which should be mentioned.

These are mainly conditions of acute inflammation involving the gingivae and perhaps other oral mucous membranes. Acute necrotizing ulcerative gingivitis, pericoronitis, and ulcerative stomatitis are examples which require, as part of the treatment, irrigation, cleansing, and instruction in oral hygiene procedures. The hygienist can be of valuable assistance to the dentist in this phase of management.

The periodontal abscess presents another emergency situation which may require surgical intervention by the dentist. The hygienist should recognize the signs and symptoms of this condition—swelling of the gingiva adjacent to a deep periodontal pocket—and call it to the dentist's immediate attention. Recognition of the possibility of this condition in telephone conversation with the patient concerning a complaint of sore gingivae can also be helpful to the dentist in arranging the emergency appointment.

THE IMPAIRED PATIENT

Patients with handicapping disease or conditions may be divided into the physically, the mentally, and the emotionally handicapped. A handicapped person may be described as one with a congenital or acquired disability which impairs or limits normal functioning. Thus the individual will probably have difficulty in adjusting to dental examination and treatment situations. It should be understood that there is considerable variation in the severity of the physical, mental, and emotional disorders affecting children and adults. Some of them can be easily treated while others may present great obstacles to treatment and effective education in oral hygiene. Each patient then will present a new challenge to both dentist and hygienist and will require imagination in handling the dental problem.

Cerebral Palsy and Cystic Fibrosis

Cerebral palsy is an example of a neuromuscular disorder which may involve uncoordinated and involuntary movement of the arms, lips, tongue, and jaws. These patients, both children and adults, may have mental retardation also, and some will be taking diphenylhydantoin sodium. Dietary regimen, of necessity, may have to be starchy in character because of uncoordinated musculature of facial muscles and tongue. Oral hygiene may be extremely difficult or impossible for these patients to perform. Caries and periodontal disease are therefore common in these patients.

If the patient can sit erect with support and hold reasonably still, the management may not be too complicated. If, however, the patient must be supported, cannot sit still, cannot expectorate, or cannot cooperate, then there will be severe management problems in spite of adjunctive equipment such as special dental chairs, seat belts, especially designed bite blocks, and suction devices. General anesthesia may then be required with dentist and hygienist working together in a hospital environment. Certain home-bound patients, if not too severely affected physically and mentally, can have dental treatments if portable equipment is available.

Many of these patients are overprotected and overindulged by family and so may not have adjusted to the handicap. Suspicion and anxiety may complicate any approach to helping them.

Cystic fibrosis is a disease due to an inborn error in the exocrine gland system. These patients produce a large amount of ropy saliva and have difficulty breathing through the mouth during dental procedures because of mucous accumulation in the throat. Recurrent respiratory infection is common. These patients may have high caries raties. Frequent recall appointments of short duration are needed in order to keep down gingival infections.

Cancer Patients

In addition to emotional aspects of coping with cancer, treatment regimens currently used frequently involve side effects which add to the pain and discomfort of the patient. Some of these involve the oral cavity. Patients who are receiving cancer chemotherapy frequently experience nausea and lack of appetite. The level of oral health may be affected by loss of incentive to practice good oral hygiene. Chemotherapeutic agents are directed against rapidly proliferating cancer cells but may also have a toxic effect on normal cells that have a high mitotic index. Oral mucosa is a major site of toxicity and ulcerations and mucositis occur in about one-third of all chemotherapy patients. Oral infections usually by opportunistic microorganisms are also frequent. The occurrence of infections is related to myelosuppression and accompanying decrease in defense mechanisms. Optimal periodontal health and maintenance of good oral hygiene during chemotherapy can significantly reduce the incidence of oral infections. Antibiotic mouthrinses are sometimes prescribed either as a preventive measure or for therapy of lesions that occur. If the patient's mouth becomes very sore, spongy swabs may be used for cleaning the teeth.

Radiation therapy for head and neck cancers may damage the salivary glands and result in highly reduced salivary flow. Carious lesions develop rapidly unless rigorous prevention measures are employed. A concern relative to periodontal health is that the presence of periodontal disease may contribute to the initiation of osteoradionecrosis, a serious potential complication of radiation therapy. Careful periodontal evaluation and treatment should ideally occur prior to radiation therapy. Extraction of periodontally-infected teeth is sometimes indicated as a preventive measure. Salivary gland damage from radiation may be permanent predisposing to lifelong xerostomia and related oral health problems. Frequent recalls with reinforcement and reassessment of good oral hygiene practices are usually needed.

Blindness and Deafness

Patients with loss of sight or hearing or both present special problems that require understanding and sensitivity on the part of the professional rendering dental service. The blind patient, for example, may need to touch the scaler or curette before it is used in scaling procedures. Special instruction or training may be helpful in preparation for handling these patients' dental needs. Having a blind patient's relative or friend remain in the operatory during dental treatment is often reassuring to the patient.

Cleft Palate Patients

Cleft palate patients who are using prosthetic appliances for closure of the palatal defect should receive special attention in the control of caries and periodontal disease. Retainer teeth for these appliances must be conserved for functional, cosmetic, and psychologic considerations. The hygienist also should look for and record any areas of irritation along the tissue and appliance borders in the palate so that the dentist may relieve these areas on the appliance.

Patients with Pacemakers and Artificial Devices

Prophylactic antibiotic coverage is often indicated when treating patients with artificial implants such as pacemakers or metallic joint replacements. The patient's physician should be consulted regarding managment for dental appointments.

An additional consideration for the pacemaker patient is that interference with the pacing system could occur during the use of ultrasonic instruments or electrical devices such as a pulp tester. The susceptibility to interference is dependent upon a number of factors such as type of pacemaker, type of ultrasonic instrument and proximity of the device to the patient. These factors should be thoroughly investigated with the patient's cardiologist prior to use of potentially dangerous instruments.

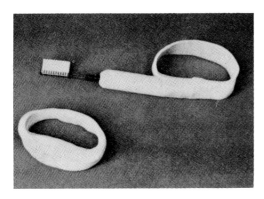

Figure 9–5. Polyform Splinting Material for the Aid of Patients with Weak Grasps. (Courtesy of Roylan.)

The Arthritic Patient

Patients with arthritis, especially when the hands and fingers are affected, have great difficulty with flossing and brushing effectively. Homemade devices can often be fashioned to aid these patients in holding a toothbrush or cleansing device (Fig. 9–5). These patients are usually not bedridden or acutely ill and therefore can be relatively independent in oral hygiene care if given the proper aids such as floss holders, electric toothbrushes, irrigating devices, and battery-powered polishing devices.

As previously discussed in this chapter, aspirin therapy in these patients may impact upon dental treatment.

Developmentally Disabled Patients

These patients, as a group, usually manifest periodontal disturbance mainly due to lack of oral hygiene and lack of regular dental care. They may or may not have physical handicaps and systemic disease. An example of this group is the Down's syndrome child who has a high incidence of periodontal involvement of the lower anterior area.

Patients who are developmentally disabled exhibit wide variation in oral health needs and ability for oral self-care. Some may possess the appropriate skills to become independently responsible for their oral hygiene, while others may require regular verbal reminders or physical assistance in performing procedures.

There is not a single approach applicable to every patient in this group that will develop optimal independent functioning. An initial assessment of individual skills, identification of potentially effective reinforcement mechanisms, and appropriate training in and evaluation of techniques are all general components of a successful oral hygiene program for the developmentally disabled patient. An effective training program involves breaking down the task to be learned into small steps that can be mastered at a rate consistent with the individual's ability.

Family members and other individuals who are responsible for the care of these patients may be involved in the training program and should participate in planning discussion.

Any additional physical or health limitations should be considered in designing an oral hygiene program for the developmentally disabled patient.

Emotionally Disturbed Patients

This group of patients may or may not have physical handicaps and systemic disease complications. Patients in this group may be exceptionally difficult to manage, depending on the nature and severity of the emotional disturbance. The oral cavity is one of the most erotic zones in the entire body and may be zealously guarded against violation by dental instruments or toothbrushes. Newer methods of treatment involving use of tranquilizers may soon enable the severely emotionally disturbed to become more receptive patients in the dental office, hospital, and home.

ORAL CARE FOR THE PHYSICALLY IMPAIRED AND CHRONICALLY ILL

Several of the conditions just described involve some degree of physical limitation in performing oral hygiene techniques.

Other conditions or accidental injury may also result in physical handicaps. Still other limitations to providing dental care or performing oral hygiene procedures may occur in chronically ill or injured patients who are institutionalized and/or bedridden on either a short-term or long-term basis.

Meeting the oral health needs of these patients is often a challenge and is frequently neglected. A variety of oral physiotherapy aids and equipment modifications have been designed to facilitate the provision of oral health care in the physically compromised patient.

Oral Hygiene Aids for Self-Care

Problems in manual dexterity may relate to difficulties in grasping or manipulating toothbrushes, dental floss, etc., or in controlling the movement of such devices. The specific impairment of a patient should be identified before attempting to make recommendations.

Frequently modifications of regular toothbrushes can be made to accommodate special needs. For patients who have difficulty grasping the handle, an alteration such as that illustrated in Figure 9–5 would be appropriate. The size of the toothbrush handle may also be increased by fitting a styrofoam ball, bicycle handle grip or a rubber ball over the end of the handle. Plastic tubing or an elastic bandage also may be used for this purpose. If these modifications are not adequate a holder such as an elastic cuff or velcro strip may be designed to hold the toothbrush against the hand. The toothbrush handle may be heated and bent to wrap around the fingers or to fit into a holder. Floss holders may be recommended and similarly modified.

For patients who have motor impairment, grasp may not be a problem but controlling the movement of the oral hygiene aid may be difficult. The toothbrush design illustrated in Figure 9–6 may be appropriate for this patient. The two brushing heads are applied to facial and lingual aspects of the teeth simultaneously and es-

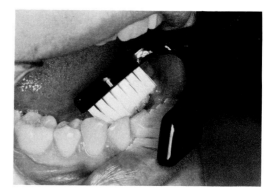

Figure 9–6. Double-Headed Toothbrush. This brush is designed to brush both facial and lingual surfaces simultaneously. This helps stabilize the toothbrush position and facilitates brushing for the patient who has problems with controlling movement.

sentially locked into position for brushing. Recommendation of electric toothbrushes or oral irrigators may be considered but skill level in manipulating these devices should first be evaluated.

Custodial Care

For patients who are institutionalized for varying lengths of time, daily oral hygiene care is frequently a low priority. In most situations, the numbers of dental personnel are inadequate to provide effective assistance and supervision of these procedures. Greater success will be realized if the dental hygienist directs primary efforts towards education and training of individuals who are responsible for daily care of institutionalized patients. Often the initial step is training these individuals in self-care techniques in their own mouths. An assessment of special needs of the patients and limitations of the facilities should be considered in designing an oral hygiene program. The use of some of the special cleaning aids just described may be indicated for some patients. For individuals who cannot sit up, a toothbrush with a suctioning mechanism would help with clearance of toothpaste and saliva during toothbrushing (Fig. 9–7). This, of course, requires some type of vacuum mechanism

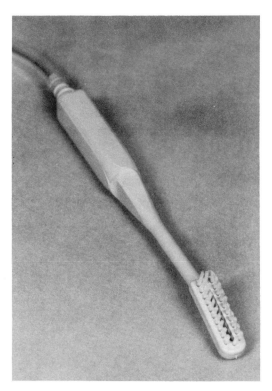

Figure 9–7. Suction Toothbrush. This tooth-brush can be attached to a suction hose to as-pirate saliva, toothpaste and debris while brushing. It is especially useful for patients who are restricted to a supine position.

to which plastic tubing can be attached. A special dental care unit has been designed that would enable quadriplegic patients to become independent in performing daily toothbrushing. This unit is designed so that each patient maintains a personal sup-ply of toothpaste, toothbrushes and straws for dispensing toothpaste and water. The unit utilizes an automatic toothbrush with easy-to-mount brushes which the patient can learn to insert with their teeth. Instal-lation alternatives include mounting the unit on a wall, suspending it from the ceil-ing or attaching it to a mobile cart. This flexibility permits access by patients with a wide variety of individual limitations.

Provision of Therapy

More frequent recalls are usually indi-cated for patients who are limited in their ability to maintain optimal oral hygiene. If handicapped patients are treated in an of-fice setting, consideration of some special needs should be considered prior to the time of the appointment. Assistance may be required in transferring a patient from a wheelchair to the dental chair. Skill levels may change between recall appointments and should be reassessed at each visit.

For treatment of patients who are insti-tutionalized, the extent of therapy depends on the extent of available facilities, equip-ment, and dental personnel. Portable units or other equipment may permit bedside treatment. Battery-powered polishing units may be used in performing dental hygiene procedures. Specialized reclinable wheelchairs have been designed so that pa-tients with spinal cord injuries or other se-vere handicaps may receive treatment that could not be rendered using a regular den-tal chair. The special design eliminates the need to transfer the patient and also pro-vides for controlling position and support for all parts of the body.

It is impossible to describe in available space the full range of special patient needs or the techniques and tools that are avail-able to facilitate meeting those needs. Oral health and the ability for self-care can be important in improving the self image and self esteem in patients who are handi-capped. Every effort should be made to identify individual patient needs and to in-vestigate means to satisfy them.

RESOURCE MATERIAL FOR AIDING THE IMPAIRED

The American Dental Association has a resource list entitled "Dentistry for the Handicapped" for both lay persons and for health professionals. The resource list and pamphlets can be obtained from the na-tional office of the American Dental As-sociation in Chicago, from the Dental Guidance Council for Cerebral Palsy in New York, and from the U.S. Department of Commerce, National Technical Information Service in Springfield, Virginia.

Audiovisuals for health professionals on Dentistry for the Handicapped can be obtained from the American Dental Association and the National Foundation of Dentistry for the Handicapped in Boulder, Colorado.

A brochure entitled "The Dental Implication of Epilepsy" can be obtained from the U.S. Department of Health and Human Services, Rockville, Maryland. It contains much useful information on prevention of dental disease, plaque control, supplemental fluoridation, and dietary counseling for the patient suffering from epilepsy.

SUMMARY

The dental hygienist plays a major role in recognizing the special needs of patients and in making modifications to accommodate those needs in order to help the patient achieve optimal oral health. Knowledge of the basic processes in many diseases or conditions is essential. Communication and counseling skills are important for achieving successful results. Patience, understanding and sometimes ingenuity are also needed in the effective management of patients with special needs. Changing state laws that permit dental hygienists to practice without direct dentist supervision, especially in some institutional settings, imposes the responsibility to be well-prepared to make professional judgments in the treatment of compromised patients.

BIBLIOGRAPHY

Baum, B.J.: The dentistry-gerontology connection, J. Am. Dent. Assoc., 109:899, 1984.

Cooley, R.L. and Lubow, R.M.: AIDS: An occupational hazard?, J. Am. Dent. Assoc., 107:28, 1983.

Council on Dental Therapeutics: Prevention of bacterial endocarditis: A committee report of the American Heart Association, J. Am. Dent. Assoc., 110:98, 1985.

Dental Implications of Epilepsy. U.S. Public Health Services Administration, U.S. Department of Health, Education and Welfare, DHEW Publication No. (HSA) 78-5217, 1977.

Douglass, C. et al.: The potential for increase in periodontal diseases of the aged population, J. Periodontol., 54:721, 1983.

Dreizen, S.: Stomatoxic manifestations of cancer chemotherapy, J. Prosthet. Dent., 40:650, 1978.

Entwistle, B.M. and Rudrud, E.H.: Behavioral approaches to toothbrushing programs for handicapped adults, Spec. Care Dentist., 2:55, 1982.

Heard, E., Jr., Staples, A.F. and Dyerwinski, A.W.: The dental patient with renal disease: Precautions and guidelines, J. Am. Dent. Assoc., 96:792, 1978.

Kalkwarf, K.L. and McLey, L.L.: Neutropenias and neutrophil dysfunction: Relationship to periodontal disease, J. West. Soc. Peridont., 32:5, 1984.

Lindquist, S.F., Hickey, A.J. and Drane, J.B.: Effect of oral hygiene on stomatitis in patients receiving cancer chemotherapy, J. Prosthet. Dent., 40:312, 1978.

Luker, J.: The pacemaker patient in the dental surgery, J. Dent., 10:326, 1982.

Manouchehr-Pour, M. and Bissada, N.F.: Periodontal disease in juvenile and adult diabetic patients: A review of the literature, J. Am. Dent. Assoc., 107:766, 1983.

Manzella, J.P. et al.: An outbreak of Herpes simplex virus type I gingivostomatitis in a dental hygiene practice, J. Am. Med. Assoc., 252:1019, 1984.

Murrah, V.A.: Diabetes mellitus and associated oral manifestations: A review, J. Oral. Path., 14:271, 1985.

Page, R.C.: Periodontal diseases in the elderly: A critical evaluation of current information, Gerodontology, 3:63, 1984.

Parvien, T., Parvien, I. and Larmas, M.: Stimulated salivary flow rate, pH and lactobacillus and yeast concentrations in medicated persons, Scand. J. Dent. Res., 92:524, 1984.

Peterson, D. and Sonis, S., eds.: Oral Complications of Cancer Chemotherapy, The Hague, Martinus Nijhoff, 1983.

Proceedings of the National Symposium on Hepatitis B and the Dental Profession, J. Am. Dent. Assoc., 110:614, 1985.

Quart, A.M.: Dental treatment for spinal cord injury patients in a specialized reclinable wheelchair, Spec. Care Dentist., 2:252, 1982.

Rommerdale, E.H., Comer, R.W. and Caughman, W.F.: University of Mississippi Dental Care Unit: Toothbrushing for the handicapped, Spec. Care Dentist., 3:108, 1983.

Sroda, R. and Plezia, R.A.: Oral hygiene devices for special patients, Spec. Care Dentist., 4:264, 1984.

van der Velden, U.: Effect of age on the periodontium, J. Clin. Periodontol., 11:281, 1984.

Wright, W.E. et al.: An oral disease prevention program for patients receiving radiation and chemotherapy, J. Am. Dent. Assoc., 110:43, 1985.

10

CONSIDERATIONS IN PERIODONTAL THERAPY

The general purpose of clinical periodontics is the same as that for most other areas of dentistry; that is, to preserve the natural dentition in a state of health, function, and comfort for the life of the individual. The significance of this goal becomes clear when it is realized that the major cause of tooth loss in adults is lack of periodontal care.

The ideal approach to the preservation of the periodontium, and thus the tooth, is by preventive procedures. Periodic scaling and polishing and adequate oral physiotherapy techniques will maintain the health of these oral tissues. As patients develop more advanced periodontal lesions, it becomes exceedingly more difficult to treat them adequately and successfully.

OBJECTIVES OF PERIODONTAL THERAPY

The ultimate goal of periodontal therapy is to cure the patient's periodontal disease. This is accomplished if all the tissue changes which occur in periodontal disease can be eliminated or corrected. If all the local irritants which cause the patho-

logic condition are eliminated, the inflammation and associated destructive processes will abate. A simple edematous gingivitis will be cured with no residual defects. Only preventive measures are indicated to keep the disease from recurring. In some cases of early periodontitis, a cure may be obtained by removing local irritants and by taking adequate preventive measures.

If the patient has periodontal pockets which cannot be sufficiently reduced by soft-tissue shrinkage occurring as the inflammatory process recedes, surgical procedures designed to eliminate pockets are employed. Periodontal pockets are areas that are difficult, if not impossible, to keep free of irritating bacterial plaque and calculus. There will be a chronic inflammatory process with associated tissue destruction at the base of the pocket. The purpose of periodontal surgery is to eliminate the pockets, or at least to reduce the depth to a maximum of 2 to 3 mm. This will enable the patient to keep the resultant crevice free of irritating substances. Concurrent with the pocket elimination procedure, every attempt is made to recontour the tissues so as to provide an area that can be easily kept clean of debris and plaque by the patient.

If occlusal trauma or bruxism is a significant factor in the etiology of the periodontal problem, adequate correction or control must be instituted to satisfy the concept of cure of periodontal disease. Occlusal adjustment may be indicated to eliminate noxious occlusal disharmonies and promote a more favorable distribution of forces on the teeth. It may be necessary to construct a bite splint for the patient to wear if he continues to grind his teeth.

Minor tooth movement may be necessary to replace migrated teeth in a more functional and esthetic position. If teeth are excessively mobile, splinting devices may have to be fabricated to stabilize the teeth to prevent secondary occlusal trauma. If teeth have been lost due to periodontal disease or caries, replacement may be needed to provide adequate function and stability to the dental arches.

To summarize, the specific objectives of periodontal therapy are:
1. To eliminate the periodontal disease by removal of the local factors causing it.
2. To teach the patient how to take care of the teeth and periodontal tissues by adequate oral physiotherapy.
3. To eliminate periodontal pockets.
4. To reproduce surgically physiologic tissue contours around the teeth.
5. To produce optimal and harmonious functional occlusion.
6. To control noxious neuroses or habits.

If these six objectives can be accomplished, the patient's periodontal disease can be cured. Of course, adequate oral physiotherapy and periodic scaling and polishing to remove plaque and calculus are necessary to prevent a recurrence of the disease. While good brushing techniques will remove much of the plaque as it forms and before it calcifies, most patients need a thorough prophylaxis at least twice yearly to keep the gingival tissues in maximal health.

It must be appreciated that many patients do not come for periodontal treatment until their problem is well advanced. It is not possible to cure periodontal disease if it has progressed to a point that the pockets cannot be eliminated or if there is insufficient bone remaining to maintain the teeth in health and function. In such cases a decision must be made clinically as to whether the involved tooth or teeth should be removed or treated palliatively.

In many situations, teeth can be retained for several years in health and function even though the periodontal condition cannot be considered to be cured. In other situations, the most practical solution is to remove the hopelessly involved teeth and replace them with either fixed or removable dental prostheses. The overall treatment plan and the patient's desire to keep his teeth are the most important considerations in regard to whether the teeth are extracted or not.

Patients who have been treated but not cured need special care by the hygienist as far as the maintenance program is concerned. Some of these patients need to be recalled every 2 or 3 months for scaling and root planing in the residual pockets. Needless to say, these patients must practice meticulous oral physiotherapy. There is increasing long term clinical evidence that active periodontal disease can be arrested and teeth maintained even when periodontal pockets persist.

ROLE OF THE DENTAL HYGIENIST

As mentioned previously, the general purpose of this book is to assist the hygienist in her many different roles as they relate to the periodontal care of patients. It is clear that periodontal care cannot be separated from health care for the entire patient. Long term success of prevention or therapy will not be obtained unless the patient is motivated to maintain adequate daily oral hygiene. The hygienist not only must be able to communicate and demonstrate the techniques of plaque removal, but must use the knowledge of behavioral sciences in such a way as to stimulate each and every patient to continually practice those techniques. Patients, of course, vary in their age, attitude, digital dexterity and disposition. Different approaches and different levels of intensity will have to be employed to be effective with the many personalities encountered in a dental practice.

Athough the opportunities for action and interaction in practice are almost limitless, the hygienist roles are primarily those of therapist, educator, consultant, advisor and assistant. In order to accomplish these many tasks, the hygienist must be an expert in the fields of preventive periodontics and knowledgeable of the entire discipline of periodontics. Chapters 11 and 12 will provide additional information for you in that regard.

PREVENTIVE PERIODONTICS

Preventive dentistry of which preventive periodontics is an important and integral part has received major consideration by dental educators and practitioners. There is enough knowledge, if exploited wisely, to control periodontal disease and dental caries effectively.

Effective use of prophylactic procedures on a regular basis plus efficient oral physiotherapy procedures can control the degree of pathologic involvement of periodontal tissues, thus prolonging the life span of the adult dentition indefinitely. The motivation of the patient to desire the preservation of the natural dentition in health lies in effective education in the local causes of periodontal disease such as calculus, bacterial plaque, and a method of oral physiotherapy which is practical and achievable in our busy culture.

True prevention is a goal of the future, realizable only through the efforts of individuals dedicated to basic investigative projects to find ways and means of eliminating entirely the local factors responsible for periodontal disease. For instance, if plaque could be prevented from forming at all on teeth, one of the local factors would be eliminated entirely in our struggle to maintain periodontal health.

Education of Patients

The hygienist by virtue of training has a key role in preventive dentistry and specifically in preventive periodontics. Although her efforts may be directed primarily to the control of periodontal disease and caries through regular periodic recall prophylaxis, she should be the dental health missionary in the most inclusive sense. For this all-important task, she needs to know how to communicate with patients in language easily understood.

The story of periodontal disease and caries can be made dramatic even to children in the following manner:

There are millions of living bacteria residing on and around the teeth and gums. These bacteria are so small that they are invisible to the naked eye. Some of them are able to penetrate the enamel of the teeth and others to cause food material to stick to the teeth and in the crevices between the teeth and soft tissues surrounding the teeth. In order for these microorganisms to live, they must have food. Some of them prefer candy and sweets and others prefer meat. As long as their favorite food is available to them, they grow and multiply and cause disease. If these bacteria can be kept to a small number, the teeth and gums can fight back and prevent trouble from beginning.

The hygienist at this point can use a disclosing agent to demonstrate the presence of these microorganisms on the teeth and gingivae. The patient, holding a hand mirror, may then ask how one can keep these microorganisms off the teeth and gums, thus preventing dental disease. A toothbrush lesson demonstrated in the patient's mouth can than be given. If the patient is a preschool child, the parent can stand behind the hygienist and learn how to instruct the child at home. The parent may need to brush the child's teeth until the child has developed his own brushing skill. Pretty teeth and gums, a pretty smile, and the satisfaction of a clean, healthy mouth free of offensive odors can be strong motivating forces for children and adults alike.

The adult patient may ask why the prevention of gingivitis is so important in periodontal disease, especially if there have been no symptoms of trouble. Here visual material of the periodontal structures in health and disease can be of assistance (Fig. 10–1). The most vulnerable areas of the gingival tissue are the interproximal areas, which are difficult to keep meticulously free of food debris and bacteria. Bacteria colonies form in these areas quickly and produce harmful substances which irritate the gingival tissue. The reaction of the body to this local irritation is inflammation that manifests itself by bleeding, swelling, and redness of the gingivae. The health of the bone supporting the teeth is affected by the health of the overlying gingivae. The bone reacts to this situation by receding away from this area of inflammation. Harmful by-products of bacteria in the gingival crevice around the tooth dissolve the connective tissue which fastens

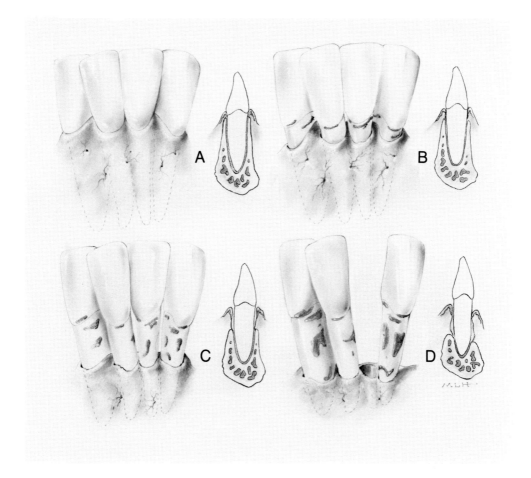

Figure 10–1. Destruction of Alveolar Supporting Bone. Drawing shows progressive destruction of alveolar supporting bone in untreated periodontitis. A, Normal bone levels. B, Beginning destruction of crestal bone. C, Marked destruction of alveolar supporting bone. D, Loss of tooth from lack of alveolar bone support.

the tooth root to the bone itself, eventually resulting in deep clefts or pockets around teeth.

The patient's own periodontal microbial flora can be demonstrated by obtaining a specimen and having the patient visualize the result on a television linkup to a phase contrast microscope (Fig. 10–2). This can be a powerful motivating factor in influencing the patient to want to learn how to prevent gingivitis and periodontitis.

At a subsequent appointment the patient will be asked to demonstrate ability to remove plaque by flossing and brushing. After the patient has flossed and brushed, the disclosing solution can be applied. The patient is given a mirror and asked to identify the surfaces or areas of teeth where plaque has not been removed. If the patient has difficulty in doing this, the hygienist can point out these areas and then review methods to help the patient do a more effective job of plaque removal. Encouragement and praise are usually rewarded by a greater effort on the part of the patient to do better.

Plaque Indexes

Since a significant relationship between clinically detectable bacterial plaque and periodontal disease has been demonstrated, several acceptable plaque scoring indexes have been developed. These indexes not only are important in epidemiological surveys of periodontal health and disease in a given population, but are helpful in monitoring the degree of plaque formation and the effectiveness of oral hygiene for individual patients.

Basically, the indexes quantitate the amount of plaque on representative teeth. The plaque may be stained artificially to assist in quantitating it. No plaque present is scored as 0 and increasing quantities of plaque receive increasing score numbers. The scores of all teeth are totaled and then divided by the number of teeth utilized in order to obtain the mouth score for the individual.

The most frequently used plaque score is the Simplified Oral Hygiene Index (OHI-S) (Green and Vermillion, 1964). This

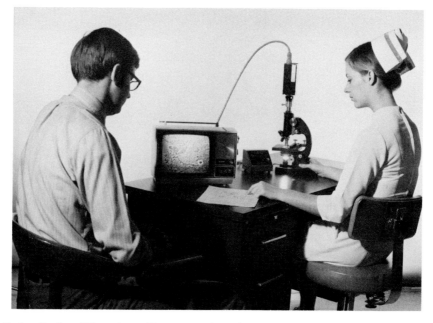

Figure 10–2. Patient Education. Demonstration of a patient's own periodontal microbial flora on television screen linkup to phase contrast microscope.

index has two components, the Debris Index—Simplified (DI-S) and the Calculus Index—Simplified (CI-S). The six teeth utilized are the facial surfaces of numbers 3, 8, 14, 24 and the lingual surfaces of numbers 19 and 30. The following scoring system is used for either the debris (plaque) or calculus score:

0—no deposit detectable.
1—no more than one third of surface covered by deposit.
2—more than one third but no more than two thirds of surface covered by deposit.
3—more than two thirds of surface covered by deposit.

The scores are totaled and divided by six to obtain respectively the debris (plaque) or calculus score. The plaque and calculus scores are combined to obtained the OHI-S.

The Periodontal Disease Index (PDI) developed by Ramfjord (1967) has a plaque index component. Teeth numbers 3, 9, 12, 19, 25 and 28 are scored 0–3 based on the amount of plaque stained by Bismark Brown. The individual plaque score is determined by totaling the tooth scores and dividing by six.

The Plaque Index (PlI) (Silness and Löe) assesses the thickness of plaque in the gingival area of the tooth. The distofacial, facial, mesiofacial and lingual surfaces of the tooth is scored on the following basis:

0—no plaque visible
1—a film of plaque recognized only by running a probe across the tooth.
2—a moderate accumulation of plaque that can be seen with the naked eye.
3—abundance of plaque on the gingival margin and adjacent tooth surface.

The PlI for each tooth is obtained by totaling the scores and dividing by four. The mouth score is determined by totaling all the individual tooth scores and dividing by the number of teeth scored.

The use of plaque scoring techniques can be informative to the hygienist as to the effectiveness of the patient's oral hygiene and can be a motivational tool for the patient. The hygienist scores the patient on the first appointment and explains the significance of the score to the patient. After instituting an oral physiotherapy program, goals are set with the patient for reducing the score. Subsequently, scoring hopefully will demonstrate to the patient that he is making progress. The patient is scored at each recall appointment to let the patient and hygienist know the effectiveness of the patient's home care regimen.

Dietary Counseling

Another method of limiting the numbers of disease-producing microorganisms on teeth, especially those causing decay, is dietary control. Sweets and carbohydrates can be reduced safely without restricting the four essential foods: milk, meat, fruit and vegetable, and bread-cereal groups (Fig. 10–3). The control of caries is necessary to the control of gingival and periodontal disease. Patients will not brush an area of the mouth where there is a sensitive carious tooth. If decay destroys a proper contact between teeth, food debris cannot easily be removed. Tooth contours are designed to protect the surrounding gingiva, and, if destroyed by caries, food will be impacted and cause local gingival irritation and inflammation.

Dietary counseling, however, should not place all the emphasis on prohibition of carbohydrate food. Positive guidance in the selection of foods is needed. Raw fruits and vegetables, which leave little food residue around teeth and gingivae, should be emphasized. In between meal snacks for children and teenagers should underline the food preference of raw fruits and vegetables and milk over candy, cookies and carbonated beverages.

Dietary Analysis and Laboratory Tests

The hygienist should be familiar with at least a qualitative evaluation of a patient's diet by examining a daily and weekly record kept by the patient of all foods consumed (Fig. 10–4). The four essential food groups—milk, meat, vegetables and fruits,

```
M_____          DIET EVALUATION SUMMARY   _____
        (patient)                                                  (Date)
```

FOOD GROUPS	1st. day	2nd. day	3rd. day	4th. day	5th. day	Ave. per day	Recommended Amts. Child	Adol.	Adults	Difference
MILK GROUP (Milk, Cheese)							3–4 serv.	4 or more serv.	2 serv.	
MEAT GROUP (meat, fish, chicken, egg dried peas or beans)							2 or more servings			
VEGETABLE–FRUIT GROUP Total No. serv. (Including those rich in Vitamin C & Vitamin A)							4 or more servings — 1 serv. daily 1 serv. every other day			
BREAD–CEREAL GROUP Enriched or whole grain							4 or more serv.			

SWEETS INTAKE

FORM	WHEN EATEN	1st. day	2nd. day	3rd. day	4th. day	5th. day	total No. Exposures
Sugar in solution	During meal						
	End of meal						
	Between meals						
Solid and Retentive sweets	During meal						
	End of meal						
	Between meals						

Grand total

Figure 10–3. Dietary Evaluation Chart. An example of a type of chart suitable for use in qualitative dietary analysis.

and cereal and whole-grain bread—should be checked against the specific dietary record of the patient as to type of food groups or overconsumption of carbohydrate type foods. Diets high in refined sugar should be recorded and referred to the dentist for further study and evaluation.

Laboratory tests, which were useful in the past, are no longer emphasized except to demonstrate to the patient the presence of acid-forming microorganisms from his own teeth by colorimetric visualization. Examples of such tests are the Albans and Grainger.

In recent years, increasingly impressive evidence has pointed to the importance of nutrition in total body health, which obviously includes the oral cavity and periodontium. Evidence of incorrect eating habits in our culture suggests that we are undernourished in spite of the accessibility of adequate and varied food supplies. This fact is tragically underlined by the prevalence of malnutrition in children and teenagers. The imbalance has been due largely to the increased intake and(or) substitution of sugar-containing foods to the detriment of the ingestion of other essential food groups and the more desirable foods such as potatoes in the carbohydrate group.

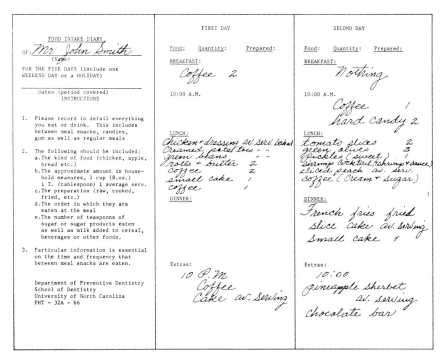

Figure 10–4. Patient Dietary Summary. There is imbalance in the diet because of overconsumption of carbohydrates and consequent inadequacy of the main protective food groups.

Periodontal disease is the result of an interplay of local and systemic influences. Refined sugar is a major source of nutriment for bacterial plaque accumulation on the teeth. By reducing the sugar intake in favor of other essential food groups we automatically reduce the plaque-forming potential on the teeth, thus helping control both caries and gingival inflammation. Thereby, in addition, we correct and reinforce the internal environment of our tissues by an intake of adequate amounts of protein, vitamins, and minerals. The integrity of the tissues of the periodontium is dependent upon this correct nutritional balance.

If the periodontal patient is instructed to reduce intake of sugar-containing foods in favor of acceptable substitutes in the four essential food groups, and if willing to cooperate, the correction of the nutritional status should not be too time consuming. Food habits, however, are difficult to modify or change. The thrust of research and

investigation is now directed at developing new, palatable, and safe sugar substitutes in order to overcome this problem. Fortunately, many non-cariogenic sugar substitutes are available and acceptable to the general public. Substitutes such as xylitol and sorbitol result in less plaque formation than sucrose (Rateitschak-Pluss, 1982).

Although the role of fluorides in oral health has been a controversial subject over the years, the overwhelming evidence is now supportive of this effective therapeutic agent in many ways. Fluorides are effective in controlling dental plaque by bacteriostatic and bactericidal properties. With fluorides over the past 30 years there have been no reports of host sensitivity, bacterial resistance, or superinfections from continuous use.

A planned regimen of fluoride therapy by topical application and daily rinses may well be the answer to suppressing plaque and resultant caries in cementum exposed by recession from improper tooth brushing or by periodontal therapy. In addition root sensitivity may well be reduced by such a regimen, thus promoting more diligent flossing and brushing.

Visual Education

There is a variety of material available for the oral health education of both child and adult patients in the values of good oral hygiene. Posters, pamphlets, slides, study casts, movies, and videotapes can be employed to instruct patients in a better understanding of periodontal disease and its prevention. There are materials from many sources now available for placement in the reception room for the instruction of patients while waiting for their appointment. The materials may be obtained from the American Dental Association and the American Academy of Periodontology. These materials alone, however, are not a substitute for the warmth of personal presentation and an interest in the welfare of the patient. Patients must be shown how a knowledge of oral disease and its prevention applies to their own oral condition and well-being.

Calling the patient's attention to the need of dental treatment and care beyond the prophylaxis can be rewarding. By letting the patient use a hand mirror, periodontal pockets can be demonstrated with the periodontal probe. Failing restorations and faulty margins can be demonstrated with an explorer. The patient's own efforts at oral physiotherapy can also be visibly demonstrated by letting him or her chew a disclosing wafer at the beginning of the appointment.

Pernicious habits on the part of the patient such as thumb-sucking in children, tongue thrust, and bruxism in adults may be observed and called to the dentist's attention. Such habits may lead to problems in occlusion and should be corrected as a part of the total program of prevention.

An extruded tooth due to the loss of an opposing member in the opposite arch can be called to the patient's attention. Ex-

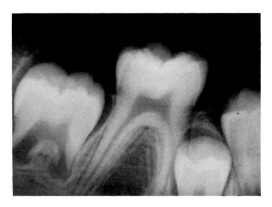

Figure 10–5. Premature Loss of Primary Molar. This radiograph of a 10-year-old child shows drifting of the first permanent molar resulting in loss of space for the eruption of the second premolar. This deformity is the consequence of premature loss of the primary molar. A space maintainer could have prevented this orthodontic problem.

truded teeth produce problems in chewing efficiency and also in hygiene as well as disruption of the dental arch. The importance of tooth replacements can be shown by suitable drawings or photographs. In children, the importance of space maintenance where a tooth has been prematurely lost can be explained to the parent in terms of resulting deformity in the secondary dentition (Fig. 10–5).

Carious teeth and the importance of restorations to prevent tooth loss and gingival disease should also be included in patient education during the dental appointment. The hygienist has an excellent opportunity to emphasize the importance of total dental care to all patients seen by her.

The hygienist's health education, talents, and efforts need not be circumscribed to individual patients. There are many opportunities for educating lay groups such as school children, parent-teacher associations, and local civic clubs. Posters, slides, and pamphlets could be integrated into a meaningful presentation to such interested groups.

REMEDIAL AND INTERCEPTIVE TREATMENT PROCEDURES

Orthodontic Considerations

When first maxillary and mandibular molars are lost during childhood or adolescence and then the space is not maintained, mesial drifting or tipping of the permanent molars usually occurs. The result is a pseudopocket (gingival) or periodontal pocket on the mesial aspect. Surgical periodontal therapy in this instance may fail to eliminate the pocket. Also restoration therapy in construction of bridges is compromised. The choice of therapy is molar uprighting by orthodontic means (Fig. 10–6). Frequent scaling and curettage are indicated during the uprighting procedure and special care must be given to oral physiotherapy.

The hygienist is heavily involved in the initial preparation of the supporting tissues before orthodontic banding of the teeth. Ideally the gingival tissues should be in a favorable state of health and free of inflammation. Frequent routine recall maintenance therapy is required during active orthodontic treatment, since bands and wires inhibit and limit the normal flossing and toothbrush regimen. Frequent routine maintenance therapy is also needed by the orthognathic surgical patient while in full bands prior to or following surgery.

When teeth are not in good alignment and are overlapped, effective oral hygiene is more difficult. Orthodontic correction can sometimes improve the dentogingival environment to a more favorable cleansing situation (Fig. 10–7).

The importance of an adequate band of attached gingiva in both children and adults before activation of orthodontic appliances has been established. This is particularly true in the mandibular anterior and premolar areas on the facial aspect. Free gingival grafts are often helpful in preventing recession of the gingival tissues during active movement of the mandibular anterior teeth (Fig. 10–8).

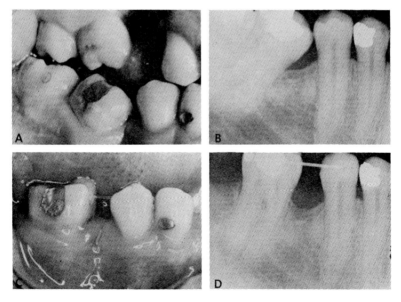

Figure 10–6. Orthodontic Uprighting to Eliminate Pocket on Mesial of Right Mandibular Second Molar. A, Clinical photograph before orthodontic correction. Third molar was extracted. B, Radiograph before uprighting. C, Clinical photograph after uprighting. D, Radiograph after uprighting. Note change in bone level on mesial of second molar. Pocket depth decreased from 6 mm to 3 mm after uprighting. (Courtesy of Drs. Howard Dorfman and John Moriarty, University of North Carolina School of Dentistry.)

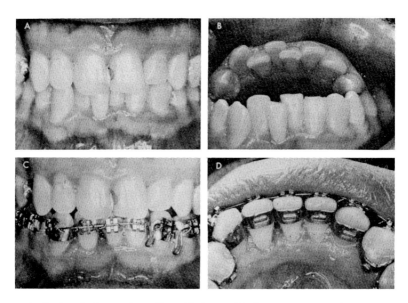

Figure 10–7.   Orthodontic Correction of Jumbled Mandibular Anterior Teeth to Facilitate Gingival Health and Oral Physiotherapy.   A & B, Clinical photographs before banding. C, After teeth were first banded. D, Active movement nearing completion. Appliance was removed at a subsequent appointment. (Courtesy of Dr. Luiz Gonzales and Department of Orthodontics, University of North Carolina School of Dentistry.)

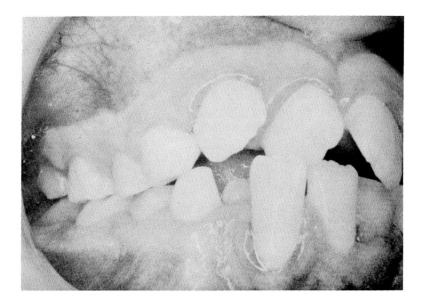

Figure 10–8.   Seven-Year-Old Child Requiring Orthodontic Correction.   Free gingival graft is needed on facial of #25 to prevent recession during active movement of mandibular anterior teeth.

Prosthetic Considerations

The maintenance of a few strategic teeth or tooth roots is now recognized as important in preservation of alveolar ridge height in removable prosthodontics. Patients with overdentures need routine maintenance recall to receive scaling and root planing of the tooth stubs under the dentures as well as instruction in oral hygiene measures when the dentures are removed after meals and at night. Cleaning full and partial dentures in order to free them of calculus and stains is part of the recall appointment and can be done either by the hygienist or the laboratory technician in the dental office. Ultrasonic machines designed for cleaning dental appliances are available in most dental offices.

Crown-Lengthening Procedures

Sometimes a carious lesion is so far advanced that restoration of the tooth crown becomes a major problem. The supporting tissues may need to be lowered by periodontal surgery measures to permit margination of the restoration above alveolar bone level. Root canal therapy is usually required where teeth are severely reduced to receive a post and core crown. The strategic importance of maintaining such a tooth plus alternate therapy such as extraction and a fixed bridge is always weighed by the dentist in making a clinical recommendation.

Pedodontic Considerations

If prevention of oral disease (caries, gingivitis, and periodontitis) is to be our goal, the logical starting place is with children. Good oral hygiene habits in children can be established early by good rapport with the therapist and easily carried forth through adolescence and adulthood.

The hygienist must deal with the child and parents in emphasizing the importance of maintaining the primary dentition in health. Should premature loss of a primary tooth occur, space maintenance for the secondary erupting teeth is not optional but mandatory. Interceptive orthodontics may be required at some point in arch and dentitional development.

Pictorial pamphlets geared to child motivation in preventive oral health care are available through the headquarters of the American Dental Association in Chicago. The hygienist is the one oral health professional who has the greatest opportunity to practice prevention of dental disease, topical fluoridation for caries prevention, and instruction in flossing and brushing to prevent gingivitis and periodontal disease.

In any unusual localized patterns of tooth attrition parafunctional habits are suspect. Bruxism is not an unusual finding in children. Pernicious habits sometimes produce abnormalities such as gingival recession by chronic fingernail trauma. The dentist should be informed so that evaluation and diagnosis can be of constructive help to the patient.

DENTAL PAIN AND SENSITIVITY

Unfortunately, the encountering of patients with pain originating from the oral cavity or sensitivity of the teeth is a daily occurrence in the routine dental practice. The study of pain—and certainly all is not understood about it—is far too broad and complex a subject to be addressed in this book. Pain is the sensation elicited in the central nervous system by noxious stimulation to certain sensory nerve endings. Dental pain is usually caused by the irritation of nerves in the pulp from chemical or mechanical reactions related to dental caries, frank pulpal exposure, or from trauma to the teeth.

Typically, chronic periodontitis does not evoke pain until it reaches the terminal stages. Gingival or periodontal pain usually results from acute inflammatory problems such as acute necrotizing ulcerative gingivitis or periodontal abscesses. Occlusal trauma or a periodontal-endodontic problem may result in pain.

Root sensitivity, or hypersensitivity as it is sometimes called, is a frequent occurrence when the root surface is exposed because of gingival recession, periodontal disease, or the results of periodontal therapy. Root sensitivity is provoked by thermal stimuli (hot or cold), by chemical stimuli (sweet or sour foods) or by mechanical stimuli (tooth brushing, root planing). The exact mechanism evoking the sensitivity is poorly understood. Part of the controversy in understanding the mechanisms lies in the lack of demonstration of whether or not sensory nerve endings are present in the dentinal tubules. Basically, there are two theories as to the mechanism of root sensitivity. One theory asserts that the noxious stimulus directly stimulates the sensory nerve endings at the exposed dentinal surface. The other theory is based on hydrodynamics. This theory asserts that the stimulus causes a rapid fluid flow in the dentinal tubules which results in a mechanical stimulation to the nerve endings in the dental pulp.

Over the decades, many substances and techniques have been employed to treat root sensitivity. None have met with success in all instances. The most consistently successful regimen witnessed by us has several components.

Firstly and most importantly, the patient must practice meticulous oral hygiene. Secondly, topical applicaitons of fluoride solutions or gels are administered at each recall appointment. And thirdly, the patient uses a toothpaste containing potassium nitrate or strontium chloride on a routine basis. This regimen will eliminate sensitivity as a problem for most patients.

Wycoff (1982) recommends the following regimen for severe cases: oral prophylaxis, burnish the specific areas with 33% sodium fluoride, have the patient use a desensitizing toothpaste which contains potassium nitrate or strontium chloride, and have the patient rinse daily with a 0.5% solution of sodium fluoride. He states that if that regimen is unsuccessful, an adhesive resin

material which does not require acid etching, such as glass ionomer cement, should be used to seal off the affected tooth structure.

An alternative approach has been successful for us. Calcium hydroxide U.S.P. (0.4 gm) is mixed in a dappen dish with sterile water to make a thick paste. The sensitive teeth are dried and isolated with cotton rolls to protect soft tissue because the medicament might cause ulceration of the gingiva. The paste is applied with a sable paintbrush to the root and allowed to remain for 5 minutes. The calcium hydroxide is then removed and the patient allowed to rinse with water. Additional applications may be required at subsequent appointments.

Local Anesthesia

Of course, it is absolutely imperative to maintain patient comfort and pain control during any periodontal procedure. For routine scaling and recall of patients it is usually not necessary to use any form of anesthetic agent to accomplish the indicated procedures. Occasionally, however, even in these situations there are areas of the gingiva or even the tooth itself where supersensitivity occurs and some topical or local anesthetic agent is needed before an adequate treatment can be rendered.

Before any form of anesthetic or other medication is employed, the medical history of the patient must be reviewed or retaken to ascertain that there is no possibility of hypersensitivity on the part of the patient to the agent.

Topical anesthetics are usually provided in the form of an ointment or a spray. The ointment is applied with a cotton applicator directly to the gingival tissue. For a few seconds it will produce a sensation of chilling and the patient may complain that it hurts the teeth. This will last only a few seconds. A period of 5 minutes should be allowed for the anesthetic to have maximal effect.

With the spray topical anesthetic, the solution is applied directly from the container to the gingival tissue.

Whenever pain control is required of the tooth itself, it is necessary to use an injectable local anesthetic. There are many satisfactory local anesthetic agents available. Most dentists have made their own selections based on the nature of their practice and their experience with local anesthetics. Usually, an anesthetic agent containing epinephrine is used, since this agent increases the duration of the pain control, and because its local constrictive action on blood vessels decreases the amount of hemorrhage.

The mechanism by which local anesthetic agents produce anesthesia is not known. It is theorized that the agent prevents the nerve membranes from changing their electric potential. A change in electric potential (depolarization) is necessary for an impulse such as pain to be conducted along the nerve membrane. Another theory is that the local anesthetic agent interferes with the production of acetylcholine at the synaptic junction of the nerve fibers. The production of acetylcholine is necessary for the electric potential of the nerve to change so that the impulse may be conducted.

The basic local anesthetic technique for the control of pain of the maxillary teeth is by supraperiosteal injection adjacent to the apices of the teeth. The area to be injected should be swabbed with a topical antiseptic agent such as iodine lotion prior to being penetrated by a needle. A topical anesthetic may be placed on the surface to allay apprehension on the part of those patients who have a phobia against needle injections. A 23- or 25-gauge needle is inserted in the alveolar mucosa several millimeters coronal to the tooth apex. The bevel of the needle should be slanted toward the tissue surface so that the very tip of the point penetrates the tissue first. The bevel slanted in this direction facilitates the anesthetic agent being injected toward the bony surface and in the direction of the

tooth apex rather than away from the bony surface into the soft tissue.

The needle is slowly inserted through the soft tissue until it approximates the periosteum, in the vicinity of the tooth apex. Care must be taken not to come directly into contact with the bone.

Approximately 0.5 ml (cc) of anesthetic is slowly injected into the area.

The maxillary bone overlying the facial surfaces of the teeth is thin and porous. The anesthetic agent diffuses through the periosteum, through the facial plate, and into the area of the apex of the associated tooth. Usually 5 minutes is necessary for the anesthetic agent to reach the appropriate nerves and invoke the pharmacologic action. All of the maxillary teeth can be anesthetized in this manner.

To anesthetize the mandibular teeth, it is necessary to administer an inferior alveolar nerve block. A review of oral anatomy in appropriate texts as to the location of the mandibular foramen on the lingual aspect of the mandible is necessary. Clinical demonstrations of locating the proper area for insertion of the needle are also mandatory before this procedure can be accomplished.

The major landmark to locate in the administration of an inferior alveolar block is the coronoid notch. This is the greatest depression on the anterior border of the ramus and may be located by gently palpating the ascending ramus with the ball of the index finger. Just lingual to the coronoid notch is a depression in the soft tissue called the pterygotemporal depression. This depression can be visualized and palpated best when the mouth is opened as wide as can be accomplished and still be comfortable.

A 1⅝-inch 25- or 27-gauge needle in an aspirating type syringe is used for an inferior alveolar nerve block. The surface area is prepared with antiseptic solution and topical anesthetic. The patient is asked to open wide so that the pterygotemporal depression can best be visualized.

The needle and syringe are carried to the site at as great an angle with the surface of the lingual aspect of the ascending ramus as is possible. That is, if the injection is to be made in the right mandible, the approach is from as far as possible toward the left side of the patient's mouth. Usually this means that when the needle is in contact with the surface of the tissue, the syringe will be in contact with the commissure of the opposite side of the lip.

The needle is inserted slowly into the tissue discharging a small amount of anesthetic as it advances. Every few seconds the plunger is pulled back on the syringe. This provides the aspirating action and, if for any reason the needle has penetrated a blood vessel, the blood will appear within the cartridge of anesthetic. If this occurs, it is necessary to withdraw the needle slightly and take a different direction so as to avoid injecting the anesthetic directly into a blood vessel.

The needle is advanced until it comes into direct contact with the periosteum on the lingual aspect of the mandible in the area of the mandibular canal. The needle then is slightly withdrawn from the surface and 1.5 to 2 ml of solution are injected slowly into the area.

The length of time taken to acquire anesthesia is dependent upon the proximity of the agent with the inferior alveolar nerve itself. The anesthesia may be acquired almost instantaneously or it may take up to 5 minutes. The lower lip begins to tingle when profound anesthesia is occurring.

A satisfactory method for checking the depth of anesthesia is by using a sharp explorer. After an appropriate amount of time has elapsed, a sharp explorer can be used to prick the area. The patient will not perceive pain (a sharp point) if the area is adequately anesthetized. He may, however, be able to perceive a blunt sensation since pressure and proprioceptive impulses are not removed by the anesthetic agent.

For many gingival procedures such as curettage, gingivectomy, and gingivo-plasty, it is not necessary to anesthetize the teeth to accomplish the procedure. Many times direct infiltration into the interdental papillae is adequate.

After the disinfectant agent and topical agent are applied, a 23- or 25-gauge 1-inch needle is inserted with the bevel toward the tissue directy into the interproximal papillae. A depth of 3 to 5 mm is adequate. A few drops of anesthetic agent are slowly injected into the interproximal papilla until it blanches. This is repeated in all papillae from both the facial and lingual or palatal aspects until the indicated area is anesthetized. Usually an entire quadrant can be anesthetized in this fashion with less than 1 ml of anesthetic agent.

OCCLUSAL ADJUSTMENT

Occlusal adjustment is a procedure by which the occlusal surfaces of the teeth are selectively ground to eliminate occlusal contacts which are placing too much force on the supporting structures of the teeth. The clinical application of this technique is indicated when a patient has traumatic occlusion, temporomandibular joint disorders related to the occlusion, facial muscle hypertonicity or spasm, or destructive bruxism.

The clinical objectives of occlusal adjustment are to eliminate centric prematurities, to eliminate interferences in eccentric movements, to improve masticatory efficiency, to place occlusal stresses within the long axis of the teeth, and to distribute the occlusal forces within the physiologic limits of the supporting structures of each tooth.

Only small amounts of tooth structure are removed. A handpiece revolving only 10,000 to 20,000 revolutions per minute is used. The areas to be reduced are usually located by the dentist with marking paper or wax strips. Small carborundum stones are used to make the reductions. After each reduction, the extraneous marks are wiped off the teeth and a new marking is made.

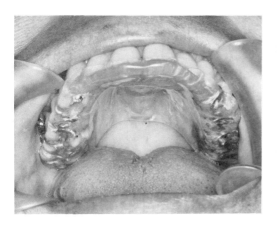

Figure 10–9. Occlusal Bite Guard. This appliance is used in the treatment of bruxism and other occlusal problems. (From Allen, D.L., Periodontics, 5:93, 1967.)

The first duty of the hygienist in occlusal adjustment is to have the instruments and materials needed for the procedure available. These usually consist of an assortment of small stones and rubber wheels, articulating paper or occlusal indicator wax, sterile sponges, and a mouth mirror. Some operators like to use a forcep to place the articulating paper between the teeth.

While the dentist is doing the adjustment, the hygienist should keep the teeth cool and the mirror clean of enamel dust by directing a jet of air on the area. After the adjustment is completed, the hygienist smooths the ground surfaces with rubber wheels, being careful not to overheat the teeth. The teeth are then polished. If any dentin has been exposed, the area is isolated with cotton rolls and a desensitizing solution of sodium fluoride or sodium silicofluoride applied.

In the case of temporomandibular joint disorder, facial muscle spasm, or bruxism, an occlusal bite splint (night guard) is often constructed in association with occlusal adjustment. The appliance prevents the patient from clinching the teeth together and relieves the amount of stress placed on an individual tooth. Figure 10–9 demonstrates a clear acrylic bite splint.

The bite splint is fabricated on stone casts. The hygienist usually mixes the impression material, fills the impression trays, and later pours the impressions in dental stone. With expanded functions the hygienist may make the impressions and deliver the appliance. When delivered, the appliance, not the opposing teeth, is adjusted as indicated so that all teeth occlude with it. Any areas which were adjusted must be repolished.

TREATMENT OF SPECIFIC PERIODONTAL DISEASES

Inflammatory Periodontal Disease

Gingivitis and periodontitis constitute, by far, the major types of periodontal disease which the therapist must treat. In general, the treatment plan consists of the removal or correction of the local irritating factors; oral physiotherapy instructions; occlusal adjustment, if indicated; and pocket elimination by the surgical procedure best designed to correct the particular problem. Restorative dentistry is extremely important in the overall treatment of many patients.

Acute Periodontal Conditions

Necrotizing ulcerative gingivitis, periodontal abscess, or pericoronitis may occur in an acute form and require systemic consideration prior to periodontal therapy. If the patient has an acute inflammatory problem as evidenced from the clinical signs and symptoms, a white blood cell differential count should be made and the patient's temperature determined.

If there is an elevation in the white blood cell count or temperature or if there is lymphadenopathy or generalized malaise, the patient should probably be placed on systemic antibiotic therapeutics prior to any local periodontal therapy. The dentist may elect to prescribe the antibiotics himself or he may prefer to refer the patient to a physician. Most patients with these acute periodontal problems will not need to be placed on antibiotic therapy.

NECROTIZING ULCERATIVE GINGIVITIS. In association with antibiotic therapy, if indicated, the patient with acute necrotizing ulcerative gingivitis is instructed to rinse his mouth vigorously every hour with a 1½% solution of hydrogen peroxide. A 3% solution of peroxide can be diluted with warm tap water or mouth wash. If it is impossible for the patient to rinse this frequently with the peroxide, tap water may be substituted part of the time. The peroxide rinse helps remove microorganisms, necrotic tissue, and debris from around the gingivae and teeth. Oxygen is released from the solution and aids in the oxygenation of the inflamed tissues. Several commercial preparations of oxygenating agents are available which may be helpful. However, it is probably the vigorous rinsing with copious amounts of solution that is of the greatest benefit.

Frequently patients with necrotizing ulcerative gingivitis are somewhat debilitated because of inadequate rest, poor diet, worry, oversmoking, or overdrinking. These problems must be realized and corrected before the best overall treatment can be rendered to the patient.

If there is a great deal of debris present, the teeth should be carefully but thoroughly polished. If the gingivae are acutely inflamed, no subgingival scaling should be attempted since they are easily traumatized. The tissues are usually so sensitive at this time that a scaling cannot adequately be accomplished.

The patient should be seen the next day to evaluate the response to the emergency treatment. After two or three days, the acute inflammatory process has usually subsided and the patient is instructed to discontinue the hydrogen peroxide rinses but to continue frequent mouth wash or tap water rinses. Oral physiotherapy instructions are given. If the acuteness has sufficiently subsided, scaling procedures may be instituted.

After all local irritants have been removed, adequate oral physiotherapy has been introduced, and the inflammation has subsided, the periodontal tissues are evaluated. The extensiveness of the tissue destruction determines the extent and type of surgical intervention which will be indicated. The rationale for surgery is to correct the interproximal defects which may accompany the disease. Defects which persist are areas that readily accumulate debris and overgrowths of microorganisms. These areas break down and result in a recurrence of the disease. Of course if the problem is treated early enough, surgery will not be necessary.

PERIODONTAL ABSCESS. A periodontal abscess is a localized accumulation of pus in the wall of a periodontal pocket. If the patient is febrile or there is an elevated white cell count, antibiotic therapy should be considered. Emergency treatment consists of incision and drainage of the abscess. The incision is made directly into the abscess and the soft tissue is massaged to express all of the suppuration. The lesion is left open so that it may continue to drain.

Frequently the involved tooth has extruded and is excessively mobile. Occlusal adjustment and temporary splinting are necessary. In most instances there is a dramatic response to the emergency procedures and, with proper definitive treatment, the tooth can remain in health and function for many years.

PERICORONITIS. This is an acute inflammation occurring in the soft tissue flap which partially covers erupting third molars. The condition is treated by irrigating under the flap with a dilute hydrogen peroxide solution. Gentian violet is applied under the flap for its antiseptic action. If systemic conditions indicate, antibiotic therapy should be instituted. These procedures may have to be repeated daily for several days before the condition clears up. The gingival flap may have to be surgically removed or the tooth extracted to prevent a recurrence of the pericoronitis.

Use of Antibiotics

Appropriate antibiotics coverage is always indicated for a patient who is susceptible to the development of subacute bacterial endocarditis, e.g., a patient with a history of rheumatic heart disease or who has a prosthetic heart valve. It has been suggested, in several places in this book, that consideration of antibiotic therapy is indicated when there is evidence of systemic complications in association with the periodontal problem. Systemic complications are manifested by an elevated body temperature, lymphadenopathy, or an elevated white blood cell count. These conditions are most likely to occur in patients with acute inflammatory diseases such as necrotizing ulcerative gingivitis, pericoronitis or periodontal abscess.

Since periodontal disease is caused by microorganisms, there is a rationale for the use of antibiotics in its treatment. Many antibiotics, including penicillin, tetracyclines, minocycline, clindamycin, and metronidazole have been shown to be effective against oral microorganisms. A short term study showed that systemic metronidazole resulted in a significant reduction in certain anaerobic organisms such as Bacteroides gingivalis and large spirochetes (Loesche et al, 1984). The virtual elimination of spirochetes was reported when tetracycline was delivered into the gingival crevice in hollow fibers (Goodson, 1979). Oral tetracycline therapy was reported to be beneficial in association with surgical treatment of four patients with juvenile periodontitis (Jaffin, 1984).

In general, there is little justification for the use of either topical or systemic antibiotics in the routine treatment of chronic periodontal disease. It has been shown that chronic gingivitis and periodontitis can be successfully treated without the use of antibiotics. Antibiotic therapy always runs the risk of developing a drug sensitivity in the patient so that they cannot take the drug again without having an allergic reaction. It also runs the danger of developing strains of bacteria that are resistant to that particular drug.

Desquamative Gingivitis and Juvenile Periodontitis

There is no specific treatment available for the degenerative aspects of these diseases. Usually inflammation is superimposed on these conditions. This is treated the same as it is for gingivitis and periodontitis. Oral physiotherapy, pocket elimination, and occlusal adjustment are important aspects of the treatment for juvenile periodontitis. Tetracycline therapy is helpful in the treatment of juvenile periodontitis. Frequent recalls are imperative. Topical applications of hydrocortisone preparations sometimes help the symptoms of desquamative gingivitis.

PERIODONTAL PROSTHESIS

In many instances, the patients with advanced periodontal disease require more than basic periodontal treatment to ensure indefinite retention of their dental arches. Many times these patients have already lost teeth or must have teeth removed prior to periodontal treatment because of inadequate periodontal support. The missing teeth must be replaced.

Many times the remaining teeth are mobile due to loss of periodontal support and have to be stabilized (Fig. 10–10). If they are not stabilized, they continue to loosen until the point is reached that they have to be removed. The replacement and splinting of teeth for the periodontal patient require the highest type of diagnostic and technical skill from the dentist.

In some cases, teeth which have migrated due to periodontal involvement need to be repositioned by orthodontic movement prior to occlusal reconstruction. After the teeth are repositioned and the occlusion is adjusted, these teeth are splinted to the more stable members of the dental arch.

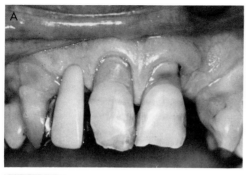

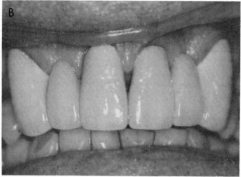

Figure 10–10. Periodontal Prosthesis. Top, These teeth have lost periodontal support, are mobile, and esthetically unpleasing. Bottom, After reconstruction. (Prosthesis courtesy Dr. M.W. Holland.)

Mobile teeth may be temporarily splinted during treatment by wire ligation, by orthodontic bands welded together, or by an acrylic bite guard. Composite restorative material, alone or reinforced with wire, is an excellent material for temporary splinting. Following periodontal treatment, the ideal method of stabilization is by the use of fixed splinting. Inlays or partial or full crowns are soldered together to provide the fixed splint. Missing teeth are replaced by pontics which are fabricated into the splint.

The primary principle involved in splinting is that the appliance will distribute the forces placed on it. The occlusal forces which would have been placed on the periodontally weakened teeth are partially absorbed by the other teeth in the splint. Splinting prevents the teeth from tilting

when laterally directed forces are applied to them and results in the maximum number of periodontal fibers functioning to support each tooth.

Patients who have extensive periodontal prostheses or splints must be instructed to practice meticulous oral physiotherapy techniques. These devices are usually more difficult to keep clean than the natural dentition. Patients with periodontal prosthesis must be recalled more frequently than other patients.

CONTINUOUS PERIODONTAL CARE

As one considers the various techniques and procedures involved in total periodontal therapy, it is obvious that the scope of periodontics is great and extends into all areas of dentistry. Periodontics is the basis for the modern practice of dentistry. To practice restorative or corrective dentistry without adequate concern for the periodontal support of the teeth is indeed like the man who built his house on the sand.

The ideal approach is to prevent the development of periodontal disease. In this realm, the hygienist can make the greatest contribution to the dental health of her patients.

All patients need periodontal care. The person who does not develop some degree of periodontal disease in the face of the local irritants which form in all mouths is rare and unpredictable. Every patient should receive regular routine oral prophylaxis and oral physiotherapy instructions. The degree and extent of treatment above this vary with the individual patient. An individual who has received periodontal treatment is in no way immune to redevelopment of the disease unless he or she is maintained on a rigid program of preventive periodontics. Patients who fail to do so will need re-treatment if there is enough periodontal tissue left to treat.

Everyone in the dental profession must recognize the full denture patient as a dental failure and employ every procedure at our command to prevent this failure from occurring.

SUMMARY

Periodontics is the basis for the practice of dentistry. The scope of periodontics is great and expands into all areas of dental practice. The various technical procedures utilized in clinical periodontics are meaningless unless their application is consistent with the patient's needs. The ultimate solution to the control of periodontal disease must be in the field of preventive dentistry. If properly indoctrinated and motivated, the dental hygienist contributes a significant service to patients in the prevention of periodontal disease.

BIBLIOGRAPHY

Addy, M., Perriam, E. and Sterry, A.: Effects of sugared and sugar-free chewing gum on the accumulation of plaque and debris on the teeth, J. Clin. Periodontol., 9:346, 1982.

Allen, D.L.: Necrotizing ulcerative gingivitis and its treatment, J. North Carolina Dent. Soc., 45:16, 1961.

Allen, D.L.: Accurate occlusal bite guards, Periodontics, 5:93, 1967.

Berman, L.H.: Dentinal sensation and hypersensitivity, J. Periodontol., 56:216, 1985.

Genco, R.J.: Antibiotics in the treatment of human periodontal diseases, J. Periodontol., 52:545, 1981.

Glickman's Clinical Periodontology, F.A. Carranza (Ed.), 6th ed., Philadelphia, W.B. Saunders Co., 1984. pp. 979 (pp. 317–321).

Goodson, J.M., Haffajee, A., and Socransey, S.S.: Periodontal therapy by local delivery of tetracycline, J. Clin. Periodontol., 6:83, 1979.

Green, B.L., Green, M.L., and McFall, W.T., Jr.: Calcium hydroxide and potassium nitrate as desensitizing agents for hypersensitive root surfaces, J. Periodontol., 48:667, 1977.

Green, J.C., and Vermillion, J.R.: The simplified oral hygiene index, J. Am. Dent. Assoc., 68:7, 1964.

Guide to Dental Health, J. Am. Dent. Assoc., Special Issue, 1985.

Jaffin, R.A., Greenstein, G., and Berman, C.L.: Treatment of juvenile periodontitis patients by control of infection and inflammation, J. Periodontol., 55:261, 1984.

Loesche, W.J., et al.: Metronidazole in periodontitis, J. Periodontol., 55:325, 1984.

McFall, W.T., Jr.: Periodontics—An old challenge revisited, Tenn. St. Dent. J., 45:28, 1965.

Ramfjord, S.P.: The periodontal index (PDI), J. Periodontol., 38:602, 1967.

Ramfjord, S.P., et al.: Longitudinal study of periodontal therapy, J. Periodontol., 44:66, 1973.

Ramfjord, S.P., et al.: Results following three modalities of periodontol therapy, J. Periodontol., 46:522, 1975.

Rateitschak-Pluss, E.M. and Guggenheim, B.: Effects of carbohydrate-free diet and sugar substitutes on dental plaque accumulation, J. Clin. Periodontol., 9:239, 1982.

Silness, J. and Löe, H.: Periodontal disease in pregnancy. II Correlation between oral hygiene and periodontal condition, Acta Odontolog. Scandi., 24:747, 1964.

Wycoff, S.J.: Current treatment for dentinal hypersensitivity, Compendium on Continuing Education in Dentistry, 3:5113, 1982.

Yeung, F.I.S., Newman, H.N., and Addy, M.: Subgingival metronidazole in acrylic resins vs chlorhexidine irrigation in the control of chronic periodontitis, J. Periodontol., 54:651, 1983.

11

PERIODONTAL SURGERY

No modality of periodontal therapy has undergone such dramatic change as periodontal surgery. From primitive beginnings in the late nineteenth century, periodontal surgical treatment has continued an evolutionary process with a wide variety of procedures introduced for specific clinical problems. Impetus for this constant alteration in periodontal surgical therapy has derived from increased understanding of the causation of periodontal diseases, of the natural history of the disease, of the histopathology of the disease, and of the wound healing phenomenon. Development of new drugs, materials, devices, and instruments have further contributed toward the introduction of new surgical methods.

HISTORIC DEVELOPMENT

In order to understand the rationale for modern periodontal surgery, it is helpful to review some of the reasons for surgical treatment in the past. Early surgical methods were designed to excise, or cut out, diseased periodontal tissues. The bone underlying periodontal pockets was thought to be necrotic (dead). When research proved that periodontal inflamma-

tion was a bodily defense and that alveolar bone was not necrotic, this rationale no longer supported that particular concept of surgical therapy.

Pocket elimination then evolved as the principal reason for periodontal surgical procedures, and this rationale has persisted to the present. By gingival surgery the progression of the disease process was thought to be stopped and further loss of bone support would not occur. In addition, the root surface could be more easily treated by the health professionals, and the periodontal patient could perform tooth cleaning procedures more easily.

Most surgical procedures of the 1930s were simple excisions of inflamed or hyperplastic gingiva. Frenulum incision was accomplished to relieve pull on the gingivae that caused recession, but this was primarily accomplished in the maxillary central incisors to aid in orthodontic closure of diastemas. It is difficult for the modern hygienist to realize the relative indifference of the dental profession in general toward periodontal disease during this period, but the emphasis was definitely on treatment of dental caries. The bacterial etiology of periodontal disease was not recognized. Calculus and stain were removed as preventive measures, and periodontal surgery was accomplished only as a last resort. Few periodontists were available and there were few hygienists to treat the population.

Another major factor in the slow development of periodontal surgery was World War II that decreased the world's efforts in dental research as attention was focused on dental health of service personnel. Interestingly, this war served valuable purposes in promoting oral hygiene, developing antibiotics, the understanding of necrotizing ulcerative gingivitis, and introducing creative periodontal surgical technics. In the 1950s and 1960s a plethora of imaginative surgical procedures emerged including periodontal flap procedures to facilitate scaling; mucogingival procedures to correct gingival deficiencies; osseous resective surgery to modify bone deformities in order to create a tissue form consistent with normal architecture, and treatment of intrabony defects to stimulate new growth of bone. Collectively, these operations represented a substantial increase in surgical periodontal therapy.

During the period of the 1970s many earlier techniques were modified and new surgical procedures developed to augment the amount of keratinized soft tissue and to enhance tooth support by implanting material in bony defects. This period of the past two decades also represents a time of unprecedented periodontal research. As a result of this effort a reappraisal of periodontal surgery has occurred with the emphasis on control of active disease and maintenance of the attachment apparatus supplanting pocket reduction as the prevailing concept.

RATIONALE FOR PERIODONTAL SURGERY

Any type of dental treatment should be predicated on sound principles and supported by appropriate clinical research. Current periodontal surgical procedures

satisfy these criteria and remain a valuable portion of the treatment of destructive disease processes. Essentially two types of periodontal surgery have evolved, resective surgery and reconstructive surgery. Resective surgery is predicated on decreasing pocket depths and reshaping soft and hard tissues to create a tissue configuration for maintenance of health. Reconstructive surgery serves to enhance the quantity and quality of soft and hard tissues to establish periodontal health. The ultimate goal of both resective and reconstructive surgery is the same, preservation of the natural dentition in a healthy environment. Only the surgical techniques differ, not the results of treatment.

Control of Active Disease

Previous chapters have stressed the role of bacteria in the etiology of periodontal disease, the importance of instrumentation in removal of plaque and calculus, and the role of bacterial control through oral hygiene. Most patients with gingivitis and early periodontitis can be successfully treated by nonsurgical means. Pocket reduction can occur by a combination of a decrease in edematous fluid in the tissue, resolution of inflammation, and reestablishment of tissue integrity. Where pocket depth is minimal, research has demonstrated that scaling and root planing are sufficient therapy. Scaling, root planing, subgingival curettage, and plaque control are also successful treatment measures, where tissue are edematous and not fibrotic, and in pockets of moderate depth (Fig. 11–1).

Nonsurgical preparation should always be accomplished prior to surgical intervention in order to control the active disease process. There are, however, limitations to the exclusive use of nonsurgical techniques. The resolution of inflammation is dependent upon removal of soft and hard microbial deposits and root preparation. With progressively deeper pockets scaling and root planing becomes increasingly dif-

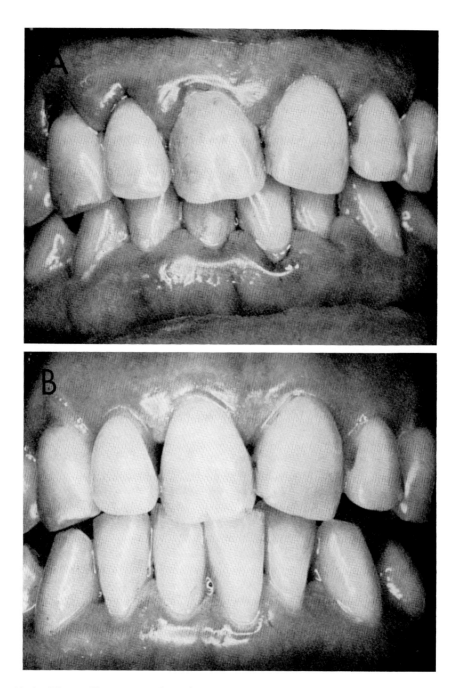

Figure 11–1. Tissue Changes Resulting from Periodontal Therapy. Positive changes in gingival texture, form, and contour have occurred from A, before treatment to B, after treatment. (From McFall, W.T.: Tenn. St. Dent. J., 45:34, 1965.)

ficult and studies have demonstrated limitations in effectiveness in pockets deeper than 5 mm. In order to achieve desired results in moderate to deep pockets, it is often advisable to perform surgery.

Periodontal surgical methods may (1) aid in control of active disease, (2) provide access for scaling and root planing, (3) establish tissue contours favorable to preservation of health, (4) provide for esthetics, (5) enhance quality and quantity of periodontal tissue, and (6) support the initiation of other treatment or repair the deleterious results of other dental therapies. Thus, periodontal surgery serves a valuable role in total patient care, and this role may become even more significant in the future if methods can be discovered to achieve a restitution of the lost attached apparatus.

Accessibility to Root Surfaces

If subgingival etiology cannot be removed by instrumentation through the pocket orifice, then periodontal surgery is indicated. Control of the disease process dictates the use of surgery to facilitate debridement. This represents a departure from the earlier rationale for periodontal surgery in which pockets were viewed as contributing to the disease process. It is now recognized that bacterial activity in the pocket with clinical evidence of altered gingival topography, bleeding, and purulent exudate represent an active disease process. Pockets, even moderately deep pockets, may represent scars of earlier disease activity and do not indicate current inflammatory change. It may be assumed that if a pocket does manifest inflammatory activity there is plaque and calculus on root surfaces.

Visualization of the root surface by surgical exposure does facilitate the removal of irritants. In deeper pockets surgery may be the only way to reach subgingival deposits. Root concavities, furcation areas, and irregular root forms provide convenient areas for plaque and calculus deposits that can only be removed by surgical exposure. Deep pockets (7 to 12 mm) have been treated surgically with greater gain in periodontal attachment than other therapies and maintained over long periods of time.

Establishing Optimal Tissue Contour

Gingival and osseous tissue deformities occur as the result of the destructive disease process. These alterations in soft tissue form are manifested as gingival overgrowths, gingival craters, or gingival recession. Such alterations in soft tissue contour invite the accumulation of microbial plaque. Further, such deformities may create difficulties for the patient in performance of oral hygiene that is essential to maintain health. Fibrosis in connective tissue of the pocket wall inhibits tissue shrinkage. Esthetics also can be compromised by such aberrations.

Changes occurring in the osseous structures due to resorption such as craters and angular defects may influence soft tissue contours and limit pocket reduction. Osseous overgrowths such as ledges and exostoses, and furcation invasion all may lead to plaque retention and impede plaque removal. Resective or reconstructive surgery can be used to correct these tissue aberrations and should be considered in achieving periodontal health.

Enhancement of Tissues

Reconstructive periodontal surgery can be accomplished in either soft or hard tissues. A loss of gingival keratinized tissue can result from gingival recession due to frenal pull, periodontal disease destruction, and deleterious habits. Gingival grafting procedures are available to augment the keratinized tissue and cover denuded root surfaces. In addition to providing a stable environment such surgery may enhance tissue health, improve esthetics, and decrease opportunities for microbial accumulation.

In modern times a number of materials, both natural and synthetic, have been suggested as implant materials to help strengthen tooth support, fill osseous voids, support overlying soft tissues, and stimulate osteogenesis. Surgical attempts to create new bone, periodontal ligament, and cemental union have unfortunately not met with much success.

It would be desirable if a successful reconstitution of tissues destroyed by disease could be achieved. Surgical procedures designed to achieve this have been termed reattachment or new attachment operations, that envision a concept of replacing lost connective tissues and the reestablishment of the attachment apparatus. Such new attachment can occur in certain circumstances such as healing following acute periodontal abscesses or in combination with pulpal-periodontal lesions. Animal models using substances that block epithelium also offer promise that a new periodontal ligament may be constituted. Most operations performed on humans have resulted in a decrease in pocket depth due to the establishment of a long epithelial attachment instead of growth of new connective tissue fibers.

Combined Therapy

A final consideration for periodontal surgery relates to the surgical tissue modifications necessary to support other dental procedures. Both resective and reconstructive surgical techniques can be used to provide a healthy periodontal foundation. Exposure of additional tooth structure may be necessary in order to treat extensive caries or tooth fracture. Sometimes simple excisional removal of excess gingival tissue is sufficient to provide this tooth structure. More commonly, flaps must be elevated and moved apically in order to gain enough clinical crown to provide adequate prosthetic retention. Bone may or may not need to be removed to accomplish this. These surgical procedures, often incorrectly termed ''crown-lengthening surgery,'' really involve an apical displacement of the periodontal attachment.

Redundant tissue may need to be removed in preparation for fixed or removable prostheses. This may involve edentulous ridges, maxillary tuberosities, or retromolar areas. Conversely, gingival augmentation may be required for esthetics or pontic adaptation. Edentulous ridges may be modified to gain additional height by vestibular deepening or placement of synthetic material on the bony ridge. Exostoses and tori may need to be removed in order to provide for placement of removable appliances.

Combination pulpal-periodontal lesions frequently require both endodontic therapy and periodontal surgery. Perforations of the root during endodontic preparation often can be strategically managed by periodontal surgical exposure.

Orthodontic movement of teeth with an insufficient amount of gingiva frequently results in serious recession. Preventive placement of keratinized grafts prior to orthodontic therapy can negate this sequelae. Removal of frenula, removal of redundant tissue, cosmetic shaping of gingiva, and severing of periodontal fibers to prevent relapse of rotated teeth are other examples of combined periodontal-orthodontic therapy. The increased use of orthognathic surgery of the mouth in order to skeletal deformities sometimes results in undesirable periodontal contours necessitating subsequent periodontal surgery.

GENERAL CONSIDERATION IN PERIODONTAL SURGERY

Periodontal surgery should never be considered until comprehensive medical histories have been secured, and the patient has been emotionally prepared for the surgical experience. A wide range of medical and neurologic conditions clearly contraindicate periodontal surgery. Included are bleeding and hormonal disorders as well as other conditions presented in Chapter 9. Certain medications necessary for treatment or control of systemic states can limit the patient's ability to undergo surgical treatment. Antibiotic prophylactic coverage may be indicated prior to surgical intervention in patients with histories of cardiovascular conditions. Appropriate consultation with physicians by the dentist is a fundamental consideration before treatment of medically compromised patients.

Even many patients in good physical health are poor candidates for periodontal surgery. Some patients are so emotionally nonstable that periodontal surgery is ill advised. All individuals exhibit some disquiet and anxiety about having to undergo surgery. These individuals can usually be successfully managed by careful explanation of the reasons for the surgery and description of anticipated discomfort. The preparatory period during nonsurgical therapy provides the opportunity to discuss this with the patient. The individual who is highly agitated, extremely nervous, resorts to alcohol or drugs, or copes poorly with life's stresses should not have periodontal surgery.

A third general class of patients for whom periodontal surgery is contraindicated are those unable to demonstrate cooperation in control of plaque. In some instances surgery may be required to enhance plaque control, but the patient who makes little effort to control their condition will not perform better oral hygiene after surgery. Indeed there is a strong tendency of patients to equate surgery with cure and there is often a concomitant reduction of oral hygiene following surgery.

We live in a time of litigation in which malpractice suits are all too common. Every patient who is to receive periodontal surgery deserves to know the benefits, limitations, and possible sequelae of such surgery. Therapists can offer advice to the patient that they feel is in the patient's best interest, but only the patient can make the decision on treatment of their bodies. Periodontal surgery should be done with the consent of a well-informed patient. Legally, this consent may be verbal, but many dentists now request written consent prior to surgery. Most intelligent patients will agree to surgical treatment when the procedural options have been thoroughly explained. Patients should understand the recurrent nature of periodontal disease and their own responsibility for their oral health before having periodontal surgery.

Except for the emergency situation such as a periodontal abscess, periodontal surgery is best delayed until nonsurgical therapy has been completed and patient cooperation has been obtained. Often a relatively long series of appointments is accomplished prior to surgical intervention. Many therapists prefer a period of 1 to 2 months after active nonsurgical preparation to judge the results of such treatment and the patient's oral hygiene effort before initiating the surgical phase. Gratifying results are often obtained negating the need for surgery that had originally been contemplated. An appointment devoted to the appraisal of the results of presurgical preparation is a sound concept.

TECHNIQUES OF PERIODONTAL SURGERY

Curettage

Curettage is a surgical procedure utilized to remove the epithelial lining from a soft tissue surface or from bodily cavities. Gingival curettage is the removal of the epithelial lining and a portion of the underlying inflamed connective tissue. This results in shrinkage of the tissue and in pocket reduction (Fig. 11–2). In situations where pockets are suprabony and the gingiva is edematous, adequate shrinkage may occur following curettage to eliminate the pocket. The procedure is accomplished under local anesthesia with a sharp curette against the soft tissue pocket wall (Fig. 11–3).

Although soft tissue curettage is still taught in many schools and is still prac-

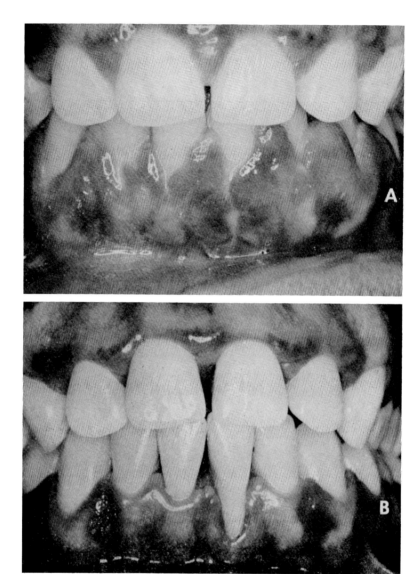

Figure 11–2. Gingival Curettage. A, Initial clinical condition with edematous gingiva. B, Gingival condition three weeks following scaling, root planing, and soft tissue curettage. The mandibular central incisor with gingival recession will require mucogingival surgical correction. (Courtesy Dr. James Antoon.)

ticed, it is not in current vogue. Research has demonstrated that thorough subgingival scaling and root planing will give the same results. If soft tissue reduction is desired, incision is a more exact method of tissue removal. Flap surgery also provides direct access to the roots for thorough debridement.

CURETTAGE FOR NEW ATTACHMENT. This procedure was designed to regain periodontal support for the tooth lost by deep, isolated pockets. The intention of the surgery was to provide an environment that would result in a reformation and new attachment of the connective tissue fibers to the tooth in an amount that would minimize the pocket. Unfortunately, evidence from research demonstrated that only a

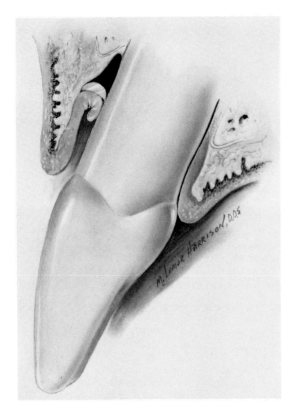

Figure 11–3. Gingival Curettage. The sharp edge of the curette is used to remove the crevicular epithelium.

long epithelial attachment was the result. Thus, this operation is seldom used.

Local anesthesia is used for the surgical procedure. A sharp curette is used to remove pocket epithelium and associated granulomatous tissue from the pocket. The root surface is planed and a blood clot allowed to form. When such a surgical approach was accomplished through the pocket orifice, it is termed closed curettage. Open curettage is a surgical method of maintaining healthy portions of attached gingiva while allowing direct access to subgingival tissues, root, and bone by elevation of a soft-tissue flap and will be discussed under the section of this chapter describing flap operations.

Gingivectomy and Gingivoplasty

Traditionally, the most utilized periodontal surgical technique has been the gingivectomy. From early in the twentieth century through the early 1960s it was the treatment of choice for suprabony pocket elimination. Gingivectomy represents a method by which suprabony pockets are eliminated by surgical resection of the diseased soft-tissue wall of the pocket. Gingivectomy is employed when the suprabony pocket persists following removal of subgingival deposits, or when the gingivae are fibrotic. Curettage is not successful when the gingivae is fibrotic. An adequate amount of attached gingiva apical to the base of the pocket must be present to provide for a physiologic topography following pocket elimination and is a major requirement for selection of this operation (Fig. 11–4A).

The gingivectomy is not a useful operation when intrabony pockets are present since a residual pocket would remain following surgery. Cosmetic considerations, such as in the maxillary anterior region, and the gain in attachment achieved with flap surgery have caused the gingivectomy to decrease in popularity. Also the gingivectomy cannot be used when osseous de-

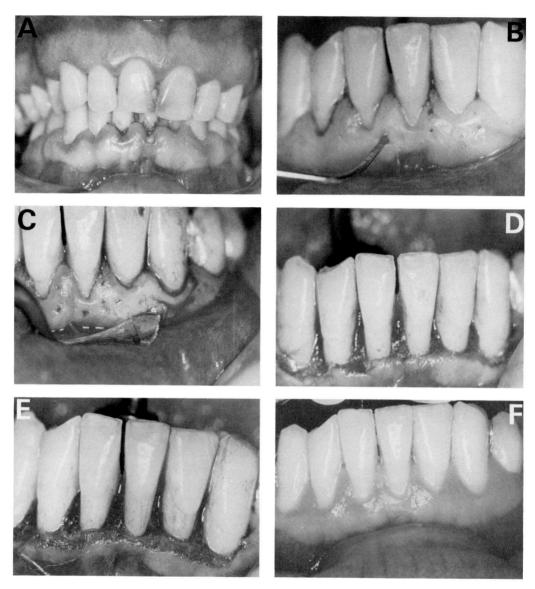

Figure 11–4. *Gingivectomy.* A, Clinical situation at initiation of therapy. Plaque and calculus have contributed to suprabony pockets and nonphysiologic contours. B, Marking pocket depths. Etiologic agents have been removed and gingival inflammation reduced. C, Primary gingivectomy incision. D, Gingival tissue has been removed. E, Gingivoplasty. F, Seven years following surgery the tissue is healthy.

formities or mucogingival problems are present.

Since the gingivectomy is a basic periodontal surgical procedure, the technique is presented in some detail so that the hygienist can understand subsequent surgical modifications. The gingival area in which

the gingivectomy is to be performed is anesthetized with a local anesthetic that firms up the tissue and aids in the control of hemorrhage. Pockets are carefully measured with a periodontal probe from the gingival margin. The depth of each pocket is then measured on the external aspect of the gingiva, and the probe is inserted horizontally into the gingiva (Fig. 11–4B). This produces a series of external markings, bleeding points, which trace the pattern of pocket depths and serve as a guide for the initial incision. An initial incision is then made with a gingivectomy knife on a coronal angle 1 to 2 mm apical to the pocket depths (Fig. 11–4C). By making the incision on an angle, a knife-edge margin is produced that facilitates physiologic form and eliminates the pocket. Care is taken to make sure that the incision is made apically enough to eliminate the pocket without removal of healthy attached gingiva. This incision is termed an *external beveled incision* (Fig. 11–4D and Fig. 11–5).

After the initial marginal incision has been made to contact with the teeth over the entire area of the operation, the papillary areas are incised with an interproximal periodontal knife and the gingival tissue is removed (Fig. 11–4E). Roots of teeth are carefully examined for residual calculus or roughness and root planing accomplished. Tags of tissue are removed, the area shaped to desired physiologic form with the edge of a periodontal knife, and the area covered with a periodontal dressing. Tissue form thus created can be well maintained for years (Fig. 11–4F).

GINGIVOPLASTY. This is a surgical procedure designed to reshape gingival tissues where pockets do not exist in order to provide contours that are more physiologic and which the patient can more readily keep clean of plaque and food debris. Goldman conceived the gingivoplasty as a means of producing knife-edged margins with appropriate interdental sluiceways. Gingivoplasty can be used to improve the rough contours left by the gingivectomy, and as a method of improving unacceptable tissue form resulting from other surgical procedures. These include bulbous interdental papillae, rolled gingival margins, interdental craters, and tissue overgrowths. The edge of a surgical knife, scalpel blade, scissors or rotary diamond stones may be used to carve the desired form. Heavy rolled hyperplastic marginal gingivae or soft-tissue craters are the main indications for gingivoplasty (Fig. 11–6).

The gingivectomy and gingivoplasty remain useful clinical surgical operations. They are used as methods for reducing excess tissue and for esthetics. Hyperplastic tissue, such as phenytoin-induced overgrowth; fibrotic tissue; or in cases of altered passive eruption, where tissue levels are coronal to the cementoenamel junction;

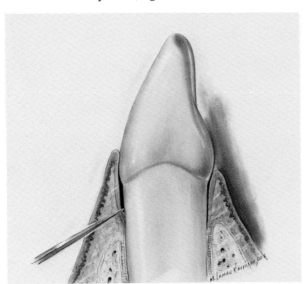

Figure 11–5. Gingivectomy. The angulation of the blade for primary gingivectomy incision results in an external bevel of the soft tissue.

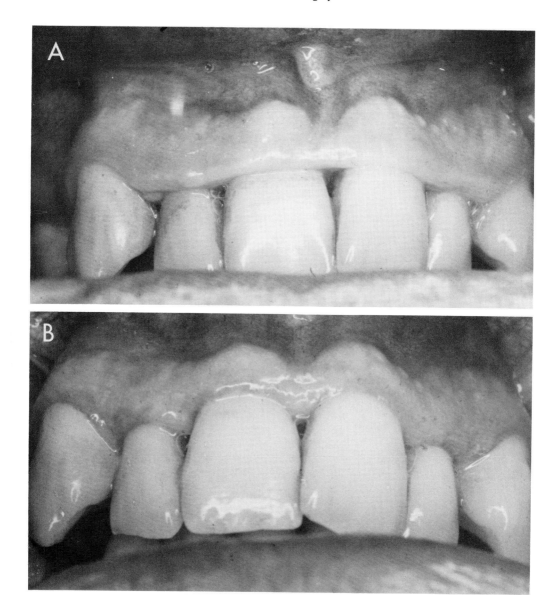

Figure 11–6. Gingivoplasty. Note changes in contour of the marginal and papillary gingival tissues from A, before surgery to B, after surgery. This patient had suffered from acute necrotizing ulcerative gingivitis.

and when additional coronal length is desired, all represent current applicability of these surgical methods.

Excisional New Attachment Procedure

A surgical procedure that represents a form of subgingival curettage performed with a scalpel blade is the excisional new attachment procedure (ENAP). The operation is really a modified flap procedure that had its antecedents in earlier surgical techniques. The procedure is accomplished by a surgical incision near the tooth sufficient to remove the epithelial lining of the suprabony pocket wall and subjacent inflamed connective tissue. Papillae are elevated and roots are thoroughly planed. The tissue is returned to its original level and sutured interproximally. No attempt is made to elevate the tissue from alveolar bone and no osseous reduction is attempted. The intention of the operation is to achieve connective tissue attachment and decrease pocket depth with more precision than closed curettage. Histologic evidence suggests that, in reality, a long, thin junctional epithelium with minimal connective tissue new attachment occurs. The name of the operation is somewhat of a misnomer, but the operation is useful in shallow and moderate suprabony defects, particularly where esthetics is a consideration (Fig. 11–7).

Periodontal Flap Procedures

Subgingival curettage gingivectomy, gingivoplasty, and ENAP are excision procedures for treatment of suprabony pockets in which the gingiva is not elevated from underlying periosteum. When access is required to reach the bone, as in intrabony defects, marginal and attached gingiva are separated from tooth structure and bone. These elevations of soft tissues are referred to as periodontal flap operations. A variety of different surgical incisions, different amounts of tissue removal, and different positioning of the flaps have resulted in different names for these flap operations.

OPEN FLAP CURETTAGE. This technique of flap surgery is advocated where preservation of tissues is important, where anatomic defects may be suitable for regeneration, where deep pockets are present and osseous resective surgery is not feasible, and for total debridement. A sharp

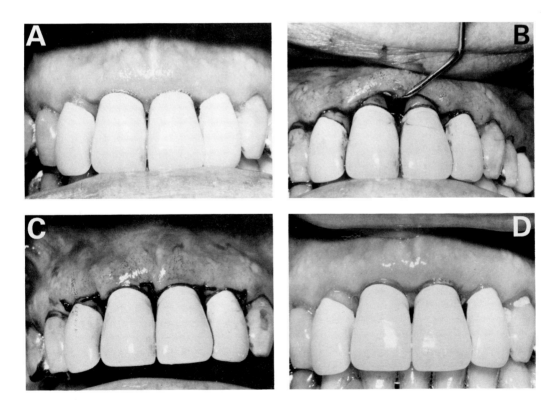

Figure 11–7. Excisional New Attachment Procedure. A, Presurgical condition. Soft tissue pockets are present. B, Incision and tissue elevation. Note calculus on facial of the central incisor. C, Sutures are placed interproximally. D, Results 6 months following surgery. (Courtesy Dr. Timothy Wahl.)

incision is made in an apical direction about 1 mm lateral to the gingival margin and extended to the alveolar crest. This was termed an inverse beveled incision by Friedman to distinguish it from the external beveled incision of the gingivectomy. A full mucoperiosteal flap is then reflected to permit thorough debridement of the tooth, removal of granulation tissue, and, in some instances, placement of inductive bone growth materials. Sutures are used to secure the flap after return to its original position.

APICALLY POSITIONED FLAP. This operation derived from an evolution in surgical methodology during the 1960s. During the 1950s resection of osseous defects had been popularized. At that time gingival tissue was excised, the bone contoured and left denuded, and a new soft tissue granulated over the bone. Research indicated that bone would be better protected by being covered by attached gingiva and surgical methods of maintaining the attached gingiva were introduced. An early article had emphasized the reposition of attached gingiva, and in 1962 Friedman introduced the term "apically-repositioned flap" to describe the technique.

A scalpel blade is used to make an inverse bevel incision in the cervical wall of marginal gingiva apicalward to the alveolar bone. Extent of the incision from the tooth is predicated on width of the gingiva, pocket depth, and extent of osseous removal projected. A full mucoperiosteal flap is then elevated from the bone and moved apicalward. Vertical relaxing incisions at the ends of the horizontal inverse bevel are placed, if desired, to facilitate placement of the flap. Any residual interdental soft tissue is freed with use of a knife. Osseous defects are recontoured or eliminated, and the flap is positioned apically to its former position and sutured. The procedure is illustrated in Figure 11–8. Apically positioned flaps are still appropriate when osseous surgery is accomplished. The procedure allows pocket elimination and

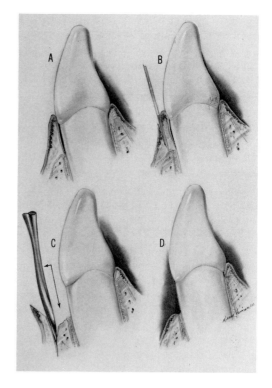

Figure 11–8. Apically Positioned Flap. A, Presurgical situation with periodontal pocket on facial aspect of tooth. B, Inverse bevel incision to remove soft tissue wall of pocket. C, Separation with periosteal elevator of mucoperiosteal flap from underlying bone. D, Mucoperiosteal flap apically positioned at bone level. Facial bone has been recontoured (osteoplasty).

modification of bone, but there is residual exposure of tooth root.

MODIFIED WIDMAN FLAP. A Scandinavian dentist, Leonard Widman, described a flap operation in 1918, but because the article was not written in English, the procedure was not widely used outside Scandinavia. A modification of this original operation was described in 1974, and was termed the modified Widman flap. The operation is not dissimilar to open flap curettage though the open flap operation is usually more extensive and less technically taxing. Maximum healing with minimal tissue loss are the objectives of the modified Widman flap.

An initial internal bevel incision is accomplished 0.5 to 1.0 mm from the gingival margin toward the alveolar crest, and then flap reflection is achieved to expose 1.0 to 2.0 mm of alveolar bone. The blade is then inserted in the bottom of the pocket and this secondary incision is carried to the alveolar bone. A curette is used to remove tissue from crestal bone. Roots are planed and bone curetted to remove tags of granulation tissue. Flaps are returned, closely approximated interproximally and sutured with an attempt being made to achieve primarily wound healing. Reports of a longitudinal study suggest a better gain in attachment in moderate and deep pockets than produced by subgingival curettage or osseous surgical pocket elimination.

Osseous Surgery

In many patients with moderate or advanced periodontal disease, the alveolar process of the mandible or maxilla is altered due to spread of inflammation, and the base of the pocket is apical to the crest of the bone. Inflammatory cells follow the loose connective tissue around interproximal blood vessels with a resultant resorption of alveolar crest and loss of cancellous bone. This, the most common osseous lesion is an interproximal crater. Generally, the alveolar process becomes progressively thicker toward the apical areas of the teeth. As crestal bone is resorbed bone ledges are created in buccal or lingual cortical plates. Interproximal bony craters occur since cancellous bone is resorbed more readily than the cortical plates. In such situations, bone may be recontoured to thin the ledges, eliminate the walls of the craters, and reduce the pocket depth.

Gingivectomy procedures cannot eliminate these bony defects, eliminate the pocket, or achieve acceptable contours. In 1949 Schluger presented a concept of surgical bone shaping to decrease pocket depth and establish an architectural form simulating normality. An inverse beveled incision is made in the gingival wall of the pocket apically at a sufficient distance from teeth to provide for apicalward positioning commensurate with extent of bone to be removed and preserve sufficient gingivae. Interproximal papillae are removed with use of surgical interproximal knives and curettes. After a full mucoperiosteal flap is elevated apical to the mucogingival junction all granulation tissue is removed.

Bone is then reshaped to desired contour with rotary burs and hand instruments. It is extremely important that sufficient coolant, sterile saline solution, or distilled water, be used with rotary instruments to prevent bone being injured by heat produced by the bur. Hemorrhage and coolant must be adequately evacuated to provide the operator a clear view of the surgical area. Roots are carefully planed, the tissue flap is placed at the bone level, and sutures are placed.

Other osseous aberrations include furcation invasions, thickened bone margins, loss of a portion of an interproximal bony septum (hemiseptal defect), and destruction of portions of cortical plates. All of these defects are amenable to osseous correction.

Flaps and ostectomy are being increasingly used to increase clinical crown lengths when extensive tooth structure has been lost due to caries, tooth fracture, or previous restorative procedures. Removal of bone facilitates placement of onlays or crowns. Crevicular or inverse beveled incisions are made, flaps retracted, and sufficient bone removed until sufficient tooth length is obtained. Usually, the resultant bone level is 2 to 2.5 mm apical to the proposed restorative margin. The soft tissue flap is then placed at the bone level and held with sutures.

OSTEOPLASTY. Recontouring of bone to enable the gingiva to assume a physiologic contour over the bone is referred to as osteoplasty. Bone overgrowths, exostoses, and tori are examples of the type of structures which can be reshaped. Like its soft tissue counterpart, gingivoplasty, osteoplasty is frequently used in conjunction with ostectomy to achieve desirable osseous form.

Considerable controversy concerning ostectomy has occurred because of the possibility that supporting bone of the teeth is sacrificed with attendant loss of attachment. Reshaping of ledges and other defects not contributing to support of teeth does not jeopardize the tooth and minimal attachment loss occurs. Since osteoplasty does not involve bone to which periodontal ligament is attached, no attachment loss occurs with this procedure. Osseous surgery does result in greater exposure of teeth and the gingiva is placed at a more apical level, but osseous recontouring remains a widely practiced surgical treatment modality because of positive benefits. Contraindications to such surgery include three-wall intrabony defects, deep periodontal pockets, bone defects associated with the external oblique ridge, moderate to deep circumferential bone defects, and isolated deep angular defects or craters. Obviously, osseous resective procedures are not needed with suprabony pockets.

RECONSTRUCTIVE SURGERY

Restoration of diseased or destroyed periodontal tissues to health is the ideal therapeutic approach. Whereas some forms of periodontal surgery result in further tissue loss because some healthy functional tissue is removed in the surgical procedure, reconstructive surgery attempts to replace all or at least part of the previously destroyed tissues. It should be understood that many of these procedures involve some excision of tissue but the overall intent is to enhance or augment periodontal tissues and tooth support. Both soft tissue and hard tissue reconstructive procedures are available.

Mucogingival Surgery

The term mucogingival surgery denotes those surgical modifications that involved both keratinized gingival tissues and alveolar mucosa. Teeth may erupt close to the mucogingival junction and have a minimal band of keratinized gingiva, restorative therapy may require additional keratinized tissue, or teeth to be moved orthodontically may require an additional band of gingiva. Frenula attachments sometimes develop close to the free gingival margin. These may occur in several areas of the mouth but are most frequently encountered in the mandibular anterior labial area. During lip or cheek movements the elasticity of these frenuli may place excessive force on the gingival margin resulting in gingival recession with associated loss of tooth support. Pockets may actually deepen so that the bottom of the pocket is apical to the mucogingival junction. Surgical procedures are available to treat all of these soft tissue aberrations and disorders.

Autogenous Free Gingival Grafts

Situations involving frenula in the lower anterior region were treated for many years by frenula removal, but this often resulted in a surgical failure. In the early 1960s a more definitive procedure was developed that effectively removed the frenum and deepened the mucobuccal fold. This periosteal fenestration procedure consisted of a vertical incision at the mucogingival junction extending laterally the width of two or three teeth on either side of the frenulum. The incision is extended 6 to 10 mm, and the mucosa was freed from the periosteum. A second incision perpendicular to the bone was made through the periosteum to the bone about half the distance between the mucogingival junction and the apical extent of the primary incision.

A periosteal flap was then raised and a window created to expose bone. The bony window created a scar (cicatrix) that helped maintain the operative depth. A periodontal dressing was placed to the depth of the incision and fastened to the teeth. After 5 to 7 days the dressing was removed and, in some instances, dressings were replaced until healing occurred. This operation

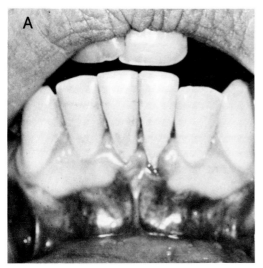

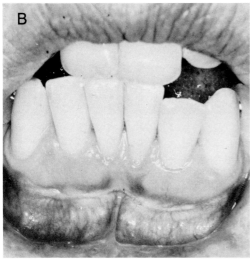

Figure 11–9. Periosteal Separation Procedure. Patient presents with an aberrant frenal attachment and an inadequate zone of attached gingiva in the mandibular anterior area. A, Before surgery. B, 40 weeks postsurgery. (From Allen, D.L. and Shell, J.H.: J. Periodontol., 39:46, 1968.)

eliminated the frenulum, deepened the vestibule, and provided a satisfactory result. A thin linear scar remained at the depth of the vestibule where the osseous fenestration was accomplished (Fig. 11–9).

Development of the autogenous free gingival graft during the late 1960s supplanted all previous methods of inducing new gin-

giva. Free grafts of palatal or gingival tissue can be obtained from the patient and placed on surgically exposed cervical bone and the cervical aspect of teeth with resultant growth of new gingiva. Such grafts have a high rate of success, wide adaptability in many parts of the mouth, and provide functional and esthetic results. The technique involves a recipient site, where the graft is placed, and a donor site, from which the mucosal graft is obtained.

Incisions of the recipient site are prepared in much the same fashion as in the periosteal separation procedure producing a thin periosteal surface or denuded alveolar bone. Research has indicated that grafts shrink less when placed on denuded bone. Measurements are made of the prepared recipient site apico-coronally and mesiodistally with a periodontal probe to ensure proper size of the graft. Some operators then prepare a template of dry foil to serve in obtaining a graft of correct size. A wet gauze is placed over the recipient area while the graft is being obtained from the donor area.

Tissue for grafting may be obtained from masticatory mucosa of the hard palate or from an edentulous area of gingival mucosa. The palate is more commonly used for such grafts as large amounts of tissue are available. The portion of the palate between rugae and second molars and midway between palatal gingiva and the palatal midline is the most appropriate source. An outline around the template is made with a scalpel blade. This incision is shallow since the obtained graft will only be about 1 mm in thickness. The tissue is then released by careful incision freeing the epithelium and a small amount of connective tissue from the donor site. Such "free" grafts are extremely thin and care must be taken to identify the epithelial side.

After careful placement of the graft in the recipient area coronal sutures are placed, and gentle, constant pressure is placed against the graft with a sponge soaked in a saline solution. This is a critical step since a fibrin clot forms beneath the graft sealing it to the underlying base. If blood pools under the graft, "take" of the graft is compromised. Periodontal dressings may or may not be placed over the recipient area and the donor area. Ointments and adhesive intraoral bandages may also be used in the donor area. Clinical healing is usually complete in 3 weeks though maturation may require months. Oral hygiene procedures should be quickly instituted, usually within 2 weeks (Fig. 11–10).

Since initial introduction of free mucosal grafts, refinements have been made and additional uses found for such grafts. When roots with recession have a narrow isthmus mesio-distally, grafts can be used to cover them with clinical success. Free grafts have been placed on roots with broader recession by treating such roots with citric acid prior to graft placement. The citric acid is thought to demineralize the root surface and expose collagen fibers. Grafts have been placed apical to teeth with recession, and, after complete take and healing, lifted as a flap and coronally positioned over the tooth roots. Though technically demanding, autogenous grafts have found wide acceptance. Unfortunately, this may have resulted in overuse. There is no reason to augment gingiva in the absence of disease, and not all teeth with recession require coverage or broader zones of gingiva.

Laterally Positioned Flaps

Even before it was known that free mucosal grafts could be used successfully for plastic reconstructive therapy, a surgical method had been developed to cover roots of isolated teeth with excessive gingival recession. This surgical procedure, originally termed a sliding flap operation, is really a pedicle flap transferred from its original site while maintaining its blood supply through attachment at its base. The procedure is dependent upon a satisfactory donor area of thick gingiva in the interdental papillae and over an adjacent tooth.

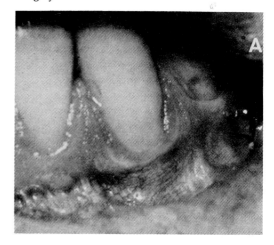

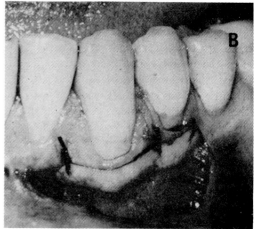

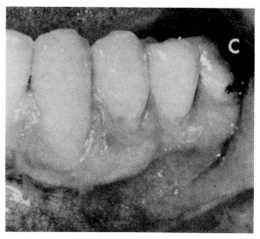

Figure 11–10. Free Gingival Graft. Tissue from the hard palate was grafted in the area of the periodontal defect associated with the mandibular cuspid. Note the minimal amount of attached gingiva on the cuspid in A, the graft sutured in place in B, and the healed site one year later in C. (Courtesy Dr. Dudley C. Chandler.)

Surrounding soft tissue of the recipient tooth is initially prepared by a removal of a U-shaped wedge of tissue to present a fresh connective tissue face for the transposed graft. The bottom of the U extends into alveolar mucosa, and if a frenulum is present this is excised. Gingival tissue around the tooth and that of the donor tissue are cut on a bevel such that close adaptation will take place. Removal of plaque and calculus is accomplished on the receptor root. Better results have been shown when the root is treated with citric acid prior to flap placement.

An incision is made in the gingiva in a coronal to apical direction distal to the adjacent donor tooth, which extends sufficiently into mucosa to provide flap mobility while preserving an adequate nutritional stalk. The flap is still attached at its base. Then the graft tissue is freed from the donor tooth and underlying bone. Full thickness mucoperiosteal flaps are easier to manage, but split-thickness grafts, in which some connective tisue remains on tooth and bone, can be employed. The flap is transposed over the recipient tooth and sutures placed through the flap into the gingiva adjacent to the recipient tooth. This leaves the donor area to granulate in with new tissue. A dressing is placed that can usually be removed in 1 week at the same time as the sutures (Fig. 11–11).

Osseous Reconstruction

Advanced periodontal disease results in creation of osseous defects and loss of periodontal attachment apparatus. With progressive inflammation tooth support is lost, the tooth is subject to secondary occlusal trauma and may eventually be lost. For years the therapist's dream has been to discover a method for regrowth of bone and reestablishment of the periodontal ligament-tooth attachment. Surgical procedures designed to accomplish this represent one of the most active areas of clinical surgical therapy. In certain instances this new growth of bone and attachment apparatus has been demonstrated to occur predictably. Implantation of autogenous bone grafts has achieved moderate success as have allografts (bone from humans). Newer, synthetic grafting materials have been developed and used with mixed results.

INTRABONY SURGERY. Configuration of the osseous defects has a significant bearing on the potential for new bone inducement and reestablishment of a functional attachment to tooth. Pritchard convincingly demonstrated that this could occur in deep bony pockets having three remaining bony walls (Fig. 11–12). For a great number of years it had been observed that a tooth extraction socket would fill in with new bone. Sockets essentially have four bony walls from which new osteogenic activity can occur. Narrow deep bony pockets provide three bony walls with osteogenic potential. The tooth presents the fourth wall. If such defects are surgically treated by removal of all soft tissue, and if epithelium can be kept from the surgical wound, then new bone and periodontal attachment can and does form. This surgical therapy is technically demanding and the three-wall defect is not as common as other defects, but the gratifying results obtained provide proof that reestablishment of the attachment apparatus can occur.

BONE AUTOGRAFTS. When the bone defect consists of only two bony walls, or is a shallow, three-wall lesion, or a hemiseptal defect, the challenge of reconstructive surgery is greater. The therapist is faced with the choice of osseous resection, or attempting to place something in the defect to induce new bone growth or fill the defect in order to support the tooth and overlying soft tissue. Cortical bone, cancellous bone, bone marrow, or combinations of these obtained from the patient can be used to attempt to meet the challenge. After flap entry cortical bone can be obtained with a bur from plates adjacent to the defect, buccal shelves, or exostoses. These small particles mixed with the patient's blood can

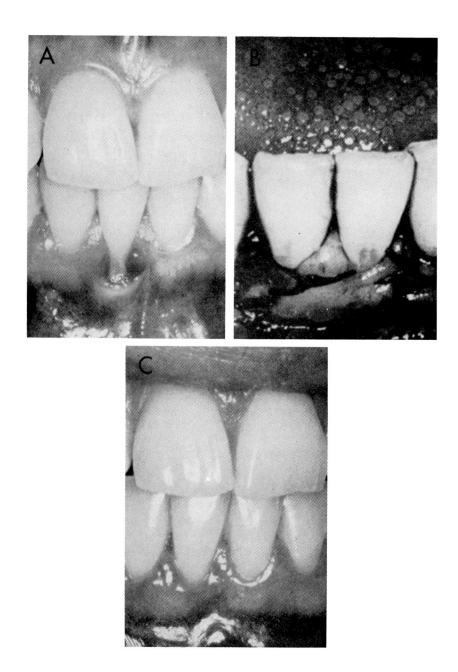

Figure 11–11.   Laterally Positioned Flap.   A, Presurgical situation with gingival recession and inflammation of facial aspect of mandibular right central incisor. B, A gingival flap has been raised on the right lateral incisor and placed over the root of the central incisor. C, Healed surgical site six months later.

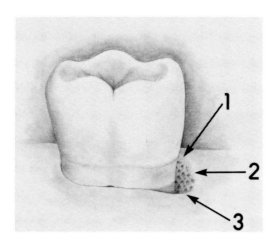

Figure 11–12. Intrabony Pocket. This illustrates the type of bone defect that contains three remaining bony walls. 1, Lingual, 2, Mesial. 3, Facial.

be introduced into the bone defect. This material is referred to as osseous coagulum. Availability of sufficient bone and the low potential for osseous induction limits the usefulness of this procedure. Cancellous bone and marrow offer greater potential for stimulation of new bone growth and can be obtained for recent extraction sockets or maxillary tuberosities. Once again the limitation is the availability of such donor sites. Extraoral sources of marrow such as the iliac crest have been used with some success, but this requires a two-stage operation and fresh marrow appears to cause root resorption.

BONE ALLOGRAFTS. Freeze-dried crushed bone obtained from human cadavers and stored in bone banks has been used extensively with reported success in regeneration of bone and decrease in pocket depth. No satisfactory demonstration of a new attachment mechanism has been shown. Problems with this material include sterility, possible antigenicity, and expense.

SYNTHETIC GRAFT MATERIAL. It would be most useful if a readily available material could be placed in bony defects. During the 1980s a number of synthetic graft products have been used in oral and periodontal surgery. These small hydroxyapatite crystals have been used with success in augmentation of bone in edentulous ridges and has been shown to fill space in periodontal osseous defects. The potential for synthetic materials to stimulate growth of host bone is problematic, and no reestablishment of an attachment apparatus has been demonstrated.

Combined Surgical Procedures

The aforementioned procedures represent the major surgical techniques utilized in current periodontal therapy. There are many modifications of each procedure. In the clinical practice of periodontal surgery, the therapist will use many variations and combinations of both resective and inductive procedures. The hygienist should recognize that concepts of periodontal surgery are in a state of change with a trend toward conservation and reconstruction of periodontal tissues. Also the skills, experience, and concepts show considerable variance between dentists. As in all medical treatment decisions, the most advantageous course of periodontal care for a given patient must rest with the therapist.

ROLE OF THE HYGIENIST IN PERIODONTAL SURGERY

The role of the hygienist, directly or indirectly, in association with periodontal treatment varies from nation to nation and office to office. Changes in dental practice acts in the United States have permitted the hygienist a more active role in periodontal surgery in some parts of the nation. Hygienists may actually participate in periodontal surgery as a therapist or surgical assistant. Regardless of the degree of the hygienist's surgical involvement, she must be knowledgeable of the nature of various procedures, the instruments utilized, the patterns of healing, and the postoperative management.

Hygienists may assume a strategic role in the physical and emotional preparation of patients destined for surgical care. Positive assurance of the worth of such planned surgery and candid explanation of the anticipated sequelae can do much to allay patient apprehension. The hygienist thus provides the calm, warm, stabilizing influence that assists the dentist in patient preparation. Ultimately, the patient treated by periodontal surgery will become the patient whose maintenance care will be managed by the hygienist.

Importance of medical histories in patient care have been previously stressed. The patient's medical history must be reviewed prior to surgery. If preoperative medications or dietary regimens have been prescribed, the hygienist should ascertain that these instructions have been followed. Both preoperative and postoperative blood pressure and pulse are regularly taken and recorded in most dental practices. Office emergency procedures should be reviewed and emergency equipment should be in place prior to the surgical appointment.

Asepsis

The exclusion of microorganisms is a desirable goal of all dental procedures, but because of the profusion of bacteria in the oral cavity, this cannot be accomplished. While it is impossible to obtain a sterile environment, every attempt should be made to reduce the number of organisms present and avoid introducing additional ones. In periodontal surgical operations, it is particularly critical that an aseptic chain be maintained.

Sterile smocks, caps, mask, and gloves should be worn by the surgical team. The patient should be draped with sterile towels and a sterile cap or towel placed over the patient's hair. All handles and switches that may be touched during the surgical procedure should be scrubbed with disinfectants or protected by sterile covers. These include the dental light, air and water syringes, saliva ejectors, dental tray or Mayo stand. All rubber tubing should be autoclaved.

Increasingly more items routinely used in surgical procedures may be obtained prepackaged as sterilized disposable products. All sterilized disposable items such as surgical sponges, cotton applicators, cotton rolls, and tongue blades should be stored in covered containers. Disinfected transfer forceps are used to remove supplies and place them on surgical trays covered with sterilized towels. Instruments must be prepared by autoclave, dry heat, or gas sterilization. No stable practical liquid disinfectant has been found satisfactory for control of hepatitis virus when used for practical lengths of time.

Rings, watches, and arm jewelry are removed prior to scrubbing and donning surgical gloves. A complete surgical scrub of hands and arms with a sterile scrub brush and disinfectant should be carried out for 2 minutes. Chlorhexidine or iodophor solutions are available commercially. After gloves are in place they must not be contaminated by touching nonsterile surfaces.

Chairside Assisting

The hygienist should be completely familiar with the duties of a surgical assistant since she may serve in that capacity or need to train dental assistants. Prior to the surgical procedure the sterile instruments are arranged on the sterile towel in an organized manner. Diagnostic instruments, probes, explorers, and mirrors are placed toward one side of the tray. Surgical instruments, scalpels, knives, curettes, and retractors are arranged in order of most common use toward the center of the tray (Fig. 11–13). Instruments used for suturing and dressing placement are placed on the side of the tray opposite the diagnostic instruments. A typical arrangement of surgical instruments is presented in Figure 11–14.

After sufficient training and experience, the surgical assistant should anticipate which instrument the operator will need and pass the instrument at the appropriate stage of the operation. As the operator re-

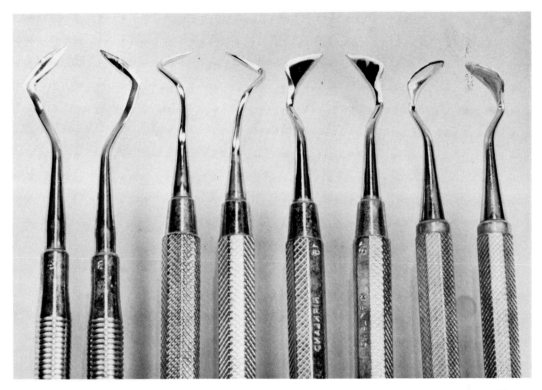

Figure 11–13. Gingivectomy Knives. From left to right are sets of Merrifield, Orban, Kirkland and Kaiser-Ward knives. The Kirkland and Kaiser-Ward knives are usually employed for making the primary incision and the others for the interdental incisions.

turns an instrument, the surgical assistant places it in its proper position on the tray. Sterile sponges are available on the tray. As sponges are used they are discarded in appropriate waste containers, and new sterile sponges are added as needed. At no time should the aseptic chain be broken. It is the surgical assistant's responsiblity to ensure this process. If the operator tends to perspire about the face, sterile towels or sponges should be used by the assistant to remove perspiration. The surgical assistant also must constantly adjust the dental light to keep it in sharp focus.

Aspiration and Irrigation

One of the most strategic duties of the surgical assistant is the maintenance of the surgical field. This is accomplished by adequate irrigation of the area and evacuation of fluid, blood, and debris produced dur-

ing the surgical procedure. Sterile water or saline is the usual irrigation solution and is most often directed toward the surgical area from a bulb syringe. The aspirator or evacuation tip is held "down stream" from the irrigating source to remove accumulated fluid and particles. It is necessary to move the aspirator tip along the entire surgical area, from time to time, as hemorrhage accumulates. The tip is also frequently placed in the posterior portions of the patient's mouth to prevent blood and saliva from entering the patient's throat. If the surgical procedure is being carried out in the maxillary arch, additional attention must be given to the floor of the mouth to aspirate fluid as it accumulates.

The side of the aspirator tip may aso be used effectively to aid in cheek reflection and protection of the patient's tongue. In procedures requiring bone removal the

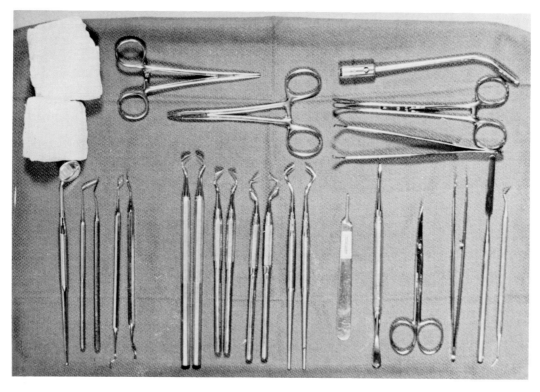

Figure 11–14. Surgical Instrument Tray Arrangement.

bone must be irrigated frequently. If a particular area is seeping much blood, a great deal of time must be spent aspirating this area. Evacuation tips should not be placed against lining mucosa of the floor of the mouth or cheek. Particular care must be exercised during grafting procedures to ensure that soft-tissue autogenous grafts or prepared bone particles are not drawn into the aspirator. At such times the tip should be held well away from the receptor area. Wet sponges are used to control bleeding in these areas.

Suturing

Sutures are usually used where soft tissue flaps or grafts are placed. The sutures provide close adaptation of wound margins and help control flap positions. Careful wound closure facilitates the healing process and diminishes the amount of secondary intention healing. Sutures permit accurate control of the position of the flap

in elimination of pockets and maintenance of adequate zones of keratinized tissue.

The surgical assistant aids in retraction of lips and cheeks and in control of the patient's tongue during suturing. Evacuation of saliva is continued during the suturing process. The operator must have good visibility and access of the area during this critical phase of therapy.

Only sharp, sterile suture needles should be used. Nontraumatic suture points are often used for delicate flaps. Suture needles in a wide variety of shapes and sizes are available as prepackaged products. These needles are secured to the basic types of suture materials, braided silk, dacron-teflon, or collagen. Braided silk is the most commonly used suture material in periodontal surgery because of the ease of use and the fact that it can be easily and securely knotted. It is also less expensive than other materials. Braided silk does have drawbacks in that it acts as a wick to carry fluid and microorganisms into the wound and does not resorb. For practical purposes, however, it remains the material of choice. Dacron-teflon does not wick, but it is difficult to knot securely and is relatively expensive. Collagen (gut) sutures have the ability to be resorbed over time by bodily fluids, but it is difficult to handle and resorption time is not predictable. Many periodontists prefer to use gut sutures because of the resorptive feature.

Suture needles are carried to the surgical area with needle holders. Typically the needle is inserted through the mobile soft tissue flap or graft from the epithelial side toward the connective tissue side. The insertion or "bite" of the needle is made far enough from the cut edge of the tissue (2 mm) to prevent tearing of the tissue when the suture is pulled taut. A length of suture material is pulled through the soft tissue but approximately 10 mm of the material is left on the epithelial side and will subsequently be used to tie the knot.

A bite is then taken with the needle in the tissue adjacent to the flap or graft from the periosteal side out toward the oral surface, the flap positioned, and a surgical (square knot) tied. Flaps are secured with additional mesial and distal sutures or by interproximal sutures in the interproximal papillae. With apically positioned flaps the wound edges usually do not meet interproximally. With the modified Widman procedure attempts are made to apposition tissues interproximally.

In tying the surgical knot the free end of the suture is grasped with a needle holder. The needle end of the suture is wrapped around the beaks of the needle holder twice in a counter-clockwise direction, and then the suture is pulled securely to form the first part of the knot. The free end of the suture is grasped again with the needle holder and the suture wrapped around the tip of the holder in a clockwise direction. Again, the suture is pulled securely. Finally, the procedure is repeated again with the needle end of the suture wrapped in a clockwise direction and the surgical knot is completed (Fig. 11–15). During this suturing procedure the aspiration of hemorrhage and saliva is continued. The surgical assistant then cuts the suture material after the knot is tied. This cut is usually made 2 to 3 mm from the knot to present slippage of the knot. This procedure is repeated as each suture is placed.

The methodology just described represent a single interrupted suture. The hygienist should be aware that a variety of sling type sutures and mattress sutures are available to control position of the flap, limit space between soft tissue and bone, and prevent necrosis of tissue edges. Sutured wounds may or may not be covered with periodontal dressings.

Periodontal Dressings

Placement of a periodontal dressing or pack was an extremely common practice when surgery left exposed surfaces as occurred with gingivectomy procedures. The dressing protected the raw wound from acid foodstuffs and liquids, helped prevent hemorrhage, and included medications for control of pain. With the flap operations the use of the dressing is more variable. When excellence in wound closure is obtained with sutures, the dressing is often dispensed with and the patient initiates oral hygiene earlier. Decisions on use of the pack are made by the operator following the surgery. Dressings may inhibit excessive granulation tissue and serve as a surgical stent. In osseous induction procedures they may actually be a deterrent by extruding into the bone defect. In the latter instance the wound may be initially covered with a foil tent prior to dressing placement. Dressings discourage patients from disturbing surgical wounds or sutures with tongue or fingers. They do tend to collect blood, food, and desquamted cells that cause a bad taste and breath.

Periodontal dressings are essentially of two types: those containing eugenol and those that do not contain eugenol. Dress-

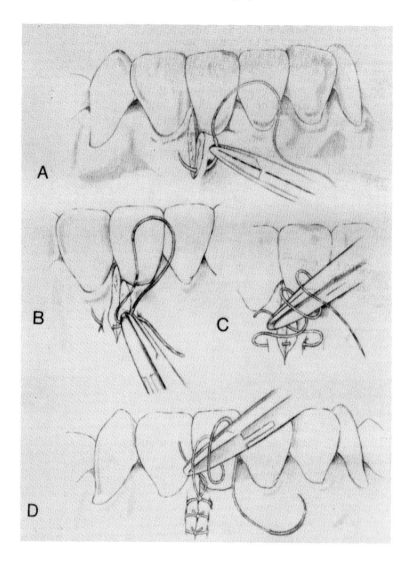

Figure 11–15. Basic Suturing Techniques. The interrupted suture is the most universal in its application. A, The needle is passed through one side of the flap and the suture pulled through. B, The needle is then passed through the other side of the incision. C, The surgeon's knot is tied approximating the edges of the flap. D, As many sutures as needed are placed.

ings containing antibiotics for topical use have been developed, but they do not offer significant advantages. Also dressings containing chlorhexidine have been suggested, but these are not in use in the United States. Liquid acrylic dressings have been used in Europe. As of this time, these have not been approved for general dental use in the United States. No definitive evidence exists that any form of dress-

ing has a positive influence on the wound healing process.

Eugenol containing dressings are available as a liquid and powder that ar mixed together. The liqid consists of eugenol, thymol, and coloring agents. Eugenol is an obtundent to cut tissues, while thymol or other aromatic oils improve the flavor. The powder contains zinc oxide, tannic acid, and powdered rosin. Zinc oxide provides bulk and tannic acid aids hemostasis. Rosin serves to increase dressing strength.

These dressings are mixed by placing the desired amounts of powder and liquid on a paper mixing pad. Extensiveness of the surgery determines the amount of ingredients. Powder is incorporated by portions into the liquid and thoroughly mixed until all of it is wet. The dressing should be mixed until all stickiness is lost and soft enough to mold around the teeth. After mixing, the dressing is rolled into a 5-mm diameter cylinder. A section of dressing, slightly longer than the surgical area in which it will be placed, is cut from the cylinder.

Eugenol dressings become extremely rigid in the oral environment, collect debris, and stain teeth. The powder components are dangerous to the lungs of dental personnel over time. For these reasons, eugenol dressings are not commonly used today. Most noneugenol dressings are commercial products with formulas protected by patents and a number of such dressings are available. One dressing is supplied in two tubes. The first tube contains metallic oxides and bithionol, while the second tube contains chlorothymol and non-ionizing carboxylic acids. Equal portions of material, 1 to 2 inches in length, are extruded from each tube on a mixing pad. A metal spatula is used to mix the material for 45 seconds. The mixture can then be manipulated with petrolatum-coated fingers. After 3 minutes the dressing loses its tackiness and can be shaped into desired form and thickness.

Other noneugenol dressings are obtainable as a paste or putty-like materials. Many of these are premixed while others require mixing. Manufacturers' instructions should be followed carefully. Operator preference and type of periodontal surgery determine selection of dressings.

Regardless of the type of dressing used, the area of surgery should be dried of saliva and hemorrhage with sterile sponges. Aspiration should be continud in order to maintain the dry environment. The dressing is carried to place and molded into interdental spaces. A carving instrument can be used to lock the material into interdental areas. The dressing should not overlap occlusal surfaces of the teeth. Manipulation of the patient's lips, cheeks, and tongue will muscle-trim the edge of the dressing and keep it from being overextended. Such overextension results in irritation and possible ulceration of the lining mucosa.

Postoperative Instructions

Patients are naturally anxious to know what to expect following periodontal surgery, and the dental hygienist should be able to answer patients' questions. Patient concerns most often relate to pain, bleeding, swelling, diet, habits, and, if present, the periodontal dressing.

Surprisingly, infections are not common sequelae following periodontal surgery, even following osseous resection. Antibiotics are often prescribed after bone surgery, particularly if extensive removal has been done in the mandibular arch. Because pain is closely related to infection, the level of pain is not great postoperatively. Patients should be told that discomfort is variable but is usually mild to moderate. The dentist will prescribe appropriate analgesics for pain. In most instances nonnarcotic analgesics are sufficient, and even when bone has been reshaped only low levels of narcotics are prescribed. For most soft tissue surgery, patients can be informed that the level of discomfort is minimal.

Slight oozing of blood occasionally is noted occasionally following surgery, but the blood clot is usually established before the patient leaves the office. Slight bleeding often can be controlled by the patient by pressure with gauze pads, which should be supplied. Patients should be cautioned to avoid vigorous rinsing of the mouth. Patients should be instructed to contact the dentist if serious bleeding persists. Uncontrolled bleeding is a true dental emergency requiring prompt therapy. Fortunately, it is a relatively uncommon occurrence.

Swelling following surgery, particularly extensive surgery, is not unusual. Some patients tend to swell more than others. Mandibular swelling is more common following surgery than is maxillary swelling. Many offices supply patients cold packs to place on the face following surgery. Ice packs should be applied to the face on the day of surgery for 15 minutes on and 15 minutes off for several hours and this cold tends to minimize swelling. Should swelling persist on the day following surgical procedure, moist heat may be used intermittently on the face in the area of swelling. Most swelling begins to disappear after 3 days.

Patients should be allowed to eat foods that they desire dependent upon how they feel. Relatively simple periodontal surgical procedures should not condemn the patient to a diet of soup. Hard, hot and sticky foods should be avoided for several hours. A nutritious diet and plenty of liquids are recommended. Food should be cut in small pieces and eating on the operated side should be avoided. Highly acidic foodstuffs such as orange juice or cola drinks may cause discomfort and should not be consumed if the surgical area is not covered by a dressing. Obviously spicy foods, barbecue sauces, pickles, or pepper sauces should not be consumed. Patient should not suck liquids through a straw since this creates intraoral pressure that may increase bleeding. Chewing gum should be discouraged.

Inconveniences related to periodontal dressings are the source of the most common patient complaints. Small pieces of periodontal dressing frequently break off, but the patient can be assured that this is not important. If a major portion, or all the dressing, is lost in less than 3 days after surgical procedure or if the patient is uncomfortable, the patient should contact the dental office. Actually, the dressing, unless needed to act as a surgical stent probably

serves its purpose prior to this time. With most mucoperiosteal flaps periodontal dressings simply delay oral hygiene. If dressings are present, the patient should be advised to avoid brushing the area. Every attempt should be made to keep the rest of the mouth free of plaque. Salt-water rinses may be used on the day following surgical procedure. When no dressing is placed, patients may brush teeth in the surgical area. Some periodontists even advise gentle interproximal cleansing with floss or interproximal brushes. This appears to provide physiologic bacterial control and emotional support. The wound area should not be traumatized.

Many offices provide written instructions for the patient following surgical therapy. Prescriptions to minimize pain or to combat infection are often provided. Specific instructions with regard to medications are provided by the dentist. It is reassuring to note that most patients have a comparatively easy postoperative course.

Dressings and Suture Removal

Periodontal dressings and silk sutures are usually removed within 5 to 7 days postoperatively. If dressings are used, they should be dislodged with care to prevent injury to the underlying healing tissue. A universal scaler is inserted under the apical edge of the dressing and pulled coronally with a light force. After the bulk of the dressing has been removed from the mouth with cotton forceps, the area may be irrigated with warm water or dilute mouthwash. Patients may rinse with dilute mouthwash in order to rid the mouth of microorganisms and desquamated cells that have accumulated under the dressing. Small fragments of dressing adhering to the teeth are removed, and the area is thoroughly inspected.

Sutures are cut with fine sterile scissors. The surgical knot is grasped with cotton forceps and the suture cut and removed. The knot of the suture should not be pulled through the tissue since this causes pain and could displace the flap from its base (Fig. 11–16). If tissue healing permits, the teeth may be polished. Proximal surfaces may be flossed or polished with linen strips. Any residual calculus uncovered by the surgery should be removed. Areas of redundant granulation tissue may be removed with a curette. This tissue is composed of capillaries and connective tissue but little nervous tissue, and anesthesia is not required for removal.

Surgical areas seldom need to be resutured, but sometimes they do need to be redressed. This is particularly true with mucogingival surgery. A topical anesthetic is applied to the surgical site prior to the application of the new dressing in order to minimize patient discomfort.

Resumption of personal oral physiotherapy following suture or final dressing removal is critical. In many instances, the gingival embrasures have been exposed by the surgical operation. Such areas invite plaque accumulation and food impaction. Hygienists must instruct the patient in proper methods of oral care including use soft toothbrushes, interdental stimula- floss or tape, and interproximal (Fig. 11–17).

s are usually reluctant to initiate therapy in a healing surgical

area for fear of doing damage. They should be told not to inflict damage but to remove all plaque. Prompt control of the causative factors can aid healing and prevent disease recurrence. Usually patients are observed for several weeks following surgery to ensure healing and plaque control.

When plaque control is quickly reinstated, root surfaces exposed by surgical procedures should not become sensitive. It is not uncommon, however, that such roots may be sensitive or susceptible to dental caries because of inadequate oral physiotherapy. Fluoride applications to the roots by the hygienist are commonly indicated. Patients can be supplied with fluoride gels for home use and fluoride containing toothpastes should be recommended.

If dentin sensitivity persists, the roots may be treated in the office with desensitizing agents. Where roots are accessible, a thick paste of calcium hydroxide U.S.P. (0.4 g) and sterile water can be applied. The sensitive tooth is dried and isolated with cotton rolls to protect soft tissues because the medicament might cause ulceration of the gingiva. The paste can be applied with a sable paintbrush or the wooden end of a cotton applicator. It should be allowed to dry for 5 minutes. The calcium hydroxide

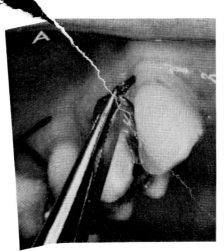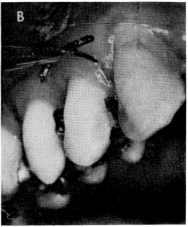

Figure 11–16. *Suture Removal.* A, Sutures are cut with surgical scissors. B, Cotton pliers are employed to grasp the knot and remove the sutures. (Courtesy Dr. James Kadi.)

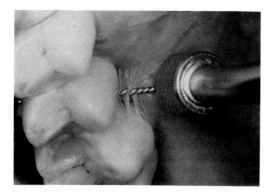

Figure 11–17. Postsurgical Cleaning. When gingival embrasures have been opened as the result of surgery, interproximal brushes can be used for plaque removal.

is then removed and the patient allowed to rinse. Additional applications of desensitizing agents sometimes may be required at subsequent appointments. Desensitizing dentifrices should be recommended for personal use to decrease sensitivity and to encourage plaque removal.

Postsurgical Care

When all surgical areas have been allowed to heal, an appointment is scheduled for postsurgical evaluation. In most offices this appointment occurs from 4 to 6 weeks following the last postsurgical appointment. The purpose of this appointment is to evaluate the results of surgical therapy, assess plaque control, gauge mobility, analyze occlusal relations, determine the need for further dental care, and establish the appropriate maintenance interval for the patient.

In most instances the general dentist or periodontist will wish to examine the patient to answer any patient questions, appraise wound healing, and determine additional dental needs. The hygienist is charged with gathering data on bleeding, pocket depths and plaque levels. A final scaling and prophylaxis is accomplished, and frequently fluoride is applied. Emphasis should be placed on patient education and motivational efforts are made with re-

gard to oral physiotherapy. The patient is reminded of their susceptibility to microbial organisms and the importance of preventive maintenance care. Patients who have received periodontal surgery must be kept on tight recall intervals.

SUMMARY

Periodontal surgery remains an essential part of periodontal therapy and probably will continue to be an important feature of future periodontal care. With development of new techniques and materials, reconstructive surgical procedures will probably become a more significant portion of the treatment designed to preserve the natural dentition. Regardless of the direction of future periodontal surgery, the hygienist will continue to occupy a position of importance in the preparation of the patient for surgery, the surgical operation itself, and the maintenance of the surgically treated patient. The next chapter discusses this critical role of the hygienist in long-term maintenance.

BIBLIOGRAPHY

Barkann, L.: A conservative surgical technique for eradication of a pyorrhea pocket, J. Am. Dent. Assoc., 26:61, 1939.

Barrington, E.P.: An overview of periodontal surgical procedures, J. Periodontol., 52:518, 1981.

Common, J. and McFall, W., Jr.: The effects of citric acid on attachment of laterally positioned flaps, J. Periodontol., 54:9, 1983.

Corn, H.: Periosteal separation—Its clinical significance, J. Periodontol., 33:140, 1962.

Crane, A. and Kaplan, H.: The Crane-Kaplan operation for elimination of pyorrhea alveolaris, Dental Cosmos, 73:643, 1931.

Echeverria, J. and Caffesse, R.: Effect of gingival curettage when performed one month after root instrumentation, J. Clin. Periodontol., 10:277, 1983.

Everette, F., Waenhaugh, J. and Widman, A.: Leonard Widman, surgical treatment of pyorrhea alveolaris, J. Periodontol., 42:571, 1971.

Friedman, N.: Mucogingival surgery. The apically repositioned flap, J. Periodontol., *33*:328, 1962.

Goldman, H.M.: The development of physiologic gingival contours by gingivoplasty, Oral Surg., *3*:879, 1950.

Grupe, H. and Warren R.: Repair of gingival defects by a sliding flap operation, J. Periodontol., *27*:290, 1956.

James, W. and McFall, W., Jr.: Placement of free gingival grafts on denuded alveolar bone, J. Periodontol., *49*:283, 1978.

Kirkland, O.: The suppurative periodontal pus pocket: Its treatment by the modified flap operation, J. Am. Dent. Assoc., *18*:1462, 1931.

Kirkland, O.: Surgical treatment of periodontoclasia, J. Am. Dent. Assoc., *21*:105, 1934.

Knowles, J., Burgett, F., Nissle, R., Shick, R., Morrison, E. and Ramfjord, S.: Results of periodontal treatment related to pocket depths and attachment levels. Eight years, J. Periodontol., *50*:225, 1979.

Knowles, J., Burgett, F., Morrison, E., Nissle, R. and Ramfjord, S.: Comparison of results following three modalities of periodontal therapy related to tooth type and initial pocket depth, J. Clin. Periodontol., *7*:32, 1980.

Mellonig, J., Bowers, G., Bright, R. and Lawrence, J.: Clinical evaluation of freeze-dried bone allografts in periodontal osseous defects, J. Periodontol., *47*:125, 1976.

Nabors, C.: Repositioning the attached gingiva, J. Periodontol., *25*:38, 1954.

Nyman, S., Gottlow, J., Karring, T. and Lindhe, J.: The regenerative potential of the periodontal ligament. An experimental study in the monkey, J. Clin. Periodontol., *9*:257, 1982.

Oschenbein, C.: Current status of osseous surgery, J. Periodontol., *45*:577, 1977.

Pritchard, J.F.: The infrabony technique as a predictable procedure, J. Periodontol., *28*:202, 1957.

Ramafjord, S., Nissle, R., Shick, R. and Cooper, H., Jr.: Subgingival curettage versus surgical elimination of periodontal pockets, J. Periodontol., *39*:167, 1968.

Ramfjord, S. and Nissle, R.: The modified Widman flap, J. Periodontol., *45*:601, 1974.

Robinson, R.E.: Osseous coagulum for bone induction, J. Periodontol., *40*:503, 1969.

Schallhorn, R.G.: Present status of osseous grafting procedures, J. Periodontol., *48*:570, 1977.

Schluger, S.: Osseous resection—a basic principle in periodontal surgery?, Oral Surg., *2*:316, 1949.

Sullivan, H. and Atkins, J.: Free autogenous gingival grafts. I. Principles of successful grafting, Periodontics, *6*:121, 1968.

Waerhaug, J.: Healing of the dento-epithelial junction following subgingival plaque control, J. Periodontol., *49*:1, 1978.

Ward, A.: The surgical eradication of pyorrhea, J. Am. Dent. Assoc., *15*:2146, 1928.

Wilderman, M.N.: Histogenesis of repair after mucogingival surgery, J. Periodontol., *31*:283, 1960.

Yukna, R., Bowers, G., Lawrence, J. and Fedi, P.: A clinical study of healing in humans following the excisional new attachment procedures, J. Periodontol., *47*:696, 1976.

Yukna, R. and Williams, J.: Five year evaluation of the excisional new attachment procedure, J. Periodontol., *51*:382, 1980.

Chapter

$$\boxed{12}$$

PREVENTIVE PERIODONTAL MAINTENANCE

Sufficient knowledge currently exists to prevent, control, and successfully treat periodontal disease to insure that the overwhelming majority of people can maintain their natural teeth for life. In order to achieve this goal of a healthy dentition for life a program of continuing periodontal care is mandatory. Such care demands effective oral hygiene practices on the part of the individual and regular periodic professional care by dental care providers.

The responsibility for maintenance of a healthy periodontium traditionally has been the responsibility of the dental hygienist. The major activity of the practicing hygienist today is oral hygiene education and health preservation through instrumentation. Every demographic study suggests that there is an increasing population that is achieving a longer life span with a greater number of remaining natural teeth. Thus more teeth will be at risk to periodontal disease in the future. Unless some undiscovered form of prevention occurs, it may be assumed that more preventive and maintenance care will be required in the future. Dental hygienists are likely to play a more significant role in these activities

than at present. No health professional is better trained or more capable of meeting this challenge.

This chapter describes the role of the hygienist in maintenance care. Presented here are the reasons for continuing care, the evidence that such procedures are effective, the methods for monitoring health, and the therapeutic measures for achieving and sustaining oral health.

RATIONALE FOR MAINTENANCE CARE

All people are susceptible to periodontal disease, and all people need periodic maintenance care by a health professional. Public awareness of this need is improving but still remains at too low a level. Throughout most of the twentieth century the major emphasis in dentistry, both in terms of professional activity and public education, has focused on dental caries. Visits to the dental office, avoidance of a cariogenic diet, and toothbrushing techniques have been directed toward treatment or prevention of dental caries. It is not surprising that the public did not recognize a need for a program of maintenance care for periodontal disease. Awareness of the magnitude of the periodontal problem is also sadly lacking among general dentists. Studies have shown that less than 2% of dental treatment is periodontal therapy and less than 1% of general practitioners' time is spent on periodontally related treatment. This is unfortunate since maintenance can prevent or successfully manage most periodontal disease states.

Microorganisms are the cause of periodontal diseases. Inflammatory changes occur in gingival tissues when pathogenic microorganisms occupy the marginal gingival area and gingival crevice. In the absence of oral hygiene, these microorganisms, in the form of plaque, will cause gingivitis in humans. If it were possible to continually remove the plaque from tooth surfaces, the inflammatory response would not occur. Indeed, the entire rationale for oral physiotherapy is based on the assumption that mechanical dispersal of the microbiota will minimize or prevent periodontal disease and dental caries. There is some evidence that oral hygiene practices are improving in the United States among young adults. Unfortunately, relatively few individuals achieve a proficiency in oral hygiene to the extent necessary to minimize the deleterious effects of plaque.

Microorganisms are constantly present in abundance in the oral cavity. The mouth provides an ideal environment for these microbiota with its moisture, warmth, and nutritional supply. Deposition of these bacteria in the gingival crevicular area is continuous. Since meticulous plaque control is infrequently realized, the process of disease occurrence or reoccurrence is likely. The cyclic phenomena of chronic disease reappearance are frustrating for both patients and practitioners. It is satisfying to know that this cycle can be broken through a program of periodic professional care. By removal of plaque and calculus on an individualized schedule, periodontal disease

can be prevented or disease progress effectively controlled.

It should be understood that the rate of periodontal destruction may not be constant over time and that there are individual variations. Gingivitis does not necessarily inevitably lead to more destructive forms of periodontal disease. Some individuals may develop gingivitis which never progresses into periodontitis or does so over a long period of time. Other individuals may experience rapid deterioration with extensive loss of support. Evidence exists that periodontal disease activity and loss of support may be episodic. In view of these variations the best philosophy is for every individual to consider that periodontal disease may affect them and seek professional care. Baseline parameters of periodontal health can be established; regular monitoring of signs of periodontal disease can be accomplished; and appropriate therapy instituted to control microbial etiology and prevent loss of support. Preventive periodontal maintenance represents the most practical insurance for the retention of the natural dentition.

STUDIES OF PERIODONTAL MAINTENANCE

An extensive body of literature now exists documenting the beneficial effects of oral hygiene and regular professional care on the prevention of inflammatory periodontal disease. Further, long-term studies of patients with periodontal disease, even in advanced stages, have shown that with proper treatment teeth can be successfully maintained for many years.

Periodontal destruction may be measured in a number of ways including classification of individuals in different categories of disease. More specific and objective measurements include extent of pocket depth or attachment loss and the loss of teeth. When these measures are conducted over a period of time on the same individuals, projections of the longitudinal nature of the disease can be presented. Longitudinal data are available for both attachment loss and tooth loss. In previous chapters the loss of periodontal support in untreated individuals with periodontal disease has been presented. Data are also available on patients who avail themselves of professional dental services.

For most of this century the dental profession encouraged people to seek dental care on a twice per year basis. The emphasis was primarily directed toward reparative services for dental caries. Another feature of this public appeal was the admonishment to "brush after every meal" that again directed attention to the dangers of dental caries. This twice per year pattern of seeing the dentist became the accepted norm, and it is still the predominant interval in general practices for both dentists and hygienists. Is this 6-month interval acceptable in the prevention and control of periodontal disease?

Studies conducted in Scandinavia on loss of periodontal support in humans reported no difference in rate of bone loss between individuals who visited the dental office sporadically and those who went for the traditional twice per year visit. Bone loss continued to occur in both groups. Other controlled clinical research studies have also demonstrated that patients who have been successfully treated for periodontal disease cannot be maintained with a 6-month interval between recall appointments. It appears that biannual dental care is not sufficient to maintain periodontal health and prevent loss of periodontal support in individuals who have shown a lack of resistance to the disease.

When careful periodontal examination, thorough cleaning and debridement, and encouragement in healthful oral hygiene practices occur at more frequent intervals excellent periodontal health can be achieved. A number of striking examples of these beneficial effects of regular maintenance visits have been reported in the literature. In 1961 Lovdal and co-workers

regularly recalled a large number of workers in an industrial plant over a 5-year period. The workers were given repeated instruction in oral hygiene, scaling, and oral prophylaxis. Their gingival conditions improved by 60%. No surgery was accomplished and instrumentation was limited in pockets in excess of 5 mm. Suomi and co-workers treated patients with gingivitis or early periodontitis by scaling and oral hygiene instruction every 3 months for 3 years. Both the inflammatory periodontal conditions and the extent of plaque accumulation were significantly reduced and minimal attachment loss occurred.

Even patients with periodontitis can be successfully treated and the favorable results sustained over considerable time periods (Fig. 12–1). A group of patients with advanced periodontitis were treated surgically by Nyman and co-workers and then received professional scaling every 2 weeks for 2 years. No further loss of attachment took place. The significance of maintenance care in the treatment of patients with advanced periodontal disease was shown by Axelsson and Lindhe. Active therapy included pocket treatment with modified Widman flaps and recall at 2-week intervals for 2 months. Patients were then placed on a 2 to 3 month program of scaling, cleaning, and reinforcement in oral hygiene. Clinically healthy gingiva, shallow pockets, and excellent plaque control were achieved over the 6-year period without attachment loss.

Long-term effects of both surgical and nonsurgical treatment followed with maintenance have been studied. After active therapy patients were placed on a maintenance program with plaque control instruction and meticulous supragingival and subgingival scaling every 3 months for 2 years. For the next 3 years the recalled interval was 4 to 6 months and therapy consisted of only supragingival cleaning and encouragement in oral hygiene. Results showed that patients with high levels of plaque-free tooth surfaces remained in

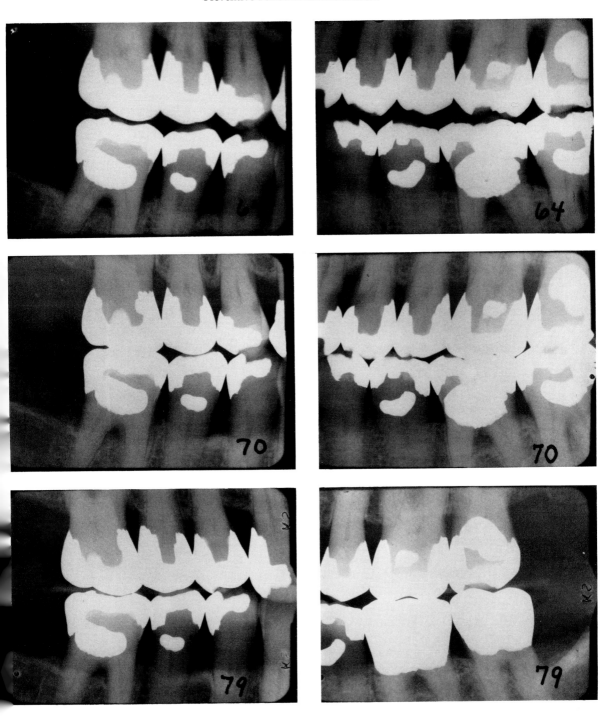

Figure 12–1. Successful Long Term Patient Maintenance. These radiographs represent the maintenance of teeth and periodontal health over a period of 17 years, It is important to note that there has been no progression of bone loss in the molar furcations in all these years. On both the right and left radiographic views the bone levels interproximally have been stable. The patient has been on periodic recall continuously.

(continued on next page.)

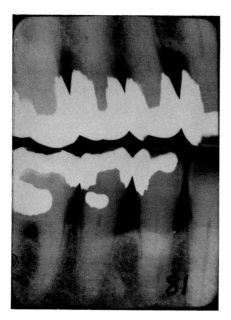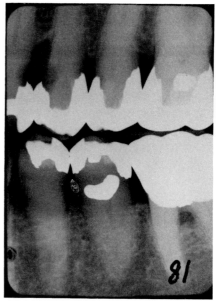

Figure 12–1.   Successful Long Term Patient Maintenance (continued).

good health, while those with poor plaque control lost attachment. The critical determinant for periodontal health appears to be debridement and control of microbiota.

In a group of patients with extremely advanced periodontal disease surgical therapy was performed and the patients placed on a 3 to 6 month recall program for a period of 14 years. Periodontal health, as measured by gingival health, pocket depth, attachment loss, and bone height was sustained during the period though a few sites in a few patients did lose attachment. Even with maintenance some periodontal disease may recur. The importance of timely recall to monitor and to promptly treat such sites is clearly indicated.

Tooth Loss Studies

The results just reviewed represent controlled clinical investigations of the effect of maintenance on loss of periodontal support. Another objective method of determining the value of maintenance is to study the number of teeth lost due to periodontal disease over a period of time. Sev-eral long-term reviews of tooth loss have been made in both untreated patients and treated patients. In adults, the major cause of tooth loss is due to destruction of the periodontal tissues. In a cross-sectional survey of adults in the United States people in the 40 to 60 age range each lost about 10 teeth due to periodontal disease. Patients with diagnosed but untreated periodontal disease lost over 7% of their teeth over a 3½-year period in another study. The annual rate of tooth loss in patients with untreated periodontal disease may approach almost one tooth per year (Table 12–1).

Conversely, long-term reports of patients whose periodontal conditions were treated by either surgical or nonsurgical methods, but all of whom were placed on maintenance, indicate only minimal loss of teeth (Table 12–2). Collectively these studies of over 1400 patients represent almost 100 years of maintenance care. All of these reports document tooth loss in patients, many with advanced periodontal destruction, referred to periodontists and maintained from 6 to 24 years. Oliver reported

Table 12–1.   Tooth Loss in Untreated Patients

Investigator	Average Years of Maintenance	Tooth Loss per Patient	Annual Rate of Tooth Loss
Marshall-Day (1955)	20.0	10.0	0.10
Löe (1978)	7.5	0.74	0.80
Becker (1979)	3.7	2.0	.61
Buckley (1984)	10.0	2.5	.25

only 0.5 teeth lost per patient over a 10-year period. Hirschfeld and Wasserman reported on 600 patients treated and maintained for an average of 22 years. In their patients classified as "well-maintained" only 0.68 teeth were lost per patient. McFall, using the same criteria as Hirschfeld and Wasserman, also reported a tooth loss of 0.68 teeth per well-maintained patient over a 19-year period. Lindhe and Nyman found only a 0.26 tooth loss in their patients maintained for 14 years. In comparison with untreated patients the rate of tooth loss would not even approach one tooth in a 10-year period (Table 12–2). It should be noted that in all these longitudinal studies a small percentage of patients continued to lose periodontal support with resultant tooth loss in spite of periodontal maintenance. These may represent patients with a rapidly progressive form of periodontal disease or those with indifferent oral hygiene practices, or that maintenance was initiated too late in the disease process (Fig. 12–2).

Cumulative evidence from clinical trials and long-term studies of tooth loss provide convincing proof of the beneficial effects of periodontal maintenance. A combination of regular individualized professional debridement and patient attention to scrupulous oral hygiene practices provides the most efficacious method for preservation of teeth.

RECALL OBJECTIVES

There are essentially two types of recall appointments. The first type, which every health provider should strive for, is the patient recall to prevent periodontal disease from developing. The second type is the maintenance recall on patients who have had periodontal therapy. The objective of both types is preservation of health and prevention of disease.

An effective recall system is an important factor not only in preventive periodontics, but also in building and sustaining a modern dental practice. In fact, the sound dental practice of tomorrow has its roots in the preventive activities of the health professionals of today. The most successful dental practices are those that have established personalized recall systems. Not surprising is the fact that such practices depend greatly on the dental hygienists to play a

Table 12–2.   Tooth Loss in Treated Patients

Investigator	Average Years of Maintenance	Tooth Loss per Patient	Annual Rate of Tooth Loss
Oliver (1969)	10.1	0.5	.05
Löe (1978)	6.4	0.11	.01
Hirschfeld & Wasserman (1978)	22.0	0.68	.03
McFall (1982)	19.0	0.68	.03
Becker (1984)	6.6	0.72	.11
Lindhe (1984)	14.0	0.26	.02

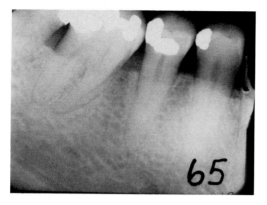

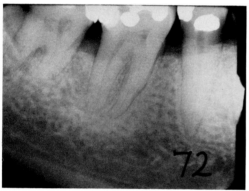

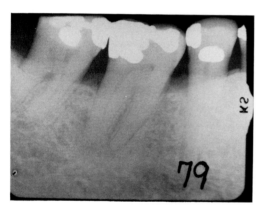

Figure 12–2. Progressive Bone Loss. Progressive bone loss can be seen interproximally in these radiographs of a patient who presented only yearly for recall maintenance. The patient has poor oral hygiene, but the recall maintenance has prevented tooth loss.

pivotal role in preventive education and therapy.

Preventive dentistry and the concept of a lifetime of preventive care cannot be delayed to the conclusion of active dental therapy but rather needs to be emphasized at the outset of dental treatment. Patients, particularly older adults, have become accustomed to view dental appointments as series of repetitive office visits in which a restorative procedure will be performed. Studies have demonstrated that people are generally unfamiliar with the term periodontal disease. Obviously, the need for public education both through the mass media and on a personal basis in the office setting is necessary for prevention of periodontal disease.

COMMUNICATION DURING THERAPY

Communication is essential in any form of interpersonal relationship. Patients must understand that they are susceptible to periodontal disease and that their teeth are at risk. During the early stages of treatment the attitude, beliefs, and behavior of patients with regard to their oral health must be ascertained. The concept of the recurrent appearance of the bacterial causation of periodontal disease must be presented in language that the patient can understand. Hygienists must develop communicative skills that can include terms such as "gum disease," "bugs," and "cleaning appointment." While such phrases might not be very scientific, they may be needed with some patients in order to educate and establish behavioral patterns.

Introduction of the recall concept to the patient can be illustrated by the following example:

"Mrs. Johnson, I believe you understand that there are millions of small bugs, we call bacteria, living on our teeth and gums. These bacteria are so small that they are invisible to the naked eye. When these bacteria accumulate in number in the critical area where the gum and teeth meet they cause changes in the gum tissues. These changes in the gum are called periodontal disease. By good brushing and flossing you can help keep these bacteria to a small number, and that is very important. But it is not enough to control the bacteria and prevent disease!

Many bacteria get between the gum and the tooth in places you can't reach with your brush and they multiply beneath the gum. Sometimes these bacteria use salts from the saliva and form hard deposits on the teeth that are called calculus. The only way to remove these bacteria under the gums and the calculus is to have your teeth cleaned on a regular basis. Many scientific studies over a long number of years have shown that this is the best way to prevent periodontal disease. When we have finished your treatment we will set up these recall appointments at times suited to your individual needs."

The example just cited is oversimplified and, purposely, not very sophisticated. The hygienist should remember that the patient knows little about the causes of their periodontal problem and that the language of dentistry is foreign to the lay public. Simple, direct and truthful explanations are the essence of professional communication. Questions from patients should be encouraged and answers provided. Patients educated in the need for recall can achieve desired levels of health and are more likely to comply well with recall appointments.

The experience of learning is a continuous process. Patients, by nature, retreat into old habit patterns of oral hygiene that may be ineffective. Individuals who have had successful preventive care tend to believe that they have some lasting immunity to periodontal disease, and patients who have undergone periodontal therapy often believe that they have been cured and will not have disease reoccurrence. Both of these concepts are fallacies. Recall appointments provide the hygienist the opportunity to continue the dialogue begun during the treatment phase. Such communication permits reinforcement of information previously presented, correction of misconceptions, introduction of new knowledge and products, and constructive nonjudg-

mental suggestions for continuing oral health. Such communication solidifies the provider-patient relationship in which both the patient and the hygienist place the primary focus upon prevention of disease.

Establishing the Recall System

Continuing preventive care is so important in maintenance of periodontal health that provision for recall must be established early in the treatment phase. Previously it has been stressed that explanation of causes of disease and methods of treatment and prevention should be introduced in the early stages of treatment. This should be a team effort by all dental care providers in the office. It is also the proper time to educate the patient to the preventive concept of recall maintenance, and it is the proper time to establish the recall system for the patient.

Many types of office recall systems have been suggested and used with varying degrees of success. The hygienist often assumes the pivotal role in developing and maintaining the office recall system. One of the simplest systems is the use of duplicate file cards, 4 × 5 inches in size. One of these cards is placed in an alphabetical file, while the other is placed in a chronologic file by the month in which the patient is next to be seen. The reason for the use of the two index cards is to promote efficiency in locating a patient's recall card should it be needed quickly for information by the dentist or for a telephone call from the patient confirming an appointment. Time would be lost if the monthly file had to be used to search out a particular recall card on short notice.

The pertinent information to be typed on the two cards is similar though the alphabetical file card is simpler than the chronologic card. It contains the patient's name and number, the patient's address, residence and business telephone number, the referring person, and the recall interval. It is also helpful to note whether the patient is on active recall, has been discontinued, has been referred, or has become inactive due to failure to keep recall appointments. The next scheduled appointment time should be noted in pencil on the card. The chronologic file card contains similar information as the alphabetical card but also contains notations on special precautions, preference for day and time of appointment, individual arrangement such as desire to have spouse's appointment on same date, and projected appointment length. Pencil notation on the date of next appointment is included. Many offices find it convenient to record on this card a history of past recall appointment dates and patient compliance in keeping recalls.

Patient recall cards are drawn from both files the month before the projected recalls, the date and time written on the card, the reminder postcard or letter prepared, and the cards replaced appropriately by month and in the alphabetical file. It is helpful for the monthly recall card to be available with the patient record at the time of the recall appointment. The next appointment often can be arranged at that time. After the patient has been seen, the chronologic card is filed in the appropriate month for the next appointment. If, for example, the patient is scheduled for a recall appointment every 4 months and is seen in the month of July, the card will be replaced in the file for the next recall under November in the monthly index file.

Recall files should be reviewed regularly and kept up to date. In many offices this recall system is managed by a receptionist, and this provides for effective appointment book control as well as updating of the recall files. The hygienist is still responsible for review of these cards on a monthly basis because only the hygienist knows the patient's needs with regard to changes in appointment interval and appointment length and individual patient considerations. Many dental practices are now utilizing computers for patient scheduling and financial transactions. Recall system management is particularly adaptable for computer use and this method will probably be increasingly incorporated in dental practice since it provides for efficient, time saving retrieval of information with provision for rapid updating. Information and advice for the file card system is equally applicable for computer utilization.

Various systems are available for notification of the patient of the recall appointment. A traditional approach has been the use of letters or postcards reminding the patient of the appointment date and time. Patients are requested to notify the office if the suggested date is not convenient. This method places responsibility for health maintenance on the patient, and, in the case of letters, also provides the opportunity to include patient educational pamphlets or office newsletters. It does have a risk in that the patient may choose to not keep the appointment resulting in loss of chair time, but experience suggests that this is not a frequent occurrence with patients educated in the importance of preventive maintenance. An example of an appointment letter, which can be printed in quantity, is shown in Figure 12–3.

Many offices prefer to remind patients of maintenance visits by a telephone call several days in advance of the appointment. While this method is more economical than use of the mailed reminder, it does have some disadvantages. Telephone calls require time of busy office personnel. Often several calls must be made in order to contact the patient. In an era in which the majority of patients have occupations, the calls often must be placed to the patient's workplace and many patients resent such intrusion. Telephone calls also provide a patient the opportunity to refuse the appointment or develop quick excuses for not keeping the appointment. A telephone system thus depends in large part upon the enthusiasm and insistence of the individual placing the call.

As patients have learned the importance of such preventive maintenance visits for their oral health, an increasing number of

```
                  H. E. SMITH, D. D. S.

                     110 North Street
                     Anytown, U. S. A.




     Mr. Ronald G. Greene
     1014 Main Street
     Anytown, U.S.A.


     Dear Mr. Greene:

            I have reserved time for a recall appointment for

     you on   Thursday, May 30,

     at 10:45 a.m.


            Please let me know if it will not be convenient for

     you to come at this time.

                              Very sincerely,



                              H. E. Smith, D.D.S.
```

Figure 12–3. Appointment Letter. An example of one type of appointment letter form that can be used for recall purposes.

offices are arranging the next recall appointment after treatment and before the patient leaves the office. An appointment date and time is entered in the appointment book and on the recall card or computer. An appointment card is provided the patient at this time and a duplicate card is prepared to be mailed a week prior to the appointment. This duplicate card can be filed in the monthly file box in a pre-addressed envelope.

Regardless of the recall method utilized, some attrition of patients will occur. Patient compliance with recall maintenance, even in patients treated for periodontitis, remains a persistent problem. The percentage of such patients lost during maintenance has been reported to range between 18 and 34%. Many factors such as economics, change in occupation, moves to new locations, indifference, stress, and changing value scales all contribute to this loss of patients. Patient compliance is enhanced by the establishment of a warm provider-patient relationship, a high quality of professional service, a sound educational program, and the personal enthusiasm and communicative skills of the hygienist.

Appointment Interval

Frequency of recall for a particular patient is dependent upon the individual needs of the patient and is variable. Some patients with essentially healthy gingiva and meticulous oral physiotherapy may not need recall appointments more than once or twice a year. Other patients who have shown a susceptibility to periodontal disease organisms in their mouths and poor oral physiotherapy may require four or five recall appointments a year. Patients who have received periodontal therapy and who may still have residual pockets obviously require more frequent therapy than patients with healthy gingiva. Because of the episodic nature of periodontal attachment loss every adult individual should be monitored at least once each year.

All too frequently patients are placed in a recall sequence interval based on a pre-established office policy. Thus patients are routinely seen at yearly or 6-month intervals. Such an approach may be efficient for the dental office, but has not proven to be of value to the patient. When such recalls are primarily directed toward discovery of recurrent caries or replacement of defective restorations, the periodontal condition is largely ignored. Unfortunately, this type of patient management has dominated dental practices in the past.

What then are the criteria upon which a proper recall interval can be established? In medicine this criteria has long been the state of the patient's health, and this standard applies equally well to the oral cavity. Preservation of health is the primary goal and the paramount reason for the recall maintenance appointmnt. The frequency of recall is determined by number of appointments in a given time period necessary to achieve this goal.

Other factors do, of course, impact upon the frequency with which the patient is seen in order to maintain health. It would be ideal if, at the conclusion of active dental therapy, all patients had obtained perfect oral health. This is our goal, but realistically such a state is not always achieved. Due to severity of destruction, medical considerations, and a host of other reasons, control of active disease rather than restoration of health may be the practical treatment result. Such compromise necessitates more frequent recall appointments. Plaque accumulation and calculus deposition are major etiologic factors in periodontal disease activity. Rates of such bacterial deposition are highly variable between individuals and dependent upon pathogenicity and host susceptibility. Gingival response varies greatly between patients. Bacterial accumulation also depends upon factors such as shape, position and number of teeth, gingival levels, furcation exposure, presence of prosthetic appliances, dietary habits, and thoroughness of oral physiotherapy. Effectiveness of oral hygiene is also influenced by variants such as patient motivation, manual dexterity of the patient, systemic medical conditions, and life situations. Collectively, these interlocking factors form a complex individual pattern that defies simplified, standardized recall intervals.

Once a recall interval has been initially established at the conclusion of the active phase of treatment, many patients assume that the time period between appointments has been permanently fixed. Hygienists must impress patients that this period is flexible and dependent upon the status of periodontal health. Patients may be assured that their efforts in their own maintenance of health through oral hygiene activities is an important determinant in the frequency of their care. One of the major purposes of the recall appointment is the assessment of the present periodontal status. Results of such assessment determines the course of future therapy and the time interval between appointments.

Recall Length

State of periodontal health is also the deciding factor in length of the recall appointment. Surprisingly, in one study of dental hygiene beliefs and activities the periodontal conditions was listed fourth behind extent of plaque, degree of calculus, and amount of tooth stain in determining length of the appointment. Removal of plaque, calculus, and stain are, of course, important in estimating the length of the recall appointment, but they are secondary to the periodontal status that controls all other procedures accomplished at the appointment. Perhaps the single most significant portion of the appointment is the acquisition of data on the current status of health. Comparison of such data with previous findings established at baseline and prior recall appointments dictates the subsequent action at the appointment.

Length of the appointment is, in part,

also predetermined by a number of factors intrinsic to the nature of the appointment itself. Thus time must be provided to seat the patient, engage in the customary amenities, obtain interim histories, document findings, dentist consultation, and patient dismissal. These customary activities require almost 12 minutes. It is totally unreasonable to accomplish these essential portions of the recall and perform therapy in a 15- or 30-minute appointment. Even patients in good health deserve the attention to detail and thoroughness which can seldom be achieved in less than 45 minutes. Exceptions to this may be children, some adolescents, and adults with only a few teeth. Most modern practices generally provide the hygienist and patient an hour to accomplish a professional recall appointment. If there has been a worsening of the periodontal condition, reoccurrence of inflammation, poor oral physiotherapy, need for additional patient education, or excessive calculus formation, the hygienist should have the prerogative to schedule additional therapy appointments soon after the recall appointment. The length of future recalls may need to be increased in such patients and the interval between appointments tightened.

Financial considerations impact upon both frequency and length of recall appointments. The increase in both has been interpreted by some patients as an economic drain on their resources because oral health has not been perceived as an essential in life quality. Many dentists have also been reluctant to recall patients too frequently because of the belief that patients will not pay for this health care service. Unquestionably, health maintenance represents a financial investment, but it is an investment that provides tremendous dividends for the patients. Such maintenance recall actually saves money by preventing development of conditions requiring costly therapy for tooth loss and replacement. The hygienist must carry this message to the patients. It is as important as any therapy rendered. Often, insurance policies will not provide for proper preventive maintenance by limiting the number of such appointments in a year to one or two. The challenge to the health provider is to attempt to preserve health. The informed patient must then determine the relative value of such health service to achieve this goal.

RECALL PROCEDURES

Patients for preventive maintenance recall may vary from those who have never had any periodontal problem to those who have undergone extensive periodontal therapy. Thus the actual amount of treatment to be accomplished at the maintenance appointment will need to be modified to suit the individual needs of the patient. Regardless of this variant in therapy certain procedures must be standard in every recall appointment. Such standardization of procedures guarantees that important criteria are not omitted and efficient use of appointment time is achieved. A list of such standard procedures would include:

1. Initial amenities
2. Medical and dental interim histories
3. Radiographic review
4. Soft tissue examination
5. Dental examination
6. Periodontal probing
7. Bleeding assessment
8. Plaque evaluation
9. Oral physiotherapy reinstruction
10. Scaling and root planing
11. Polishing teeth
12. Chemical therapy
13. Doctor examination
14. Dismissal and reappointment

Even if a patient required only minimal scaling, the combined standard procedures would require better than 30 minutes. The "rubber cup prophylaxis" of the past is no longer acceptable if the goals of preservation of health and prevention of disease are to be realized. Patients should receive ex-

cellence in care and attention to detail accomplished by these standard recall procedures. The dental hygienist who conscientiously adheres to this regimen will find satisfaction in the knowledge that the highest standards of the dental hygiene profession have been realized. Those who do not include such a pattern in the preventive maintenance appointment will find only frustration. Every patient deserves this type of exhaustive assessment. To do less is to render inadequate care.

It must again be emphasized that such effective recall procedures must be presented to the patient during active phases of therapy not just at the conclusion of treatment. This is particularly true for the patient with periodontal disease who will receive extensive treatment. Both the hygienist and the dentist are usually involved in such treatment, and both must emphasize the limitations of active therapy without continued maintenance care. Ogilvie has likened this patient to the treated diabetic who must guard their health to survive. In the patient with moderate to advanced periodontal disease it is survival of the natural dentition that is at risk.

INITIAL AMENITIES. Every person appreciates the courteous acts and manner of polite social behavior. This initial time spent with the patient sets in motion the entire tone of the maintenance appointment. Ideally, the hygienist should personally greet the patient in a warm professional manner, in the reception area (Fig. 12–4). It is not acceptable to simply shout out the patient's name in a crowded reception room. The hygienist should go to the patient and start the conversation. It may be necessary to remind the patient of your name. This is particularly true with older patients, patients with extended interval between recalls, or child patients.

The patient is then escorted to the dental operatory, comfortably seated, properly draped, and the supporting headrest properly positioned. Conversation should begin on neutral subjects such as activities

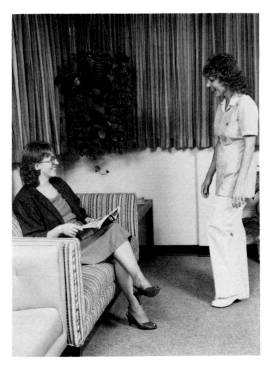

Figure 12–4. Greeting Patient in the Reception Area. Rapport is established on the maintenance appointment by meeting the patient outside the dental operatory.

since the last office visit, family, travel, occupation, and hobbies. If proper records have been obtained during active therapy such patient interests should have been noted in the patient's records. It is also permissible to comment briefly on your own activities. This type of interpersonal verbal exchange is invaluable in cementing the provider-patient relationship. It does take some time, perhaps 5 minutes, but it is quality use of time. Some dentists feel that time spent talking to the patient is wasted and not economically practical, but the most successful practices are those that encourage the patient to express themselves. Information on the patient's future plans should be written in the chart for the doctor's attention.

MEDICAL AND DENTAL INTERIM HISTO-RIES. A natural verbal shift from preliminary conversation to the professional de-velopment of the appointment is achieved through questioning the patient concerning their medical and dental status. If a thorough health history has been obtained previously, it is only necessary to update this through brief questions. Examples include: "Have you been in good health since your last visit?" "Have you had any change in your general health?" "Have you seen your physician since you were last here?" "Are you taking any new medications?" If a particular patient has a significant medical history, the status of this condition should be determined. In many modern dental practices blood pressure determinations have become a regular part of the recall appointment. Such determinations are required in patients with a history of hypertension or coronary heart disease, but this is a valuable service to perform for all patients. Unrecognized high blood pressure is one of the major undiagnosed diseases and patients often seek dental maintenance care more commonly than medical services. Older patients, who often have periodontal disease, also may have undiagnosed hypertension.

Review of the interim dental history is often simple and brief, but it is essential to establish the current patient profile. Questions should include: "Are you aware of any tooth or gum problems?" "Have you had any discomfort in your face, jaws, or neck?" "Are any of your teeth sensitive?" Most commonly such questions will receive a negative response, but if specific complaints are elicited, the area should be observed during clinical examination. The complaint should be recorded and the doctor informed when he appraises the patient. Under a total health concept all health providers perform their professional responsibilities in a combined effort to maintain health for the patient. If conditions warrant consultation with the patient's physician, the dentist will make the needed contact. The medical and dental review is a short, but essential, portion of the preventive maintenance appointment and it is another step in the concept of continuous patient monitoring.

RADIOGRAPHIC REVIEW. Before the advent of preventive dental care and fluoridation, bitewing radiographs were considered an essential part of every recall examination. With the decrease in dental caries and the public's and dental profession's concern with excess radiation this is currently less common. Radiographic full series of films probably need not be required more often than at 5-year intervals. Vertical bitewing radiographs probably should be acquired at year and one-half intervals. The hygienist should place the most recent radiographs on the viewbox and note the date of their acquisition. If an extended time has elapsed since the radiographs have been obtained, this should be called to the attention of the doctor. If the patient has poor oral hygiene practices, high plaque scores, recurrent caries, or progressive periodontal destruction, radiographs may be indicated more frequently. If the patient reports pain or specific discomfort in any area of the mouth, immediate consultation with the dentist concerning the problem is mandatory early in the appointment. The radiograph will then be available for the dentist for immediate appraisal, and appropriate action can be taken. Periodontal attachment loss occurs clinically many months prior to appearance of bone changes observable on radiographs. Routine acquisition of radiographs is not in the best interest of the patient.

SOFT TISSUE EXAMINATION. Both extraoral and intra-oral inspection of soft tissues represents a significant procedures in the recall appointment. It is not necessary to palpate the masticatory musculature unless the patient has reported discomfort, but it is important to visually inspect the patient's face, neck, and lips for changes from the norm. Changes in size, texture, color and consistency in skin features should be noted. Often this can be accomplished during the conversational portion of the appointment. Dryness of lips, angular cheilitis, herpetic lesions, and pigmented skin changes should be visually inspected. Lips should be carefully palpated as part of the clinical examination. Glandular structures should also be palpated, particularly if the patient reports discomfort in this region. Any condition differing from normal should be recorded and called to the attention of the doctor.

Intraoral inspection of oral soft tissues including cheeks, vestibule, throat, tongue and palate constitute the first phase of the clinical examination. All of the features of gingival examination previously described must be repeated at the recall appointment. Changes in color, form, texture, level, and amount of gingiva must be compared with data obtained at post-treatment evaluation and previous recalls.

DENTAL EXAMINATION. This phase of the clinical examination includes occlusal analysis, patterns of tooth mobility, and tooth by tooth assessment of health. It is probably not necessary to perform a complete occlusal analysis unless the patient has lost considerable bone support around the teeth, has had previous occlusal therapy, or has been identified as having a clenching or bruxing habit. Mobility should be evaluated by palpation of teeth as the patient brings the teeth together in both centric and eccentric movements. Then in a systematic manner each tooth should be tested for increased mobility in the manner previously described. All mobility above physiologic should be recorded on the recall chart.

Careful inspection of the teeth for caries, cuspal fracture, and defective restorations is then accomplished. Changes from previous findings are entered on the chart. Some hygienists prefer to delay this until the time of instrumentation, but this does not provide the proper attention to this step in the examination. Further, it is inconvenient and time wasting to have to stop and record information while scaling. Recall maintenance may occur for many years after active therapy, and gingival recession with root exposure may result in root caries; recurrent decay may occur; and even the finest restorations are subject to wear and failure. All of these reasons dictate careful adherence to this portion of the examination.

PERIODONTAL PROBING. No portion of the recall examination is more important than the standardized probing of the gingival crevices. Monitoring of the separation of soft tissues from the tooth when compared with measurements previously obtained provide a significant determinant in assessment of periodontal health. In Chapter 6 on clinical determinations the measurement of attachment loss was emphasized. It would be ideal if measurements from a fixed reference point such as a stent or the cemento-enamel junction could be routinely employed in the recall examination. From a practical standpoint such determinations require time that is not available at recall appointments. Thus periodontal probings must be made from the variable gingival margin level. While admittedly such measurements lack accuracy, they do provide a method of monitoring disease progression when compared with previous findings. A continuous record of such measurements can help determine overall periodontal health and provide an alert to specific sites which are demonstrating change. This type of change in health is easily visualized on a chart with sufficient space for multiple entries (Fig. 12–5). Detection of such changes may be indicative of disease activity and directs the course of therapy at the recall appointment.

BLEEDING ASSESSMENT. Bleeding upon gentle probing is an objective method for monitoring periodontal status. It is an earlier sign of gingivitis than tissue changes that can be observed visually. It may be of more value in monitoring disease activity at the gingivitis stage than in more advanced states. In all stages of the disease, however, bleeding represents an alert to the therapist that pathologic destruction is taking place in a site. Because bleeding is

such an important indicator of inflammation, it should be noted prior to the use of plaque disclosing agents which might obscure its detection. This dictates that periodontal probing and evaluation of bleeding be accomplished prior to obtaining a plaque record. Following the systemic probing of the facial or lingual of a sextant of teeth, bleeding should be determined. A bleeding record can be maintained and a bleeding index recorded if desired. Another method is to simply circle the pocket measurement obtained at the bleeding site (Fig. 12–5). Bleeding upon probing at the recall appointment dictates immediate, appropriate therapy.

PLAQUE EVALUATION. Determination of plaque and calculus are significant measures of the patient's efforts in control of periodontal etiology. For reasons mentioned earlier these measures are properly delayed until critical analysis of gingival changes, probing and bleeding have been accomplished. Extent, location, and amount of supragingival calculus should be observed and recorded (Fig. 12–6). By reference to data entries noted on prior appointments, it can be determined if the patient is improving or relapsing in efforts for control. The Plaque Control Record is a direct and objective measure of the plaque level at the time of examination, and it can be used with or without a disclosing agent. Monitoring of patient progress in plaque management can easily be related to previous evaluations (Fig. 12–7).

There are, however, some variables that must be considered in interpretation of these data. The plaque score obtained at the recall appointment reflects the extent of plaque at the time of examination only and cannot monitor patient performance during the interval between recalls. Bleeding and probing are better ways to measure the true activity over time. Patients often increase their oral hygiene efforts before the recall examination in an attempt to make the tissues healthier and "fool" the

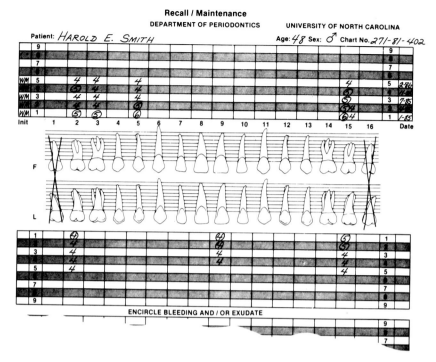

Figure 12–5. Recall Maintenance Record. A continuous record of changes in pocket depths at maintenance appointments should be kept. Areas that bleed are designated by circling the pocket depth number.

health provider that they have been complying with preventive suggestions.

ORAL PHYSIOTHERAPY REINSTRUCTION. Almost all patients presenting for recall examination have some plaque accumulation. Patients exhibiting periodontal health and satisfactory plaque control require minimal reinstruction in oral physiotherapy. What is demanded is strong encouragement to reinforce patient motivation. Patients should be complimented on their fine efforts and urged to make an even better effort in those areas where plaque is located.

It is particularly helpful if the dentist, when examining the patient, will reemphasize the positive tone set by the hygienist. This can be accomplished by statement such as, "Mrs. Connor, your oral health is excellent and we are so pleased with what we have accomplished together. You are doing a superb job in keeping plaque off your teeth. We really enjoy having someone like you in our practice." An increase in the interval between maintenance appointments may be the reward for such fine patient effort.

Patients who appear at recall with demonstrably poor plaque control require more effort and time on the part of the hygienist. It does little good to severely scold such patients. Instead, the hygienist should seek to determine the cause for such poor patient behavior and attempt to motivate the individual. Many of these patients are aware of their poor oral hygiene performance, and this lack of plaque management may have been the initiating factor in their original periodontal condition. Skill and tact are required to determine why the patient is lax in plaque control. Patients are often under stressful conditions that overshadow concern for oral health. Some individuals are naturally lazy and use the recall appointment as an opportunity to remedy their own lack of self-

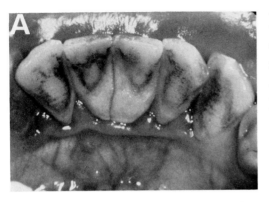

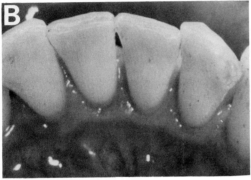

Figure 12–6. Calculus and Calculus Removal. Some patients with indifferent oral hygiene practices can accumulate plaque and calculus between recall appointments. This patient had not attended to recall for more than a year. A, Presentation at recall. B, Two weeks following maintenance appointment. (Courtesy of Dr. David Simpson)

care. The hygienist, who would be teacher, should ask leading questions, "Are you setting aside time every day for brushing?"; "Do you attempt to get the bristle down to gums?"; or "Are you trying to use floss?" By listening to the patient's answer the hygienist can adapt the proper therapeutic and motivational approaches. Extensive reeducation, reinstruction, and encouragement may be required. Changes in brushing methods or oral physiotherapy aids may be indicated.

Reviewing the Plaque Control Record and indicating to the patient sites where plaque is present is a good instructional approach. The use of the graph on the Plaque Control Record provides a dramatic

way to illustrate lack of progress (Fig. 12–7). Sequential entries of plaque levels trace a patient's progress or lack of progress in control of plaque. A challenge or goal can be established for the patient to achieve for himself or herself. Competing with oneself to reach a better score can be an effective motivational aid, especially if encouragement is given and compliments for good achievement are forthcoming from the hygienist. With the patient observing in a mirror, the hygienist then must demonstrate plaque containing areas in the patient's mouth. Use a toothbrush and floss to demonstrate the ease with which the plaque can be removed. Then have the patient remove the plaque by brushing their own teeth. Review with the patient the progress made by their own efforts, and praise the effort. This type of education is time consuming, but the motivational stimulus is strong and well worth the time expended.

Great personal and professional satisfaction is gained when patients who have been poor oral hygiene performers demonstrate improvement in plaque control. Unfortunately, some patients will never comprehend their own role in their own physical health and will never alter their poor behavior. Hygienists must accept the reality that sometimes their best attempts at education will not succeed. Such patients must be recalled at frequent intervals since only the professional care rendered by the hygienist can help control inflammatory disease. Poor patient attitude or performance by the patient must be entered in the patient record and called to the doctor's attention. All of the best efforts of health professionals may not help an individual who will not help themselves toward better health.

SCALING AND ROOT PLANING. Procedures accomplished to this point in the recall appointment should have identified those sites that require additional therapy. Conventional wisdom, in the past, has suggested that every surface of every tooth

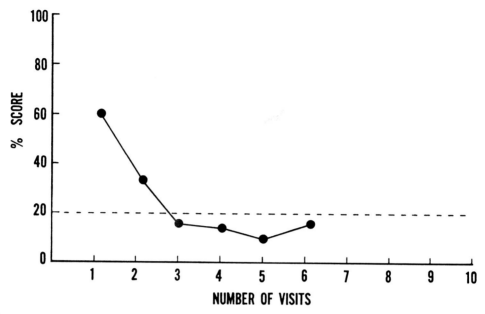

Figure 12–7. Graph Showing Patient Progress in Reducing Plaque. Note the patient's progress over successive appointments in controlling plaque after instruction in oral hygiene practices. This graph is useful in encouraging patient self-care.

must be thoroughly scaled at every recall. This may not be the most helpful way to treat patients at recall. If the majority of sites in a mouth appear to be in good health, it is unnecessary to meticulously scale and root plane them. Scaling and root planing should be directed toward sites where active inflammatory changes are occurring. In these sites scaling should remove irritants. In many instances root planing with sharp curettes should be accomplished to accomplish debridement and smooth the root surface. Where deep pockets or extensive bleeding is present, local anesthesia is a useful adjunct to control hemorrhage, alleviate patient discomfort, and facilitate proper instrumentation. Control of the active disease process and minimization of further attachment loss is the desired goal.

This approach does not imply that supragingival calculus and plaque at healthy sites is ignored, rather it is suggested that primary effort should be given to disease areas. All calculus, plaque, and stain should be removed. Increasingly, hygien-

ists are finding the use of ultrasonic instrumentation a convenient way of accomplishing such therapy. When hand instruments are used in healthy sites, only removal of etiologic agents should be accomplished. Aggressive scaling and root planing of healthy sites may cause tissue damage and result in attachment loss. Though the concept of confining meticulous instrumentation to only disease site represents a departure from traditional therapy, it is a reasonable approach supported by clinical research.

POLISHING TEETH. Both patients and hygienists always have placed a high value on the removal of stain and the esthetically pleasing vision of clean teeth. The term "oral prophylaxis" is a standard chart entry by many hygienists to describe the entire recall appointment. Patients have stains and these should be removed, though the effect of stain in the development of inflammatory disease is probably not significant. While esthetically pleasing teeth is a happy by-product of the polishing procedure, it is not the principal reason for polishing teeth. The fundamental goal of polishing is to remove plaque and prevent its recurrence. Plaque levels should approach zero at the conclusion of the maintenance appointment. This point should be stressed to the patient in order to emphasize that plaque accumulation occurring between maintenance visits are the patient's responsibility. In order to complete the plaque removal flossing of the interproximal surfaces by the hygienist should follow the polishing procedure.

Because abrasive substances are used in the polishing process, some tooth structure is removed. Polishing has been shown to remove fluoride from the teeth. Use of a fluoride containing polishing paste may be helpful in restoring some of this lost protection. It is appropriate to restore the fluoride by application of fluoride containing solutions following the polishing phase.

CHEMICAL THERAPY. Fluoride agents and products for treatment of sensitive teeth are currently widely used as a final clinical procedure in the maintenance appointment. An increasing number of new chemical agents are becoming available for topical application to control bacterial growth. It is probable that in the near future the hygienist will conclude the recall with the topical application of bacteriostatic or bactericidal substances.

Through preventive professional care and the use of fluorides dental caries has dramatically declined, and more people are retaining their teeth. Gingival recession, due to multiple causes, often is seen in older patients. Roots are thus exposed to the oral environment and are susceptible to dental caries. Many older individuals live alone and tend to eat convenience foods with a high content of refined carbohydrates. In order to protect against root caries the hygienist should accomplish a fluoride treatment. Research has demonstrated that stannous fluoride is an effective agent in control of some plaque containing bacteria. Because of the proven efficacy of fluoride as a caries preventive

agent and potential for plaque inhibition, a fluoride treatment is a recommended portion of the maintenance appointment.

Antiseptic agents that suppress oral flora have been previously reviewed, and may be used during the scaling portion of the recall. Effective scaling and polishing probably are sufficient to reduce the bacterial level, but the future may hold the possibility of an application of some agent that can be applied at the maintenance appointment to inhibit growth of destructive microorganisms. Antibiotics in the form of localized pocket placement are already a clinical reality. In the future antibiotics may be placed in deep pockets with recurrent active inflammation as a preventive measure between maintenance visits.

Sensitive root surfaces inhibit oral physiotherapy on the part of the patient. The hygienist can apply agents to minimize this discomfort. In Chapters 8 and 10 these measures were discussed and the reader should refer to these in selecting an approach for the recall management of this vexing condition.

Chlorhexidine, a bisbiguanide, is an effective antiplaque agent and may be of value in selected patients. Widely used in Europe, chlorhexidine will be used in the United States as a prescription drug.

DOCTOR EXAMINATION. At the completion of the clinical phase of the recall the doctor should be requested to examine the patient. The hygienist should inform the dentist of significant findings revealed during the recall appointment as well as relevant events in the patient's life (Fig. 12–8). Such information provides the dentist with a conversational entree and provides a status report on the patient's health. The time the dentist spends with the patient may be brief but it is an important reinforcement of the doctor-patient relationship and the dental provider team concept (Fig. 12–9). Specific dental concerns or other health concerns may be expressed by the patient that only the dentist can answer. The dentist should make a clin-

TREATMENT RECORD

Date'	Plaque Score		ADA CODE & FEE
2-5-86	14%	Bleeding score 6%. Reviewed oral hygiene	4910.
		and floss use in #2-#3, and #14-#15 area.	
		Light supragingival calculus lower anteriors,	
		coffee stains. Scaled and polished teeth. Root	
		plane max. molars. New periapical. Caries	
		distal #5. Oldest daughter, Pam, getting	
		married in April. Recall scheduled for May.	

Figure 12–8. Chart Entry for Recall Appointment. Information recorded on the patient's record provides a permanent representation of the patient's condition and alerts the dentist to the patient's health, oral status, and personal concerns.

ical examination of the patient to review findings accumulated by the hygienist. Some hygienists resent this examination by the dentist because they feel the dentist is grading their performance. Hygienists with more perception will realize that the dentist examination is an extension of the concept of maintaining optimal patient health. It is most satisfying if the dentist comments favorably on the hygienist's performance in front of the patient. Successful dental practices use mutual praise between providers as a strategic part of internal marketing.

DISMISSAL AND REAPPOINTMENT. Following the departure of the dentist, the patient is dismissed from the operatory. Many offices provide the patient with a new tooth-

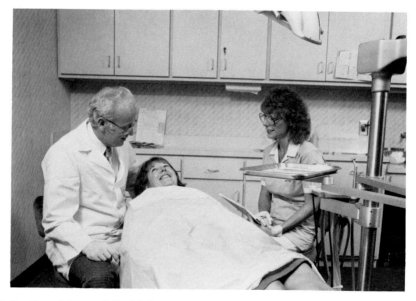

Figure 12–9. Completion of the Maintenance Appointment. The success in preserving health results in mutual satisfaction for the patient, hygienist, and doctor.

brush or other oral hygiene aids and preventive literature during this period. This provides another opportunity for oral physiotherapy motivation. Arrangements for future maintenance appointments are solidified during this period. If possible, the hygienist should escort patients back to the reception area and bid them farewell.

THE DENTAL TEAM

Throughout this book the concept of a group of dental health providers working in concert to preserve patient oral health has been stressed. The era of the solo dentist, often even without a dental assistant, is thankfully vanishing. If the goal of preservation of the natural dentition in comfort, health, and function is to be realized, a cooperative professional effort is required. Each individual in the office, dentist, hygienists, assistant, and receptionist, brings particular skills and talents to the team concept, but only the dentist and the hygienist bring the professional experience to render therapy. There is little doubt that practices with hygienists can provide a higher level of patient care with greater efficiency.

The maintenance appointment procedures outlined in this chapter are demanding on the hygienist. When added to the task of operatory maintenance, appointment control, instrument sharpening, surgical participation, and sterilization they may appear overwhelming. Certainly, they do require time to accomplish at a high level of quality. Human patients are not a product that can be processed through the dental office in order to reach a productivity level. The most successful dental practices are established on quality not quantity. Service to the patient must always be the central focus. Wise dentists provide adequate time for hygienist to achieve quality results both during active therapy and during recall appointments. Hygienists deserve the right to reschedule patients in order to ensure the finest level of care.

Mutual respect is the essence of the dental team concept. The hygienist should realize that the dentist possesses knowledge and skills beyond that of the hygienist. In turn, the dentist must appreciate that the hygienist possesses unique skill as a health educator and therapist. When competent, compassionate dentists and energetic, enthusiastic, technically skilled hygienists work together for their patients' health, the results are greater than either can accomplish alone.

Education is a life-long continuous process. The hygienist who graduates today will be a better hygienist with years of patient experience. Too often the formal process of education stops with graduation. Hygienists must constantly update their knowledge and skills. Reading professional journals, attendance at dental meetings, and acquisition of new knowledge through continuing education courses and active participation in professional organizations are all necessary qualities of the superb hygienist. Communication with the dentist on new techniques, new agents, and new products awakens interest and strengthens the bonds of mutual trust and respect in the dental team. Dental hygiene is a rewarding career, but it can become drudgery unless there are periods of professional renewal. In the best of possible worlds, such renewal is found in the team concept.

PATIENT RIGHTS OF EXPECTATION. All dentral providers at some time are dental patients as well. Consider what you desire in your own dental care and whether you are satisfied with the dental service you are provided. Every individual needing dental treatment should have some expectation of what care they should receive. There are several basic rights which all patients deserve. These include the right to courtesy and honesty. Emergencies and relief of pain should receive prompt attention. At the conclusion of active therapy clinical assessment and the patient record should indicate that procedures accepted as therapeutic have been accomplished. Active periodontal disease must have been arrested. Therapy should have left the mouth free of detectable etiologic agents and gingival areas should be healthy. No bleeding on light probing or exudate should be present. Sometimes anatomic restrictions, cosmetic considerations, morphology of periodontal lesions, and patient desires may place limitations on obtaining optimal results. Patients should have been fully informed of the causation of their disease and their current status. All patient questions should have been factually answered. The patient should have been carefully instructed in oral hygiene procedures. An appropriate recall maintenance program should have been recommended to the patient. Many of these patient rights are adopted from guidelines of the American Academy of Periodontology, but they are appropriate to all dental practices.

FUTURE PROJECTIONS

Change is a constant over all the ages, but never in history has change occurred with the speed of this century. In this time of the computer a literal knowledge explosion is taking place in science. This book represents the latest information available, but even as you read this sentence new products, new drugs, and new concepts are replacing those presented here.

All health professionals look forward to the day when periodontal disease is diminished to the same extent as dental caries. We have no crystal ball, but we can foresee an increasing emphasis on periodontics in education and research. Specific microorganisms causing various periodontal diseases will probably be identified and appropriate measures for control of these organisms will surely follow. It is exciting to contemplate a victory over this widespread disease. Until this time arrives the ideas and procedures presented in these chapters provide the best of modern therapy. No matter what the future holds the

dental hygienist will always occupy a strategic role as a health care educator and therapist.

SUMMARY

Periodontics is the basis for the practice of dentistry. The scope of periodontics expands into all areas of dental practice. The various technical procedures utilized in clinical periodontics must be consistent with individual patient needs. This chapter has emphasized the importance of continuing periodontal care. Patients have the right to expect excellence in their dental treatment. The ultimate solution to the worldwide control of periodontal disease will be in the field of preventive research. Knowledgeable and motivated dental hygienists contribute a significant service in the prevention of periodontal disease.

BIBLIOGRAPHY

Axelsson, P. and Lindhe, J.: The effect of controlled oral hygiene procedures on caries and periodontal disease in adults. Results after 6 years, J. Clin. Periodontol., 8:239, 1981.

Badersten, A., and Nilveus, R. and Egelberg, J.: Effect of nonsurgical periodontal therapy. III. Single versus repeated instrumentation, J. Clin. Periodontol., 11:114, 1984.

Bawden, J.W. and DeFriese, G.H.: *Planning for Dental Care on a Statewide Basis: The North Carolina Dental Manpower Project*, Chapel Hill, Dental Foundation of North Carolina, 1981.

Becker, W., Berg, L.E. and Becker, B.E.: Untreated periodontal disease: A longitudinal study, J. Periodontol., 50:234, 1979.

Becker, W., Berg, L. and Becker, B.E.: The long term evaluation of periodontal treatment and maintenance in 95 patients, Int. J. Perio. and Rest. Dent., 2:55, 1984.

Buckley, L.A. and Crowley, M.J.: A longitudinal study of untreated periodontal disease, J. Clin. Periodontol., 11:523, 1984.

Developing Communication Themes for Increasing Awareness, Detection and Treatment of Periodontal Disease, A report to the American Academy of Periodontology, Chicago, Market Facts, Inc. 1980.

Douglas, C.W. and Day, J.M.: Cost and payment of dental services in the U.S., J. Dent. Educ., 43:330, 1979.

Douglas, C.W., Gillings, D., Sollecito, W. and Gammon, M.: The potential for increase in the periodontal diseases of the aged population, J. Periodontol., 54:721, 1983.

Greenstein, G.: The role of bleeding upon probing in the diagnosis of periodontal disease. A literature review, J. Periodontol., 55:684, 1984.

Guidelines for Periodontal Therapy, Chicago, The American Academy of Periodontology, September, 1983.

Hirschfeld, L. and Wasserman, B.: A long-term survey of tooth loss in 600 treated periodontal patients, J. Periodontol., 49:225, 1978.

Lindhe, J., Westfelt, E., Nyman, S., Socransky, S.S. and Haffajee, A.D.: Long-term effect of surgical-nonsurgical treatment of periodontal disease, J. Clin. Periodontol., 11:448, 1984.

Lindhe, J. and Nyman, S.: Long-term maintenance of patients treated for advanced periodontal disease, J. Clin. Periodontol., 11:504, 1984.

Löe, H., Theilade, E. and Jensen, S.B.: Experimental gingivitis in man, J. Periodontol., 36:177, 1965.

Löe, J., Anerud, A., Boysen, H. and Smith, M.: The natural history of periodontal disease in man. Tooth mortality rates before 40 years of age, J. Perio. Res., 13:563, 1978.

Lovdal, A., Arno, A., Schei, O. and Waerhaug, J.: Combined effect of subgingival scaling and controlled oral hygiene on the incidence of gingivitis, Acta Odont. Scand., 19:537, 1961.

Marshall-Day, C.D., Stephens, R.G. and Quigley, L.F., Jr.: Periodontal disease: Prevalence and incidence, J. Periodontol., 26:185, 1955.

Mazza, J.E., Newman, M.G., and Sims, T.N.: Clinical and antimicrobial effect of stannous fluoride on periodontitis, J. Clin. Periodontol., 8:203, 1981.

McFall, W.T., Jr.: Tooth loss in 100 treated patients with periodontal disease. A long-term study, J. Periodontol., 53:539, 1982.

McFall, W.T., Jr., Hutchens, L.H., Jr., Marshall, T.W. and Holland, J.C.: Periodontal activities and attitudes of dental care providers, A.A.D.R. Abstract #529, J. Dent. Res., 63:228, 1983.

McFall, W.T., Jr. and Simpson, D.M.: Impact of periodontal continuing education on dental hygienists' practices, I.A.D.R. Abstract #1229, J. Dent. Res., 63 (special issue):307, 1984.

National Institute of Dental Research: Prevalence of dental caries in the United States' children. 1979–1980. National dental caries prevalence survey, National Institute of Dental Research: pp. 1–12, 1981.

Nyman, S., Rosling, B. and Lindhe, J.: Effect of professional tooth cleaning on healing after periodontal surgery, J. Clin. Periodontol., 2:80, 1975.

Ogilvie, A.L.: Recall and maintenance of the periodontal patient, Periodontics, 5:198, 1967.

Oliver, R.C.: Tooth loss with and without periodontal therapy, J. West. Soc. Perio., 17:8, 1969.

Ramfjord, S.P., Knowles, S.W., Nissle, R.R., Burgett, F.G. and Shick, R.A.: Results following three modalities of periodontal therapy, J. Periodontol., 46:522, 1975.

Schallhorn, R.G. and Snider, L.E.: Periodontal maintenance therapy, J. Am. Dent. Assoc., 103:227, 1981.

Simpson, D.M., McFall, W.T., Jr., and Jewson, L.G.: Periodontal practice patterns of dental hygienists, I.A.D.R. Abstract #1228, J. Dent. Res., 63 (special issue):307, 1984.

Socransky, S.S., Haffajee, A.D., Goodson, J.M. and Lindhe, J.: New concepts of destructive periodontal disease, J. Clin. Periodontol., 11:21, 1984.

Suomi, J.D., Greene, J.C., Vermillion, J.R., Doyle, J., Chang, J.J. and Leatherwood, E.C.: The effect of controlled oral hygiene procedures on the progression of periodontal disease in adults. Results after the third and final year, J. Periodontol., 42:152, 1971.

Tinanoff, S., Wei, S.H.Y. and Parkins, F.M.: Effect of a pumice prophylaxis on fluoride uptake in tooth enamel. J. Am. Dent. Assoc., 88:384, 1974.

United States National Center for Health Statistics: Basic data on dental examination findings of persons 1–74 years, United States, National Center for Health Statistics, series 11, no. 223, 1981.

GLOSSARY OF
PERIODONTAL TERMS

Abrasion . . . . The wearing away of teeth or gingiva by abnormal mechanical pressure.

Abscess . . . . A localized collection of purulent exudate in the periodontal tissue.

Acute . . . . The sudden onset and swift course of a disease.

Alveolar bone (proper). . . The perforated layer of compact bone that forms the alveolus

Alveolar mucosa . . . . That portion of the nonkeratinized lining mucous membrane which extends from the attached gingiva to the vestibular fornix.

Alveolar process . . . . Bony processes of the mandible or maxilla that surround and support the teeth.

Alveolus. . . . . The bony socket surrounding the root or roots of a tooth.

Antibiotic. . . . . Products of certain organisms used against infections caused by other organisms

Arthritis . . . . Inflammation of the joints due to infectious, metabolic or constitutional causes.

Asepsis. . . . . Exclusion of microorganisms and avoidance of infection.

Attached gingiva . . . . The portion of the masticatory mucosa which is firmly connected to the teeth and alveolar process.

Attachment apparatus . . . The tissues consisting of the alveolar bone, cementum, and periodontal ligament which support the teeth.

Atrophy . . . . A decrease in size and number of cells of a tissue or organ.

Attrition . . . . A wearing away of tooth structure such as results from mastication or bruxism.

Autograft . . . . A piece of tissue transferred from one location to another within the same individual.

Autogenous gingival graft (free graft) . . . . A portion of masticatory mucosa surgically removed and transferred to another area in order to increase the amount of keratinized tissue.

Automatic toothbrushes. . Motor-driven instruments used for cleaning the teeth. Power is provided by battery or electricity.

Bacterial plaque (micro-bial, dental plaque) . . . .   An accumulation of microorganisms on the surface of the tooth or gingiva, or in the gingival crevice

Bevel. . . . .   The slope of a surface at an angle less than a right angle.

Bite guard (occlusal guard, night guard) . . . .   An appliance worn on the teeth to relieve excessive occlusal forces; usually used in association with the treatment of bruxism or occlusal trauma.

Bruxism . . . .   The habitual grinding or clenching of the teeth.

Buccal mucosa . . . .   The lining mucous membrane of the cheek.

Calculus (tartar) . . . .   An abnormal mineralized deposit found on the surfaces of teeth.

Canine-guided occlusion   In lateral functional movements, the canines assume functional contacts, thus disarticulating the premolars and molars.

Cementum . . . .   The hard tissue covering the anatomical root of the tooth.

Centric occlusion . . . .   Maximum intercuspation or contact of the teeth of opposing arches. Also called acquired centric and habitual centric.

Centric relation . . . .   The relation of the mandible to the maxilla (and other cranial structures) at any given vertical dimension when the condyles are in the most superior, posterior, unstrained position in the glenoid fossae.

Chisel . . . .   An instrument with the blade in the same general plane as the shank.

Chronic . . . .   A disease continuing over a long period of time.

Cicatrization . . . .   A scar produced in the healing process.

Citric Acid . . . .   A highly acidic medicament used to dimineralize root surfaces.

Cleft . . . .   A vertical groove or fissure in the gingiva.

Col . . . .   A depression between the facial and lingual peaks of the interdental papillae.

Crater . . . .   A saucer-shaped defect of soft tissue or bone in the interdental area.

Crossbite . . . .   A reverse occlusal arrangement between antagonizing maxillary and mandibular teeth in which the facial cusps of the maxillary teeth and the lingual cusps of the mandibular teeth act as supporting cusps for the occlusal vertical dimension.

Curettage. . . . .   The surgical removal by scraping of the epithelial lining of soft-tissue surfaces such as that in periodontal pockets.

Curettage for new attach-ment (renewed attach-ment, reattachment) . . .   The surgical removal of the pocket wall by scraping in an attempt to obtain pocket elimination by re-formation of the lost periodontium.

Curette. . . . .   An instrument with a double-edged spoon-shaped blade which is used to scrape the lining or surface of tissue or to remove deposits from teeth.

Cytotoxic . . . .   Damaging or lethal to body cells.

Debridement.............   Removal of foreign material or devitalized or contaminated tissue.

Dehiscence ....   A vertical loss of alveolar bone over the facial or lingual aspect of a tooth's radicular surface.

Dental abrasion ....   The mechanical wearing of the teeth such as that which results from incorrect toothbrushing.

Dentogingival junction...   Union of gingiva to the tooth by the junctional epithelium and gingival collagen fibers.

Desquamative gingivitis..   An unusual dystropic disease of the gingiva characterized by shedding of the epithelium.

Disuse atrophy..........   A decrease in the size of tissues due to inadequate stimulation.

Edematous gingivitis ....   An inflammatory disease of the gingivae characterized by swelling of the part.

Endotoxin ....   Component of cell walls of Gram-negative bacteria that becomes absorbed in or on cementum or calculus and is irritating to periodontal tissues.

Exudate ....   Fluid, cells, or cellular debris that has escaped from blood vessels, usually due to inflammation, and been deposited in or on tissues.

Fenestration ....   A windowlike opening through the alveolar bone over prominent root surfaces.

File ....   An instrument with several short blades at right angles to the shank.

Fistula.................   A tract transmitting fluid or pus from an area of infection.

Flap...................   A portion of masticatory mucosa separated by incision from surrounding tissue except at its base.

Free gingivae ....   Portion of gingivae not directly attached to tooth or bone; marginal gingiva and interdental papillae.

Free gingival groove ..... A linear depression intervening between the free marginal gingiva and the attached gingiva.

Freeway space ....   The difference between rest vertical and occlusal vertical.

Frenectomy ....   The surgical elimination of frenal attachments.

Frenulum..............   A small fold of oral mucosa attached to the gingiva.

Functioning side ....   That side toward which the mandible is projected in eccentric lateral movements.

Furcation invasion.......   Resorption of interradicular bone as the result of periodontitis.

Gingiva ....   That portion of the masticatory mucosa which is attached to the teeth and alveolar process and surrounds the cervical area of the teeth.

Gingival abrasion........   A superficial wound of the gingiva resulting from scraping or rubbing.

Gingival crevice (sulcus)	The physiologic space, either actual or potential, between the surface of the tooth and the free gingiva.
Gingival recession	Loss of gingiva in an apical direction resulting in exposure of the root of the tooth.
Gingivectomy	The surgical resection of the gingivae to eliminate periodontal pockets.
Gingivitis	An inflammatory disease of the gingivae.
Gingivoplasty	The surgical reshaping of the gingivae to produce physiologic form.
Graft	A portion of tissue transposed from one location to another to correct a defect.
Group function occlusion	Lateral forces are distributed to as many of the posterior teeth as possible.
Hereditary gingival hyperplasia	An inheritable disease characterized by gingival overgrowth.
Herpetic stomatitis	An inflammatory disease of oral mucous membranes caused by the herpes simplex virus.
Hoe	An instrument with a single blade usually at a right angle to the shank.
Hyperplastic gingivitis	An inflammatory condition of the gingiva characterized by enlargement due to an increased number of tissue elements.
Immunity	The formation of antibodies or sensitized lymphocytes to an irritant so that the body is protected from subsequent exposure.
Implant	A tissue graft or nonvital substance used to correct an anatomic defect.
Incisal guidance	This term refers to the influence of mandibular movement brought about by guidance of the mandibular anterior teeth against the lingual surfaces of the maxillary anterior teeth.
Index	A system of measurement that quantitates the extent of etiologic agents or the extent of tissue change.
Infection	Invasion of the body by pathogenic microorganisms and their toxic products resulting in disease.
Inflammatory response	Nonspecific response of body tissues to an irritant that is mediated by leukocytes.
Intercellular	Occurring between cell boundaries.
Interdental stimulation	Massage of the interproximal gingiva.
Interference	A disharmony in tooth-to-tooth or jaw-to-jaw relationships in the lateral range of movement.
Interproximal	Between the proximal surfaces of adjoining teeth.
Intrabony pocket	A periodontal pocket the base of which extends apical to the crestal alveolar process.
Intracellular	Occurring within the cell.

Junctional epithelium	Epithelium forming the union of the gingival connective tissue and the tooth surface at the base of the gingival crevice.
Juvenile periodontitis	An atypical disease of the periodontium characterized by intrabony pocket formation primarily involving incisors and first molars in young individuals.
Lamina dura	A radiopaque line which is the radiographic image of the alveolus.
Lamina propria	The connective tissue portion of the mucous membrane immediately adjacent to the basement membrane.
Laterally positioned flap	A soft-tissue flap displaced over an adjacent anatomic tooth defect with maintenance of connective tissue blood supply.
Lining mucosa	A type of nonkeratinizing oral mucous membrane.
Marginal gingiva	That portion of the free gingiva located on the facial and lingual aspects of the teeth.
Masticatory mucosa	A division of the oral mucous membranes consisting of the gingival tissues and the covering mucosa of the hard palate.
Mucobuccal fold (vestibular fornix)............	The depression between the alveolar mucosa and labial or buccal mucosa.
Mucobuccal fold extension	A surgical procedure employed to increase the depth of the vestibular fornix (mucobuccal fold).
Mucogingival junction ...	The wavy border between the attached gingiva and the alveolar mucosa.
Mucogingival surgery....	Plastic operative procedures designed to correct or modify defects involving both gingiva and lining mucosa.
Necrosis	Death of cells or tissues.
Necrotizing ulcerative gingivitis (Vincent's infection, ANUG)..........	An inflammatory disease of the gingivae characterized by cratering of the interdental papillae and sloughing of surface tissue.
Nonfunctioning side	That side away from which the mandible is projected in eccentric lateral movements.
Occlusal adjustment	The technical procedure of reshaping the teeth for the purpose of elimination of prematurities and interferences in the occlusion.
Occlusal interference	Contact relationship of opposing teeth in lateral and protrusive movements which results in excessive pressure to the attachment apparatus.
Occlusal prematurity	Contact relationship of opposing teeth in centric before full jaw closure is reached.

Occlusal trauma . . . .   An injury to the periodontium which results from excessive occlusal contact of the teeth or from excessive forces applied to the teeth.

Occlusion. . . . .   The relation of the maxillary and mandibular teeth in all jaw positions and movements.

Oral physiotherapy . . . . . .   Those procedures practiced by the individual to maintain mouth hygiene.

Oral prophylaxis . . . .   The removal by instrumentation of deposits and debris from the surfaces of the teeth for the purpose of preventing gingival and periodontal diseases.

Osseous implant . . . .   A bony graft used to fill a defect in alveolar bone.

Ostectomy . . . .   The surgical removal of bone adjacent to a tooth for the purpose of periodontal pocket elimination.

Osteoplasty . . . .   The surgical reshaping of the bone around the teeth to produce physiological form.

Overbite . . . .   Vertical overlap. The extension of the maxillary teeth over the mandibular teeth in a vertical direction when the opposing teeth are in centric occlusion.

Overjet . . . .   Horizontal overlap. The projection of the maxillary teeth beyond the mandibular teeth in a horizontal direction when the opposing teeth are in centric occlusion.

Pack . . . .   See Periodontal dressing.

Panolipse or panorex radiograph. . . . .   Panoramic radiograph requiring special equipment which moves the film and tube-head around the patient.

Papillary gingiva . . . .   That portion of the marginal gingival tissue which occupies the interdental embrasure apical to the contact areas of the teeth.

Pericoronitis . . . .   Acute inflammation of the soft tissue adjacent to a partially erupted tooth.

Periodontal abscess . . . . . .   An accumulation of pus in the gingival wall of a periodontal pocket.

Periodontal chart . . . .   A graphic record of clinical findings of the periodontal disease at the time of examination.

Periodontal disease . . . . . .   Any abnormality or pathologic state involving the gingiva or supporting tissues of the teeth; commonly used to designate collectively the inflammatory and degenerative diseases of the periodontium.

Periodontal dressing . . . . .   A protective anodyne material that is placed over an area of periodontal surgery.

Periodontal ligament (periodontal membrane) . . .   The fibrous connective tissue between the alveolus and the cementum of the tooth.

Periodontal pocket . . . . . .   A defect between the surface of the tooth and the diseased gingivae associated with an apical migration of junctional epithelium.

Periodontal probe . . . .   A calibrated instrument used to locate and measure the depth of periodontal pockets.

Periodontal prosthesis . . .   An appliance used to replace and stabilize teeth for patients who have had advanced periodontal destruction.

Periodontics	That aspect of clinical dentistry involved in the prevention and treatment of diseases of the periodontium.
Periodontitis	An inflammatory disease of the supporting structures of the teeth characterized by pocket formation and bone loss.
Periodontium	A collective term for the tissues that surround and support the teeth, i.e., gingivae, cementum, periodontal ligament, and alveolar bone.
Periodontopathogens	A bacterial species that contributes to or causes periodontal destructive processes.
Phenytoin enlargement ..	Overgrowth of gingival tissue due to the drug diphenyl-hydantoin sodium.
Physiologic rest position	The position the mandible assumes with mandibular musculature exhibiting minimal tonic contraction against the force of gravity with the head itself in an upright position.
Plaque	See Bacterial plaque.
Polishing	The removal by instrumentation of stains and nonmineralized deposits from the surface of the teeth; the creation of a smooth, glossy surface on a tooth, dental restoration, or dental prosthesis.
Premature contact	An occlusal contact that occurs before a balanced and stable jaw-to-jaw relationship is reached to either centric relation or centric occlusion, or in the area between these two positions.
Protrusion	A position of the mandible forward to (in front of) centric occlusion.
Pyorrhea alveolaris	An archaic term for periodontal disease.
Reattachment	A misnomer. Actually a new attachment of connective tissue or epithelium to tooth surface.
Recession	Gradual atrophy or abrasion of the gingival tissue from its normal position on the necks of the teeth.
Reconstructive periodontal surgery	Surgical procedures by which periodontal tissues are restored to physiologic states, usually by grafting bone or soft tissue into the defect.
Repositioned gingival flap	A surgical procedure in which masticatory and alveolar mucosae are positioned so as to eliminate periodontal pockets.
Resolution	Return of a diseased tissue to health.
Resorption	Loss of bone or tooth structure due to a physiologic or pathologic process.
Retrusion	Posterior movement of the mandible from centric occlusion.
Root planing	The smoothing by instrumentation of the roots of the teeth.
Scaler	An instrument used to remove deposits from the surfaces of the teeth.

Scaling . . . . The removal by instrumentation of deposits from the surfaces of the teeth.

Sickle scaler . . . . An instrument with a triangular-shaped blade employed to remove calculus from the tooth surface.

Splint . . . . A device or appliance used to stabilize mobile teeth and redistribute occlusal forces.

Specialized mucosa . . . . . . The dorsum of the tongue which is modified for taste reception.

Stain . . . . A pigmented substance, either on the surface of or within the tooth, which results in an abnormal discoloration of the tooth.

Sterilization . . . . A process that kills all forms of life.

Stippling . . . . The pitted appearance of the attached gingiva.

Stomatognathic system . . The physiologic group of organs which performs the functions of mastication, deglutition, and speech.

Subgingival . . . . The area apical to the free gingival crest within the gingival crevice or pocket.

Submucosa . . . . The layer of connective tissue that attaches mucous membrane to subjacent structures.

Suprabony pocket . . . . A pocket, the base of which is coronal to the crestal alveolar process.

Supragingival . . . . The area coronal to the gree gingival crest.

Temporomandibular joint disorder . . . . A general term used to describe diseases of or impaired function of the temporomandibular joints.

Trabeculation . . . . The anatomic pattern of the spicules of cancellous bone.

Trauma . . . . A wound or injury of tissue.

Ultrasonic scaler . . . . An automatic device utilized for removal of calculus and stain on the teeth employing the principle of high-frequency vibration and cavitation.

Vestibular fornix . . . . See Mucobuccal fold.

Working side (functional side) . . . . The side toward which the mandible moves in lateral excursion.

Xerostomia . . . . Dry mouth. Decrease in salivary flow resulting from effects of some medications or diseases or from radiation treatments to the head and neck area.

INDEX